Nutrition for Anemia

Nutrition for Anemia

Editor

Javier Diaz-Castro

MDPI • Basel • Beijing • Wuhan • Barcelona • Belgrade • Manchester • Tokyo • Cluj • Tianjin

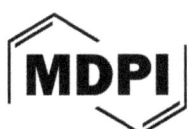

Editor
Javier Diaz-Castro
University of Granada
Sapin

Editorial Office
MDPI
St. Alban-Anlage 66
4052 Basel, Switzerland

This is a reprint of articles from the Special Issue published online in the open access journal *Nutrients* (ISSN 2072-6643) (available at: https://www.mdpi.com/journal/nutrients/special_issues/Nutrition_Anemia).

For citation purposes, cite each article independently as indicated on the article page online and as indicated below:

LastName, A.A.; LastName, B.B.; LastName, C.C. Article Title. *Journal Name* **Year**, *Article Number*, Page Range.

ISBN 978-3-03936-936-2 (Hbk)
ISBN 978-3-03936-937-9 (PDF)

© 2020 by the authors. Articles in this book are Open Access and distributed under the Creative Commons Attribution (CC BY) license, which allows users to download, copy and build upon published articles, as long as the author and publisher are properly credited, which ensures maximum dissemination and a wider impact of our publications.

The book as a whole is distributed by MDPI under the terms and conditions of the Creative Commons license CC BY-NC-ND.

Contents

About the Editor vii

Preface to "Nutrition for Anemia" ix

Jorge Moreno-Fernandez, María J. M. Alférez, Inmaculada López-Aliaga
and Javier Díaz-Castro
Role of Fermented Goat Milk on Liver Gene and Protein Profiles Related to Iron Metabolism
during Anemia Recovery
Reprinted from: *Nutrients* **2020**, *12*, 1336, doi:10.3390/nu12051336 1

Teresa Nestares, Rafael Martín-Masot, Ana Labella, Virginia A. Aparicio,
Marta Flor-Alemany, Magdalena López-Frías and José Maldonado
Is a Gluten-Free Diet Enough to Maintain Correct Micronutrients Status in Young Patients with
Celiac Disease?
Reprinted from: *Nutrients* **2020**, *12*, 844, doi:10.3390/nu12030844 15

Takana Mary Silubonde, Jeannine Baumgartner, Lisa Jayne Ware, Linda Malan,
Cornelius Mattheus Smuts and Shane Norris
Adjusting Haemoglobin Values for Altitude Maximizes Combined Sensitivity and Specificity to
Detect Iron Deficiency among Women of Reproductive Age in Johannesburg, South Africa
Reprinted from: *Nutrients* **2020**, *12*, 633, doi:10.3390/nu12030633 25

Shuichi Shibuya, Toshihiko Toda, Yusuke Ozawa, Mario Jose Villegas Yata
and Takahiko Shimizu
Acai Extract Transiently Upregulates Erythropoietin by Inducing a Renal Hypoxic Condition
in Mice
Reprinted from: *Nutrients* **2020**, *12*, 533, doi:10.3390/nu12020533 39

Javier Diaz-Castro, Jorge Moreno-Fernandez, Ignacio Chirosa, Luis Javier Chirosa,
Rafael Guisado and Julio J. Ochoa
Beneficial Effect of Ubiquinol on Hematological and Inflammatory Signaling during Exercise
Reprinted from: *Nutrients* **2020**, *12*, 424, doi:10.3390/nu11102424 49

Chiao-Ming Chen, Shu-Ci Mu, Chun-Kuang Shih, Yi-Ling Chen, Li-Yi Tsai, Yung-Ting Kuo,
In-Mei Cheong, Mei-Ling Chang, Yi-Chun Chen and Sing-Chung Li
Iron Status of Infants in the First Year of Life in Northern Taiwan
Reprinted from: *Nutrients* **2020**, *12*, 139, doi:10.3390/nu12010139 65

Lucía Iglesias Vázquez, Victoria Arija, Núria Aranda, Estefanía Aparicio, Núria Serrat,
Francesc Fargas, Francisca Ruiz, Meritxell Pallejà, Pilar Coronel, Mercedes Gimeno and
Josep Basora
The Effectiveness of Different Doses of Iron Supplementation and the Prenatal Determinants of
Maternal Iron Status in Pregnant Spanish Women: ECLIPSES Study
Reprinted from: *Nutrients* **2019**, *11*, 2418, doi:10.3390/nu11102418 77

Jorge Moreno-Fernández, Inmaculada López-Aliaga, María García-Burgos,
María J.M. Alférez and Javier Díaz-Castro
Fermented Goat Milk Consumption Enhances Brain Molecular Functions during Iron
Deficiency Anemia Recovery
Reprinted from: *Nutrients* **2019**, *11*, 2394, doi:10.3390/nu11102394 97

Genny Raffaeli, Francesca Manzoni, Valeria Cortesi, Giacomo Cavallaro, Fabio Mosca and Stefano Ghirardello
Iron Homeostasis Disruption and Oxidative Stress in Preterm Newborns
Reprinted from: *Nutrients* **2020**, *12*, 1554, doi:10.3390/nu12061554 . . . . **111**

Rafael Martín-Masot, Maria Teresa Nestares, Javier Diaz-Castro, Inmaculada López-Aliaga, Maria Jose Muñoz Alférez, Jorge Moreno-Fernandez and José Maldonado
Multifactorial Etiology of Anemia in Celiac Disease and Effect of Gluten-Free Diet: A Comprehensive Review
Reprinted from: *Nutrients* **2019**, *11*, 2557, doi:10.3390/nu11112557 . . . . **133**

Sajidah Begum and Gladys O. Latunde-Dada
Anemia of Inflammation with An Emphasis on Chronic Kidney Disease
Reprinted from: *Nutrients* **2019**, *11*, 2424, doi:10.3390/nu11102424 . . . . **149**

About the Editor

Javier Diaz-Castro is Professor at the Department of Physiology from the University of Granada. His research has been developed in the area of Physiology and Nutrition, participating in 14 funded research projects. He has published more than 80 research articles, 2 books, and 13 scientific book chapters. He has presented 60 communications to national scientific conferences and 61 communications to international scientific conferences. He has directed 12 doctoral theses, 40 Final Master's Projects, and 52 Final Degree Projects and has been awarded with several scientific awards.

Preface to "Nutrition for Anemia"

ANEMIA: A PUBLIC HEALTH PROBLEM. The World Health Organization (WHO) reports that anemia affects around 800 million children and women. In fact, 528.7 million women and 273.2 million children under the age of 5 were anemic in 2011, and about half of them were also iron-deficient. Malnutrition and micronutrient malnutrition have serious economic consequences, with an estimated cost of 2.3% of the world's gross domestic product (GDP) per year. Investment in prevention and treatment of micronutrient malnutrition results in improved health status and reduced infant and maternal mortality. Iron deficiency is the most widespread micronutrient deficiency in the world, often resulting in chronic iron deficiency or iron deficiency anemia. Taking into account background, it is important to address the causes of iron deficiency to mitigate the serious health consequences; however, excessive iron intake or overload can be harmful, potentially leading to iron overload and blood disorders. In order to implement efficient and feasible strategies as a solution to iron deficiency anemia, it is important that each country addresses the recommendations of experts in iron nutrition and the WHO in a systematic way, including legislation and research, bioavailability and provision of iron fortification, and educate the population about iron deficiency and conduct tests on individuals using clinical pathways to measure serum or plasma ferritin concentration as an index of iron deficiency and overload. This important health problem is addressed in this book, reporting nutritional strategies and the consequences for the organism of excessive iron consumption, in an attempt to raise awareness of the importance of this health problem with repercussions on health and economic policies worldwide.

Javier Diaz-Castro
Editor

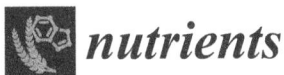

Article

Role of Fermented Goat Milk on Liver Gene and Protein Profiles Related to Iron Metabolism during Anemia Recovery

Jorge Moreno-Fernandez [1,2,3], María J. M. Alférez [1,2], Inmaculada López-Aliaga [1,2,*] and Javier Díaz-Castro [1,2]

1. Department of Physiology, University of Granada, 18071 Granada, Spain; jorgemf@ugr.es (J.M.-F.); malferez@ugr.es (M.J.M.A.); javierdc@ugr.es (J.D.-C.)
2. Institute of Nutrition and Food Technology "José Mataix Verdú", University of Granada, 18071 Granada, Spain
3. Nutrition and Food Sciences Ph.D. Program, University of Granada, 18071 Granada, Spain
* Correspondence: milopez@ugr.es; Tel.: +34-958-243880; Fax: +34-958-248959

Received: 6 April 2020; Accepted: 30 April 2020; Published: 8 May 2020

Abstract: Despite the crucial role of the liver as the central regulator of iron homeostasis, no studies have directly tested the modulation of liver gene and protein expression patterns during iron deficiency instauration and recovery with fermented milks. Fermented goat milk consumption improves the key proteins of intestinal iron metabolism during iron deficiency recovery, enhancing the digestive and metabolic utilization of iron. The aim of this study was to assess the influence of fermented goat or cow milk consumption on liver iron homeostasis during iron-deficiency anemia recovery with normal or iron-overload diets. Analysis included iron status biomarkers, gene and protein expression in hepatocytes. In general, fermented goat milk consumption either with normal or high iron content up-regulated liver DMT1, FPN1 and FTL1 gene expression and DMT1 and FPN1 protein expression. However, HAMP mRNA expression was lower in all groups of animals fed fermented goat milk. Additionally, hepcidin protein expression decreased in control and anemic animals fed fermented goat milk with normal iron content. In conclusion, fermented goat milk potentiates the up-regulation of key genes coding for proteins involved in iron metabolism, such as DMT1, and FPN1, FTL1 and down-regulation of HAMP, playing a key role in enhanced iron repletion during anemia recovery, inducing a physiological adaptation of the liver key genes and proteins coordinated with the fluctuation of the cellular iron levels, favoring whole-body iron homeostasis.

Keywords: fermented cow and goat milk; anemia; iron homeostasis; iron repletion; gene and protein expression

1. Introduction

Iron deficiency anemia (IDA) is a highly prevalent pathology and a medical condition in the clinical practice, affecting more than two billion people worldwide. This public health problem has a negative impact on the lives of infants and fertile women worldwide [1]. Daily, in the duodenum and proximal jejunum, 2 mg of iron is absorbed. The non-heme iron in the diet is in Fe^{3+} form and it must be reduced to ferrous form before it can be absorbed by the action of duodenal cytochrome B. Fe^{2+} is then transported across the apical membrane of enterocytes by the divalent metal transporter 1 (DMT1). This protein transports some divalent cations including ferrous iron. Iron crosses the basolateral membrane of intestinal enterocytes by the action of ferroportin, an iron exporter, entering into systemic circulation. After that, iron can be stored in the liver joined to ferritin, which is an iron storage protein. The mechanisms regulating systemic iron homeostasis are largely centered on the liver and involve two molecules, hepcidin and ferroportin, that work together to regulate the flow of iron from cells into the systemic circulation [2].

Due to the key role of iron in many physiological cell functions, including replication, ATP, DNA synthesis and the heme group in hemoglobin [3], and as a constituent of essential cofactors such as iron–sulfur (Fe-S) clusters [4], the organism has evolved to conserve body iron stores; however, it does not have an efficient mechanism for removing excess iron, iron-overload being highly deleterious to many physiological mechanisms. In addition, defects in molecules related to regulating iron homeostasis are usually a cause of genetically inherited iron overload, called hereditary hemochromatosis (HH) [2]. Therefore, it is essential to tightly regulate iron homeostasis, a function performed mainly by the liver [5].

The liver is one of the most functionally and metabolically active organs in the body. In addition to roles in detoxification, digestion, protein synthesis, gluconeogenesis, and fat metabolism, the liver also plays a significant role in iron homeostasis. It is responsible for approximately 8% of plasma iron turnover and it is the major site for iron storage, acting also as the key regulator of iron homeostasis [6]. The liver synthesizes hepcidin, a peptide which binds to and induces the internalization of ferroportin [7], reducing the amount of iron released into the bloodstream, therefore being the major contributor to systemic regulation of iron status [8]. The noteworthy influence of the liver on body iron regulation can be attributed to the expression of many liver-specific or liver-enriched proteins, which play an important role in the physiological regulation of iron metabolism [6].

On the other hand, it has been previously reported that fermented goat milk consumption improves the key proteins of intestinal iron metabolism during IDA recovery, enhancing the digestive and metabolic utilization of iron [9]. However, in spite of the crucial role of the liver as a central regulator of iron metabolism, to date, no studies have directly tested the modulation of hepatic gene and protein expression profiles during anemia recovery, including divalent metal transporter 1 (DMT1), ferritin light chain 1 (FTL1), ferroportin 1 (FPN1), and hepcidin antimicrobial peptide (HAMP). Taking into account all these considerations, the aim of this study was to contribute to a better understanding of iron metabolism during IDA recovery, by studying how fermented goat vs. cow milk (the most commonly consumed milk worldwide) consumption affects liver iron homeostasis during nutritional iron repletion in animal models with severe, induced iron-deficiency anemia and overload.

2. Material and Methods

2.1. Animals and Experimental Design

One hundred male Wistar rats aged 3 weeks and weighing about 34.56 ± 6.35 g, purchased from the University of Granada Laboratory Animal Service (Granada, Spain), were included in this study. The animals were maintained under standard animal housing conditions with a 12-hour light/dark cycle (lights on at 9:00 A.M.), temperature (23 ± 2 °C) and humidity (60 ± 5%). All animal experiments were carried out in accordance with Directive 2010/63/EU on the protection of animals used for scientific purposes.

In the pre-experimental period (PEP), 100 rats were randomly divided into two groups; a control group received the AIN-93G diet (n = 50) [10] and an anemic or experimental group received a low Fe diet (n = 50) for 40 days [11]; deionized water and diet were available ad libitum. In the experimental period (EP), control and anemic groups were fed for 30 days with either fermented cow milk or fermented goat milk diet, with normal Fe (4.5 mg/100 g) or high Fe content (45.0 mg/100 g) (Fe citrate) [12]. Deionized water was available ad libitum, and dietary intake pattern induced by pair feeding (80% of the average intake) (Figure 1). At the end of the PEP and EP, hematological parameters and serum iron, total iron binding capacity (TIBC), transferrin saturation, ferritin, serum hepcidin and transaminases were determined. Furthermore, the liver was removed (at the end of the PEP, in 10 animals per group and in all the animals in the EP), for measurement of hepatosomatic index (HSI), and a fraction of the liver was snap-frozen in liquid nitrogen and keep in a −80 °C freezer for subsequent mineral analysis (liver iron content). Subsequently 1 g of liver was stored overnight at 4 °C with RNA-later (Thermo Fisher Scientific, Waltham, MA, USA), the solution was removed and stored at −80 °C until isolation of total RNA.

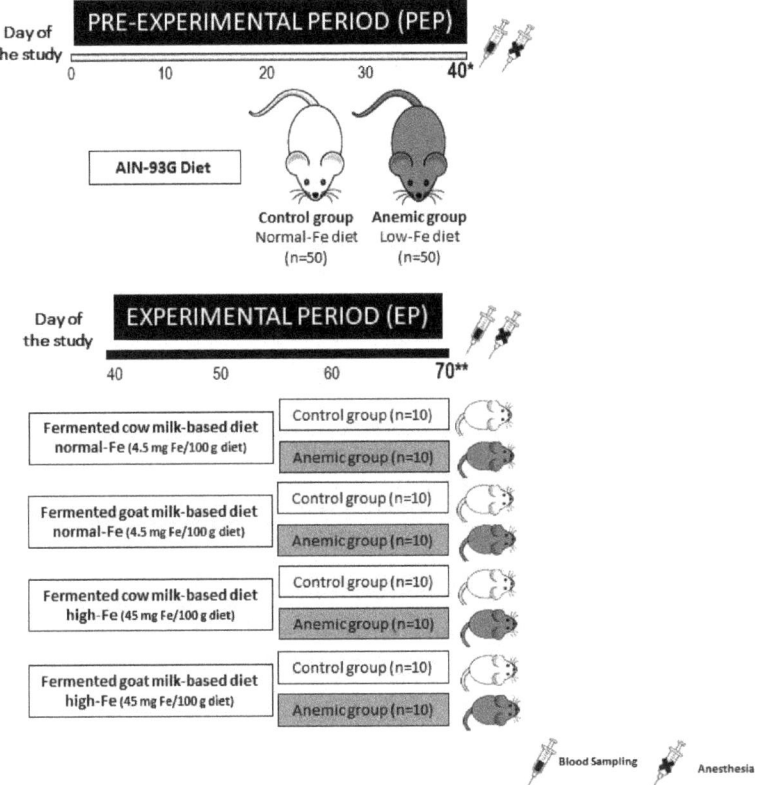

Figure 1. Experimental design of the study. * 10 animals per group and ** all the animals were anesthetized, peripheral blood samples from caudal vein were analyzed for hematological and biochemical parameters and the liver was removed.

2.2. Diets Preparation

Diets were prepared with fermented cow or fermented goat milk. *Lactobacillus bulgaricus* subsp. *delbrueckii* and *Streptococcus thermophilus* were inoculated to an initial concentration of 1×10^{11} CFU/mL (10 mL/L inoculum) in goat or cow milk, and then the samples were incubated at 37 °C for approximately 24 h. Subsequently, fermented milk samples were dehydrated by a smooth industrial process to obtain products with a moisture content ranging between 2.5% and 4.5%. Sufficient amounts of fermented dehydrated cow or goat milk were utilized in the experimental diets to provide 20% of protein and 10% of fat. The constituents and nutrient compositions of the experimental diets are presented in Table 1.

Table 1. Composition of experimental diets.

Constituents	Pre-Experimental Period	Experimental Period	
g/100 g Diet		Fermented Milk Diets [2]	
	AIN-93G [1]	Cow Milk	Goat Milk
Protein	20.00	20.50	20.60
Lactose	-	29.50	29.10
Fat	10.00	10.00	29.10
Wheat starch	50.00	20.00	20.30
Constant ingredients [3]	20.00	20.00	20.00

[1] Normal iron content for control rats (4.5 mg Fe/100 g diet) [10], or low iron content (0.5 mg Fe/100 g diet) [11] for the anemic group. [2] Specific vitamin and mineral premix supplements for fermented goat and cow milk diets were to meet the recommendations of the AIN-93G for diets with normal iron (4.5 mg Fe/100 g diet) [12] or diets with high iron content (45 mg Fe/100 g diet) (Raja et al., 1994). [3] Fibre (micronized cellulose) 5%, sucrose 10%, choline chloride 0.25%, L-cystine 0.25%, mineral premix 3.5%, vitamin premix 1%.

2.3. Hematological Tests

Hematological parameters were measured at the end of PEP and EP using a fully automated hematology analyzer (Mythic 22CT, C2 Diagnostics, Grabels, France).

2.4. Transferrin Saturation, Serum Iron, Total Iron Binding Capacity (TIBC), Serum Ferritin and Serum Hepcidin

Transferrin saturation, serum iron and TIBC were determined using Sigma Diagnostics Iron and TIBC reagents (Sigma-Aldrich Co., St. Louis, MO). Serum ferritin was measured by the Elisa method using a standard kit (rat ferritin ELISA Kit) supplied by Biovendor GmbH, Heidelberg (Germany). Hepcidin-25 was determined using a DRG ELISA Kit (DRG Instruments GmbH, Germany).

2.5. Hepatosomatic Index, Hepatic Iron Concentration and Transaminases Analysis

The HSI was determined by the use of the following equation:

$$HSI = (\text{weight of the liver}/\text{weight of the body}) \times 100$$

Prior to iron analysis, liver fractions were mineralized by wet digestion in a sand bath (Selecta, Barcelona, Spain) using nitric acid followed by a mixture of $HNO_3:HClO_4$, 1:4 v/v (69%:70%, v/v; Merck, Darmstadt, Germany) until the total elimination of organic matter. Finally, the samples were diluted with Milli Q (Millipore S.A., Bedford, MA, USA) ultrapure water. Iron analysis was undertaken using a PerkinElmer Optima 8300 inductively coupled plasma-optical emission spectrometer (ICP-OES) (Waltham, MA, USA) with a segmented-array charge-coupled device (SCD) detector. Multi-elemental Atasol calibration solution (Analytika, Khodlova, Prague) was used to calibrate the apparatus. For the calibration curve, diluted standards were prepared from concentrated standard solutions. After each series of 5 samples, an internal standard solution of 10 mg/L was used. The acceptable result was assessed as 10%. Three replicates of each sample were analyzed.

Alanine aminotransferase (ALT) and aspartate aminotransferase (AST) were measured by standard colorimetric and enzymatic methods using a BS-200 Chemistry Analyzer (Shenzhen Mindray Bio-Medical Electronics Co. Ltd., Shenzhen, China).

2.6. RNA Extraction and Quantitative Real Time PCR

From liver samples, total RNA was extracted with TRIsure lysis reagent (Bioline, Luckenwalde, Germany) following the manufacturer's instructions. The RNA quantity and purity were measured using a spectrophotometer (NanoDrop 1000, Thermo Fisher Scientific, Waltham, Massachusetts, USA) at 260/280 nm. Reverse transcription was performed on 1 µg of total RNA in a 20 µL reaction to synthesize complementary DNA (cDNA), using an iScript cDNA Synthesis kit (Bio-Rad). Quantitative real-time PCR was performed in a total reaction volume of 20 µL using the CFX96 Touch Real-Time PCR Detection System (Bio-Rad) and SYBR Green detection using Sso Avdvanced Universal SYBR Green Supermix (Bio-Rad). Primer sequences of divalent metal transporter 1 (DMT1), ferroportin 1 (FPN1), ferritin (FTL1) and hepcidin antimicrobial peptide (HAMP) for quantitative real-time PCR are shown in Table 2 and were obtained from Eurofins MWG Biotech (Ebersberg, Germany). The expression of the target genes was normalized to the housekeeping gene β-actin. All the measurements were done in duplicate and, to confirm PCR product size, melt curve analysis and gel electrophoresis were conducted.

Table 2. Primers, annealing temperatures, and product sizes for PCR amplification.

Gene	Direction	Primer Sequence (5′→3′)	Annealing Temperature	Size (bp)
β-Actin	Forward	GGGGTGTTGAAGGTCTCAAA	57 °C	165
	Reverse	TGTCACCAACTGGGACGATA		
DMT1	Forward	GGCATGTGGCACTGTATGTG	59 °C	163
	Reverse	CCGCTGGTATCTTCGCTCAG		
FPN1	Forward	GAACAAGAACCCACCTGTGC	57 °C	191
	Reverse	AGGATGGAACCACTCAGTCC		
HAMP	Forward	CCTATCTCCGGCAACAGACG	59 °C	121
	Reverse	GGGAAGTTGGTGTCTCGCTT		
FTL1	Forward	GCCCTGGAGAAGAACCTGAA	59 °C	247
	Reverse	AGTCGTGCTTCAGAGTGAGG		

2.7. Western Blotting and Immunocytochemistry

Liver samples were mechanically homogenized in tissue protein extraction reagent (T-PER) (Thermo Scientific Inc., Hanover Park, IL, USA) supplemented with a protease inhibitor cocktail (Sigma-Aldrich, St. Louis, MO, USA) under ice-cold conditions. On 4%–20% Criterion TGX (Tris-Glycine extended) gels (Mini-PROTEAN TGX Precast Gels; Bio-Rad), 12 µg of total protein was separated in a vertical electrophoresis tank (Mini-PROTEAN System; Bio-Rad) at 250 V for 20 min Separated proteins were transferred onto a polyvinylidene difluoride membrane (Bio-Rad) by wet transfer for 60 min at 120 V. Thereafter, the membranes were blocked with 5% dry milk in Tris-buffered saline (TBS) plus Tween-20 (TTBS) (Bio-Rad) solution for 1 hour at room temperature. After three washes in TBS, membranes were incubated with rabbit anti-DMT1 polyclonal, dilution 1:400 (Santa Cruz Biotechnology Inc., Santa Cruz, CA, USA), rabbit anti-SLC40A1 polyclonal antibody (FPN1), dilution 1:800, hepcidin polyclonal antibody, dilution 1:500, and mouse anti-β-actin monoclonal, dilution 1:1000 (Abcam, UK) as primary antibodies, in 5% dry milk in TTBS overnight at 4 °C with shaking. β-actin was used as the loading control. Then, the membranes were washed 3 times in TTBS and incubated for 1 h at room temperature with the appropriate secondary conjugated antibody Immun-Star Goat Anti-Rabbit (GAR)-HRP; Bio-Rad Laboratories; 1:40,000 amd ImmunStar Goat Anti-Mouse (GAM)-HRP; 1:80,000 in TTBS. Immunoblots were detected with a chemiluminescence Luminata forte western HRP Substrate (Merck KGaA, Darmstadt, Germany) and visualized with chemiluminescence using ImageQuant LAS 4000 (Fujifilm Life Science Corporation, USA). All results were analyzed with Image J software.

2.8. Statistical Analysis

Data are presented as mean ± standard error of the mean (SEM) and statistical analyses were performed using SPSS 26.0 (SPSS Inc., Chicago, IL, USA). Differences between groups (control versus anemic during the PEP and normal Fe versus high Fe during the EP) were tested for statistical significance with Student's t-test. Following a significant F-test ($p < 0.05$), individual means were tested by pairwise comparison with Tukey's multiple comparison test when main effects and interactions were significant. Two-way analysis of variance (ANOVA) was used to determine the effect of the type of diet supplied to the animals, anemia, and iron content in the diet. Statistical significance was set at $p < 0.05$ for all comparisons.

3. Results

3.1. Effect of Iron Deficiency on Hepatosomatic Index, Liver Iron Content and Serum Levels of Aspartate Aminotransferase and Alanine Aminotransferase

Iron deprivation impaired all the hematological parameters studied [9], and these parameters are detailed in Supplementary Table S1. Additionally, body weight and liver iron content were lower in the anemic group ($p < 0.001$); however, liver weight remained unchanged, and, as a consequence, HSI was higher in anemic group ($p < 0.05$). Transaminases were significantly higher in the anemic group ($p < 0.001$) (Table 3).

Table 3. Hepatosomatic index, liver iron content and serum levels of aspartate aminotransferase and alanine aminotransferase from control and anemic rats in the pre-experimental period (PEP).

	Control Group (n = 20)	Anemic Group (n = 20)
Body weight (g)	239.7 ± 3.9	201.15 ± 2.9 **
Liver weight (g)	6.324 ± 0.31	6.129 ± 0.31
HSI (%)	2.55 ± 0.07	2.89 ± 0.09 *
Liver iron content (µg/g dry weight)	615.25 ± 31.10	432.31 ± 24.07 **
AST (UI/L)	103.58 ± 8.93	228.04 ± 18.45 **
ALT (UI/L)	24.57 ± 1.16	52.28 ± 2.73 **

Values are means ± SEM (n = 10). HSI, hepatosomatic index; AST, aspartate aminotransferase; ALT, alanine aminotransferase. * Significantly different from the control group (*, $p < 0.05$) Student's t-test). ** Significantly different from the control group (**, $p < 0.001$) Student's t-test).

3.2. Effect of Fermented Milk-Based Diets on Hepatosomatic Index, Liver Iron Content and Serum Levels of Aspartate Aminotransferase and Alanine Aminotransferase during Anemia Recovery

After supplying both fermented milk-based diets during a month, all the hematological parameters were recovered, either with normal Fe or high Fe content. The results were described [9] and are shown in Supplementary Table S2. Fermented goat milk reduced body weight in control and anemic animals, either with normal Fe or high Fe content ($p < 0.001$) compared to animals fed fermented-cow-milk-based diets. Body weight was significantly lower in anemic animals fed both fermented milks with normal Fe content ($p < 0.01$). Body weight was lower a with high Fe content diet than with a normal Fe content diet in animals fed with fermented-cow-milk-based diets in both groups (control and anemic) ($p < 0.05$). HSI was higher in both groups of animals (control and anemic) fed fermented-goat-milk-based diets, either with normal Fe or high Fe, compared to animals fed fermented-cow-milk-based diets ($p < 0.001$). Liver iron content was increased in animals fed with fermented goat milk compared to animals fed with fermented cow milk with normal Fe content diets ($p < 0.01$). In contrast, liver iron content was lower in animals fed fermented goat milk compared to fermented cows' milk with high Fe content ($p < 0.01$). Liver iron content was lower in anemic animals compared to the control group, irrespective of the iron content in both types of fermented milks ($p < 0.01$). As expected, dietary high Fe content increased the liver content of this mineral in control and anemic animals fed fermented cow milk ($p < 0.001$), this increase being lower in the animals fed fermented goat milk ($p < 0.05$). AST and ALT were lower in rats fed with fermented-goat-milk-based diets compared to rats fed with fermented-cow-milk-based diets in all experimental conditions ($p < 0.01$). High Fe content did not affect the transaminases when supplying both milk-based diets (Table 4).

Table 4. Hepatosomatic index, liver iron content and serum levels of aspartate aminotransferase and alanine aminotransferase, from control and anemic rats fed for 30 days with fermented cow- or goat-milk-based diets with normal Fe or high Fe content in the experimental period (EP).

		Fermented Cow Milk		Fermented Goat Milk		2-WAY ANOVA		
	Fe Content	Control Group	Anemic Group	Control Group	Anemic Group	Diet	Anemia	Fe Content
Body weight (g)	Normal	365.23 ± 8.61 a	347.21 ± 8.39 A,*	278.98 ± 3.70 b	255.41 ± 2.85 B,*	<0.001	<0.01	<0.05
	High	339.42 ± 5.18 a,c	329.22 ± 5.81 A,C	287.27 ± 4.92 b	267.57 ± 4.03 B	<0.001	NS [1]	
Liver weight (g)	Normal	6.528 ± 0.24 a	6.269 ± 0.10 A	8.391 ± 0.23 b	8.521 ± 0.21 B	<0.001	NS	<0.05
	High	6.764 ± 0.2 a	6.555 ± 0.12 A	7.692 ± 0.22 b,c	7.934 ± 0.22 B,C	<0.01	NS	
HSI (%)	Normal	1.84 ± 0.04 a	1.77 ± 0.02 A	2.95 ± 0.03 b	3.27 ± 0.05 B	<0.001	NS	NS
	High	1.79 ± 0.03 a	1.82 ± 0.03 A	2.65 ± 0.04 b	3.12 ± 0.04 B	<0.001	NS	
Liver iron content (µg/g dry weight)	Normal	559.56 ± 28.72 a	401.56 ± 24.50 A,*	666.45 ± 33.21 b	489.32 ± 29.64 B,*	<0.01	<0.01	<0.01
	High	832.25 ± 32.56 a,c	782.32 ± 33.55 A,C,*	735.67 ± 29.33 b,c	657.15 ± 29.22 B,C,*	<0.01	<0.01	
AST (UI/L)	Normal	107.62 ± 4.29 a	80.86 ± 4.25 A,*	67.99 ± 2.75 b	61.11 ± 2.12 B	<0.01	<0.05	NS
	High	82.92 ± 4.15 a,c	78.19 ± 3.82 A	60.43 ± 1.10 b	68.47 ± 2.03 B	<0.01	NS	
ALT (UI/L)	Normal	28.91 ±1.34 a	27.77 ± 3.91 A	23.14 ± 1.9 b	16.49 ± 0.76 B,*	<0.01	<0.01	NS
	High	24.0 ± 1.73 a	19.00 ± 1.21 A	19.47 ± 0.53 b	14.48 ± 0.35 B,*	<0.01	<0.01	

Values are means ± SEM (n = 10). [1] NS, not significant. HSI, hepatosomatic index; AST, aspartate aminotransferase; ALT, alanine aminotransferase. * Significantly different from the control group ($p < 0.05$) Student's *t*-test). a,b Mean values among groups of controls rats fed with different diets; different lower-case letters in the same row indicate a significant difference by two-way ANOVA (Tukey's test). A,B Mean values among groups of anemic rats fed with different diets; different upper-case letters in the same row indicate a significant difference by two-way ANOVA (Tukey's test). C Mean values of controls rats were significantly different from the corresponding group of rats fed with normal Fe content at $p < 0.05$ by Student's *t*-test. c Mean values of anemic rats were significantly different from the corresponding group of rats fed with normal Fe content at $p < 0.05$ by Student's *t*-test.

3.3. Effect of Fermented Milk-Based Diets on Liver Iron Homeostasis during Anemia Recovery

Fermented goat milk up-regulated liver DMT1 gene expression in control and anemic rate fed with high Fe content ($p < 0.01$) and in control groups fed with a normal Fe diet, and previously induced anemia reduced DMT1 expression in the animals fed fermented goat milk with normal Fe content ($p < 0.05$) (Figure 2A). Similarly, DMT1-relative protein expression was higher in control and anemic animals fed fermented goat milk with normal Fe ($p < 0.001$). Induced anemia increased liver DMT1 protein expression in animals fed both fermented milk with normal Fe content ($p < 0.001$). High Fe content increased DMT1 protein expression in all groups of animals fed fermented goat or cow milk ($p < 0.001$), except in control animals fed fermented goat milk, which showed a decrease ($p < 0.05$) (Figure 2B).

Expression of FPN1 mRNA increased in control and anemic animals fed fermented goat either with normal Fe ($p < 0.001$) or high Fe content ($p < 0.01$) (Figure 2C). Protein expression of FPN1 increased in control and anemic animals fed fermented goat milk with normal Fe content ($p < 0.001$). Anemia decreased FPN1 protein expression in animals fed fermented goat milk with normal Fe ($p < 0.01$) and increased in animals fed both fermented milks with high Fe content ($p < 0.001$). High Fe content increased liver FPN1 protein expression in all groups of animals fed fermented goat or cow milk ($p < 0.001$), except control animals fed fermented goat milk, which showed a decrease ($p < 0.001$) (Figure 2D).

HAMP mRNA expression was lower in control and anemic animals fed fermented goat milk with normal Fe ($p < 0.05$) and also in control and anemic animals fed fermented goat milk with high Fe content ($p < 0.001$). Anemia increased HAMP mRNa expression in animals fed fermented cow milk with high Fe content ($p < 0.01$). High Fe content increased HAMP gene expression in anemic animals fed both fermented milks ($p < 0.001$) and in control groups fed a fermented cow milk diet ($p < 0.01$) (Figure 2E). Hepcidin protein expression decreased in control and anemic animals fed fermented goat milk with normal Fe content ($p < 0.001$). Anemia decreased hepcidin protein expression in animals fed fermented cow milk with normal Fe content ($p < 0.001$) and increased in animals fed fermented goat milk with normal Fe content ($p < 0.05$); however, with high Fe content, anemia increased hepcidin protein expression in the animals fed both fermented milks ($p < 0.001$). High Fe content increased hepcidin protein expression in all groups of animals fed fermented cow or goat milk ($p < 0.01$) but decreased in control animals fed fermented cow milk ($p < 0.001$) (Figure 2F).

In general, fermented goat milk induced an up-regulation of mRNA FTL1 expression in control and anemic animals fed either with normal Fe or high Fe content ($p < 0.01$). Anemia up-regulated liver mRNA FTL1 expression in animals fed fermented cow milk with high Fe content ($p < 0.01$). High Fe content up-regulated FTL1 mRNA expression in the anemic groups fed both fermented milks ($p < 0.001$) and in the control group fed fermented cow milk ($p < 0.01$) (Figure 3).

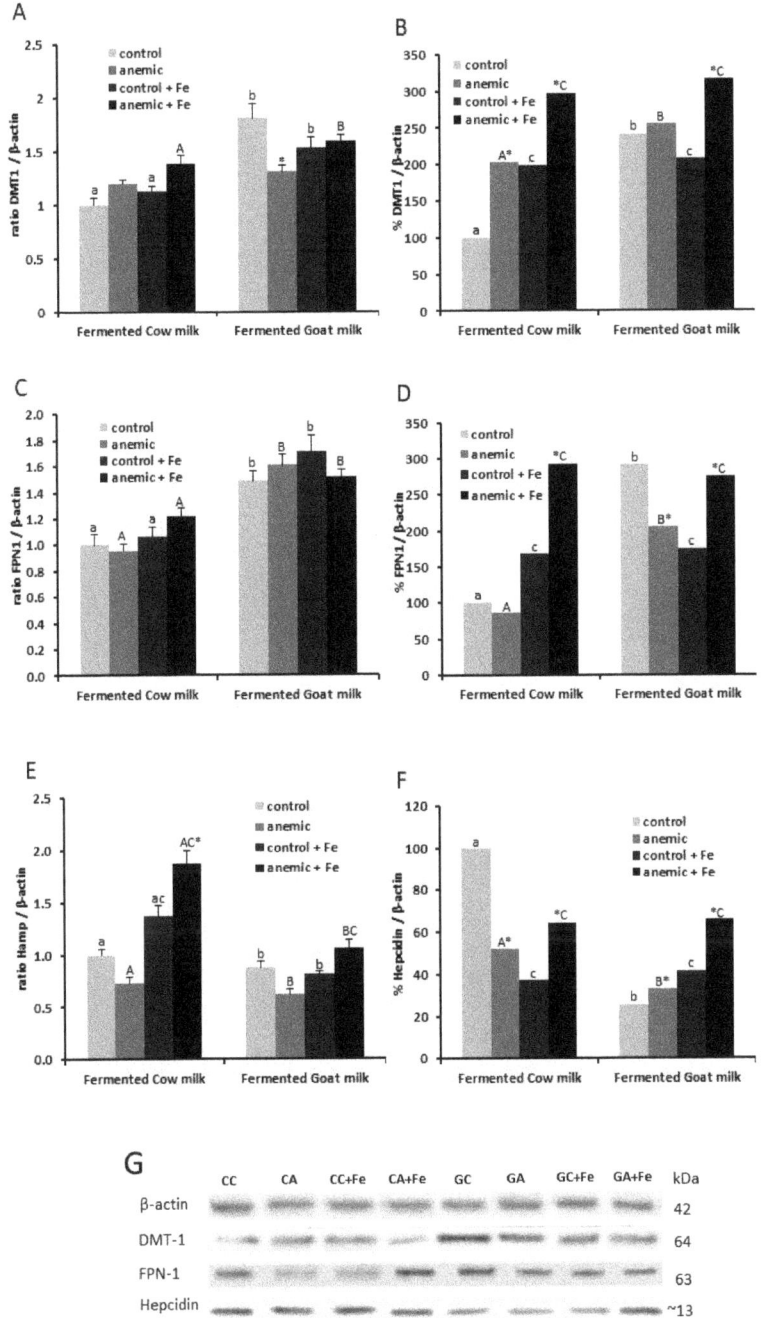

Figure 2. mRNA levels (**A**,**C**,**E**) and protein expression levels (**B**,**D**,**F**) of DMT-1, FPN1 and hepcidin in livers of control and anemic rats, fed normal Fe or high Fe content fermented cow or goat milk-based diets. Values are represented as mean ± SEM (n = 10). For protein expression, values are expressed as % vs β-actin. a,b: mean values among groups of control rats fed with different diets; different lower-case

letters in the same row indicate a significant difference by two-way ANOVA (Tukey's test). A,B: Mean values among groups of anemic rats fed with different diet; different upper-case letters in the same row indicate a significant difference by two-way ANOVA (Tukey's test). * Significantly different ($p < 0.05$) from the control group by Student's *t*-test. c: Mean values of control rats were significantly different from the corresponding groups of rats fed with normal Fe content at $p < 0.05$ by Student's *t*-test. C: Mean values of anemic rats were significantly different from the corresponding group of rats fed with normal Fe content at $p < 0.05$ by Student's *t*-test. (**G**) Representative immunoblots. Abbreviations: cow control (CC), cow anemic (CA), cow control high Fe content (CC+Fe), cow anemic high Fe content (CA+Fe), goat control (GC), goat anemic (GA), goat control high Fe content (GC+Fe), goat anemic high Fe content (GA+Fe).

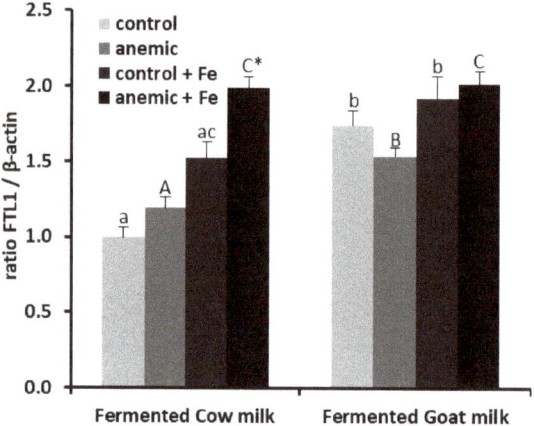

Figure 3. mRNA levels of FTL1 in the liver of control and anemic rats, fed normal Fe or high Fe content fermented cow- or goat-milk-based diets. Values are represented as mean ± SEM ($n = 10$). a,b: mean values among groups of controls rats fed with different diets; different lower case letters in the same row indicate a significant difference by two-way ANOVA (Tukey's test). A,B: mean values among groups of anemic rats fed with different diets; different upper case letters in the same row indicate a significant difference by two-way ANOVA (Tukey's test). * Significantly different ($p < 0.05$) from the control group by Student's *t*-test. c: mean values of controls rats were significantly different from the corresponding group of rats fed with normal Fe content at $p < 0.05$ by Student's *t*-test. C: mean values of anemic rats were significantly different from the corresponding group of rats fed with normal Fe content at $p < 0.05$ by Student's *t*-test.

4. Discussion

Anemia reduced body weight in the PEP, due to the impairment of hematological parameters and the depletion of the hepatic iron levels. These negatively affect the weight gain of animals during the growing period, since the hypoxia induced by the lack of iron limits ATP production and decreases levels of thyroid hormones and ghrelin, inducing cachexia and leading to reductions of lean mass [13]. In a previous study, we reported that serum total bilirubin was increased in hepatocellular damage. In that study, bilirubin was increased and AST and ALT activities were also found elevated in IDA. The increase of transaminase release into the bloodstream could be due to the impairment of the hepatic function induced by the iron deficiency [13,14].

During the EP, body weight was statistically lower in the animals fed fermented goat milk. This finding can be explained because, as previously reported [15], fermented goat milk consumption influences adipose tissue depot homeostasis during iron deficiency recovery, reducing adiposity, increasing leptin elevation and reducing ghrelin, and, therefore, diminishing appetite and increasing basal metabolic rate. Additionally, fermented goat milk consumption reduces adiponectin levels and shows an inverse correlation with non-esterified fatty acids, indicating increased lipolysis rates in adipose tissue [15].

Liver iron homeostasis is tightly regulated to maximize the iron supply when anemia is established and to promote storage when iron status is adequate. Intracellular iron content is regulated by the relative rate of cellular import, via DMT1, versus export, via FPN1 [16].

Fermented goat milk improves iron metabolism, because, as previously reported [15], it increases expression of duodenal key proteins in intestinal iron metabolism, improving iron absorption after induced anemia. However, in spite of the role of the liver as the central regulator of iron homeostasis, a better characterization of the hepatic events in the pathophysiology of iron deficiency instauration and recovery leads to new nutritional strategies to improve liver molecular functions related to iron homeostasis.

After supplying the fermented-milk-based diets, iron repletion was more efficient with fermented goat milk, a fact that is corroborated by the recovery of hematological parameters and the liver iron content recorded in the current study. This fact can be explained due to the beneficial increase in the liver DMT1 iron-transport gene and protein expression, enhancing iron metabolism and storage compared with fermented cow milk. DMT1 is localized both to the plasma membrane and in the cytosol of hepatocytes [17]. In addition to its role in endosomal iron export, the presence of DMT1 on the microvillous membrane of hepatocytes reveals that the liver is capable of absorbing non-heme, non-transferrin-bound iron. Contrary to the duodenal DMT1, hepatic DMT1 expression parallels iron status [17], playing a key role by regulating iron homeostasis in the liver. Therefore, the increased liver DMT1 protein levels faithfully reflect the increased liver iron storage after dietary iron repletion [18] and, this way, the increase in DMT1 protein expression in anemic animals fed fermented goat milk reveals that iron repletion is more efficient, a finding that is supported and corroborated by the higher iron storage in the rats fed fermented goat milk compared with fermented cow milk. As previously reported, goat milk fat is richer in medium-chain triglycerides, which are oxidized in the mitochondria, providing fast energy discharge used in several metabolic pathways [19] and thus contributing to increasing the synthesis of carrier proteins such as DMT1 [20]. On the other hand, goat milk has more than twice the vitamin A content of cow milk [19], and this vitamin increases liver DMT1 protein expression by posttranscriptional regulation via increased protein translation or decreased degradation [18].

Hepcidin is a key indicator of iron status and metabolism. This hormone regulates iron levels and location in response to nutritional status. High hepcidin levels block intestinal iron absorption and macrophage recycling, causing anemia. Low hepcidin levels favor bone marrow iron supply for hemoglobin synthesis and erythropohiesis. Multiple factors regulate the expression of hepcidin in the liver. As expected, low serum hepcidin levels were recorded in the PEP due to the increased expression of key duodenal proteins involved in iron absorption [20], favoring red blood cell production during insufficient dietary iron supply. On the other hand, inflammation is a strong inducer of hepcidin production and release from the liver [21–23], resulting in reduced iron release from stores and macrophages, thereby reducing iron in the circulation and disrupting iron homeostasis [24]. In the current study, a down-regulation of liver hepcidin has been recorded in animals consuming fermented goat milk, a fact that increases the iron efflux from the hepatocytes to the serum, due to the inverse correlation between hepcidin expression and the FPN1 activity [9,25].

In addition, we have previously reported that fermented goat milk consumption decreased pro-inflammatory cytokines and increased anti-inflammatory cytokines [25], due to the anti-inflammatory activities of its biologically active lipid fractions, such as sphingomyelin, phosphatidylcholine, and phosphatidylethanolamine lipid derivatives [26,27]. Moreover, fermented goat milk has a higher content in conjugated linoleic acid than fermented cow milk, featuring a putative role modulating anti-inflammatory responses [25]. All these anti-inflammatory properties of fermented goat milk would contribute to the decrease in liver hepcidin expression. This decrease in hepcidin, together with the increase in DMT1 and FPN1 gene and protein liver expression recorded when fermented goat milk is supplied, would led to the mobilization of iron from hepatic storage to sustain erythropoiesis and improve iron status, even under Fe-overload conditions. These data indicate a not only a better hematological recovery but also improved iron mobilization for liver storage to target organs.

Although, in physiological conditions, hepatocytes have a high capacity for iron storage, the liver is also the main organ affected by the oxidative stress caused by Fe-overload toxicity due to its high propensity to induce reactive oxygen species (ROS) [28]. As mentioned above, the increase in DMT1 and FPN1 gene and protein liver expression recorded with fermented goat milk lead to lower amounts of iron stored in the hepatocytes during the dietary Fe overload in comparison with fermented cow milk, reducing the evoked oxidative stress. In this sense, fermented goat milk has positive effects on enzymatic antioxidant hepatic defense, even in a situation of Fe overload, which limits the processes of lipid peroxidation in comparison with cow milk, due to the improvement of zinc bioavailability (with antioxidant capacity) and the better lipid quality in comparison to fermented cow milk, reducing the generation of ROS [29]. Additionally, these findings are supported by the previous results [30], reporting a clear diminishment of transaminase release into the bloodstream, corroborating the hepatoprotective effect of goat milk during Fe overload and reducing hepatocellular damage, a fact that could avoid, at least partially, the progression of Fe-overload-related diseases [31].

FTL1 is the intracellular iron storage protein that stores and releases iron in a controlled way, and its expression greatly increases when cellular iron concentrations rise, providing the cell with an enormous ability to sequester iron. When intracellular iron content is low, iron-responsive element-binding protein 2 (IRP2) represses FTL1, mRNA translation, while intracellular iron accumulation promotes IRP2 degradation and allows FTL1 mRNA translation [32]. As previously mentioned, the increased DMT1 and FPN1 expression levels when fermented goat milk is supplied improve iron storage, also explaining the higher levels of mRNA FTL1. In addition, Fe overload increased FTL1 gene expression, probably as a compensatory mechanism to avoid the liver oxidative damage induced by Fe overload, because intracellular iron redox activity is controlled by ferritin [33].

5. Conclusions

Fermented goat milk consumption potentiates the up-regulation of key genes and proteins involved in iron metabolism, such as DMT1 and FPN1, and downregulates liver hepcidin, enhancing and improving iron repletion during anemia recovery. In addition, taking into account the better iron storage in the liver during anemia recovery, the reduction in the iron accumulation during Fe overload, and the improvement of the hematological parameters, fermented goat milk consumption induces a hepatic physiological adaptation of the key genes and proteins that regulate the fluctuation of the cellular iron levels, favoring whole-body iron homeostasis.

Supplementary Materials: The following are available online at http://www.mdpi.com/2072-6643/12/5/1336/s1, Table S1: Hematological parameters of control and anemic rats in the pre-experimental period (PEP); Table S2. Hematological parameters from control and anemic rats fed for 30 days with fermented cow or goat milk-based diets with normal-Fe content or Fe-overload in the experimental period (EP).

Author Contributions: Research Design, I.L.-A. and J.D.-C.; Methodology, J.M.-F., J.D.-C., I.L.-A., and M.J.M.A.; Formal Analysis, Investigation and Software, J.M.-F. and J.D.-C.; Writing—Original Draft Preparation J.M.-F., I.L.-A., J.D.-C. and M.J.M.A.; Supervision and Project Administration, I.L.-A. All persons designated as authors qualify for authorship, and all those who qualify for authorship are listed. All authors have read and agreed to the published version of the manuscript.

Funding: This study is funded by the Excellence Project (P11-AGR-7648) from the Regional Government of Andalusia.

Acknowledgments: J.M.-F. was supported by two fellowships from the Ministry of Education, Culture and Sport (Spain), FPU and Traslados Temporales FPU (University of King´s College of London). J.M.-F. is grateful to the Excellence Program "Nutrición y Ciencias de los Alimentos" from the University of Granada. The authors are grateful to Susan Stevenson for her efficient support in the revision with the English language.

Conflicts of Interest: The authors declare no conflict of interest.

References

1. McLean, E.; Cogswell, M.; Egli, I.; Wojdyla, D.; de Benoist, B. Worldwide prevalence of anaemia, WHO Vitamin and Mineral Nutrition Information System, 1993–2005. *Public Health Nutr.* **2009**, *12*, 444–454. [CrossRef] [PubMed]
2. Wallace, D.F. The Regulation of Iron Absorption and Homeostasis. *Clin. Biochem. Rev.* **2016**, *37*, 51–62.
3. Hentze, M.W.; Muckenthaler, M.U.; Galy, B.; Camaschella, C. Two to tango: Regulation of Mammalian iron metabolism. *Cell* **2010**, *142*, 24–38. [CrossRef] [PubMed]
4. Maio, N.; Jain, A.; Rouault, T.A. Mammalian iron-sulfur cluster biogenesis: Recent insights into the roles of frataxin, acyl carrier protein and ATPase-mediated transfer to recipient proteins. *Curr. Opin. Chem. Biol.* **2020**, *55*, 34–44. [CrossRef] [PubMed]
5. Weiss, G.; Goodnough, L.T. Anemia of chronic disease. *N. Engl. J. Med.* **2005**, *352*, 1011–1023. [CrossRef] [PubMed]
6. Rishi, G.; Subramaniam, V.N. The liver in regulation of iron homeostasis. *Am. J. Physiol. Gastrointest. Liver Physiol.* **2017**, *313*, G157–G165. [CrossRef]
7. Ross, S.L.; Tran, L.; Winters, A.; Lee, K.J.; Plewa, C.; Foltz, I.; King, C.; Miranda, L.P.; Allen, J.; Beckman, H.; et al. Molecular mechanism of hepcidin-mediated ferroportin internalization requires ferroportin lysines, not tyrosines or JAK-STAT. *Cell Metab.* **2012**, *15*, 905–917. [CrossRef]
8. Vyoral, D.; Jiri, P. Therapeutic potential of hepcidin—The master regulator of iron metabolism. *Pharmacol. Res.* **2017**, *115*, 242–254. [CrossRef]
9. Moreno-Fernandez, J.; Diaz-Castro, J.; Pulido-Moran, M.; Alferez, M.J.; Boesch, C.; Sanchez-Alcover, A.; Lopez-Aliaga, I. Fermented Goat's Milk Consumption Improves Duodenal Expression of Iron Homeostasis Genes during Anemia Recovery. *J. Agric. Food Chem.* **2016**, *64*, 2560–2568. [CrossRef]
10. Reeves, P.G.; Nielsen, F.H.; Fahey, G.C., Jr. AIN-93 purified diets for laboratory rodents: Final report of the American Institute of Nutrition ad hoc writing committee on the reformulation of the AIN-76A rodent diet. *J. Nutr.* **1993**, *123*, 1939–1951. [CrossRef]
11. Pallares, I.; Lisbona, F.; Aliaga, I.L.; Barrionuevo, M.; Alferez, M.J.; Campos, M.S. Effect of iron deficiency on the digestive utilization of iron, phosphorus, calcium and magnesium in rats. *Br. J. Nutr.* **1993**, *70*, 609–620. [CrossRef] [PubMed]
12. Raja, K.B.; Simpson, R.J.; Peters, T.J. Intestinal iron absorption studies in mouse models of iron-overload. *Br. J. Haematol.* **1994**, *86*, 156–162. [CrossRef] [PubMed]
13. Moreno-Fernandez, J.; Diaz-Castro, J.; Alferez, M.J.M.; Lopez-Aliaga, I. Iron Deficiency and Neuroendocrine Regulators of Basal Metabolism, Body Composition and Energy Expenditure in Rats. *Nutrients* **2019**, *11*, 631. [CrossRef] [PubMed]
14. Tolman, K.G.; Re, J.R. Liver function. In *Tietz Textbook of Clinical Chemistry*; Burtis, C.A., Ashwood, E.R., Eds.; W.B. Saunders: Philadelphia, PA, USA, 1999; pp. 1125–1177.
15. Diaz-Castro, J.; Moreno-Fernandez, J.; Pulido-Moran, M.; Alferez, M.J.M.; Robles-Rebollo, M.; Ochoa, J.J.; Lopez-Aliaga, I. Changes in Adiposity and Body Composition during Anemia Recovery with Goat or Cow Fermented Milks. *J. Agric. Food Chem.* **2017**, *65*, 4057–4065. [CrossRef]
16. Blankenhaus, B.; Braza, F.; Martins, R.; Bastos-Amador, P.; Gonzalez-Garcia, I.; Carlos, A.R.; Mahu, I.; Faisca, P.; Nunes, J.M.; Ventura, P.; et al. Ferritin regulates organismal energy balance and thermogenesis. *Mol. Metab.* **2019**, *24*, 64–79. [CrossRef]
17. Trinder, D.; Oates, P.S.; Thomas, C.; Sadleir, J.; Morgan, E.H. Localisation of divalent metal transporter 1 (DMT1) to the microvillus membrane of rat duodenal enterocytes in iron deficiency, but to hepatocytes in iron overload. *Gut* **2000**, *46*, 270–276. [CrossRef]
18. Kelleher, S.L.; Lonnerdal, B. Low vitamin a intake affects milk iron level and iron transporters in rat mammary gland and liver. *J. Nutr.* **2005**, *135*, 27–32. [CrossRef]
19. Alférez, M.J.M.; López-Aliaga, I.; Nestares, T.; Díaz-Castro, J.; Barrionuevo, M.; Ros, P.B.; Campos, M.S. Dietary goat milk improves iron bioavailability in rats with induced ferropenic anaemia in comparison with cow milk. *Int. Dairy J.* **2006**, *16*, 813–821. [CrossRef]

20. Diaz-Castro, J.; Pulido, M.; Alferez, M.J.; Ochoa, J.J.; Rivas, E.; Hijano, S.; Lopez-Aliaga, I. Goat milk consumption modulates liver divalent metal transporter 1 (DMT1) expression and serum hepcidin during Fe repletion in Fe-deficiency anemia. *J. Dairy Sci.* **2014**, *97*, 147–154. [CrossRef]
21. Nemeth, E.; Valore, E.V.; Territo, M.; Schiller, G.; Lichtenstein, A.; Ganz, T. Hepcidin, a putative mediator of anemia of inflammation, is a type II acute-phase protein. *Blood* **2003**, *101*, 2461–2463. [CrossRef]
22. Ganz, T. Hepcidin and iron regulation, 10 years later. *Blood* **2011**, *117*, 4425–4433. [CrossRef]
23. Ueda, N.; Takasawa, K. Impact of Inflammation on Ferritin, Hepcidin and the Management of Iron Deficiency Anemia in Chronic Kidney Disease. *Nutrients* **2018**, *10*, 1173. [CrossRef] [PubMed]
24. Peng, Y.Y.; Uprichard, J. Ferritin and iron studies in anaemia and chronic disease. *Ann. Clin. Biochem.* **2017**, *54*, 43–48. [CrossRef] [PubMed]
25. Lopez-Aliaga, I.; Garcia-Pedro, J.D.; Moreno-Fernandez, J.; Alferez, M.J.M.; Lopez-Frias, M.; Diaz-Castro, J. Fermented goat milk consumption improves iron status and evokes inflammatory signalling during anemia recovery. *Food Funct.* **2018**, *9*, 3195–3201. [CrossRef] [PubMed]
26. Nasopoulou, C.; Smith, T.; Detopoulou, M.; Tsikrika, C.; Papaharisis, L.; Barkas, D.; Zabetakis, I. Structural elucidation of olive pomace fed sea bass (Dicentrarchus labrax) polar lipids with cardioprotective activities. *Food Chem.* **2014**, *145*, 1097–1105. [CrossRef] [PubMed]
27. Tsorotioti, S.E.; Nasopoulou, C.; Detopoulou, M.; Sioriki, E.; Demopoulos, C.A.; Zabetakis, I. In vitro anti-atherogenic properties of traditional Greek cheese lipid fractions. *Dairy Sci. Technol.* **2014**, *94*, 269–281. [CrossRef]
28. Maras, J.S.; Maiwall, R.; Harsha, H.C.; Das, S.; Hussain, M.S.; Kumar, C.; Bihari, C.; Rastogi, A.; Kumar, M.; Trehanpati, N.; et al. Dysregulated iron homeostasis is strongly associated with multiorgan failure and early mortality in acute-on-chronic liver failure. *Hepatology* **2015**, *61*, 1306–1320. [CrossRef]
29. Diaz-Castro, J.; Perez-Sanchez, L.J.; Ramirez Lopez-Frias, M.; Lopez-Aliaga, I.; Nestares, T.; Alferez, M.J.; Ojeda, M.L.; Campos, M.S. Influence of cow or goat milk consumption on antioxidant defence and lipid peroxidation during chronic iron repletion. *Br. J. Nutr.* **2012**, *108*, 1–8. [CrossRef]
30. Alferez, M.J.; Rivas, E.; Diaz-Castro, J.; Hijano, S.; Nestares, T.; Moreno, M.; Campos, M.S.; Serrano-Reina, J.A.; Lopez-Aliaga, I. Folic acid supplemented goat milk has beneficial effects on hepatic physiology, haematological status and antioxidant defence during chronic Fe repletion. *J. Dairy Res.* **2015**, *82*, 86–94. [CrossRef]
31. Knutson, M.D. Iron transport proteins: Gateways of cellular and systemic iron homeostasis. *J. Biol. Chem.* **2017**, *292*, 12735–12743. [CrossRef]
32. Muckenthaler, M.U.; Rivella, S.; Hentze, M.W.; Galy, B. A Red Carpet for Iron Metabolism. *Cell* **2017**, *168*, 344–361. [CrossRef] [PubMed]
33. Gozzelino, R.; Soares, M.P. Coupling heme and iron metabolism via ferritin H chain. *Antioxid. Redox Signal.* **2014**, *20*, 1754–1769. [CrossRef] [PubMed]

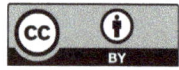

© 2020 by the authors. Licensee MDPI, Basel, Switzerland. This article is an open access article distributed under the terms and conditions of the Creative Commons Attribution (CC BY) license (http://creativecommons.org/licenses/by/4.0/).

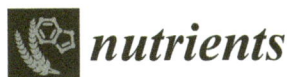

Article

Is a Gluten-Free Diet Enough to Maintain Correct Micronutrients Status in Young Patients with Celiac Disease?

Teresa Nestares [1,*], Rafael Martín-Masot [2], Ana Labella [3], Virginia A. Aparicio [1,4], Marta Flor-Alemany [1], Magdalena López-Frías [1] and José Maldonado [5,6,7,8]

1. Department of Physiology and "José MataixVerdú" Institute of Nutrition and Food Technology (INYTA), University of Granada, 18071 Granada, Spain; virginiaparicio@ugr.es (V.A.A.); martadelaflor@correo.ugr.es (M.F.-A.); maglopez@ugr.es (M.L.-F.)
2. Pediatric Gastroenterology and Nutrition Unit, Hospital Regional Universitario de Malaga, 29010 Málaga, Spain; rafammgr@gmail.com
3. Pediatric Clinical Management Unit., "San Cecilio" University Hospital, 18016 Granada, Spain; alnestares92@gmail.com
4. Sport and Health University Research Institute (iMUDS), 18071 Granada, Spain
5. Department of Pediatrics, University of Granada, 18071 Granada, Spain; jmaldon@ugr.es
6. Biosanitary Research Institute, 18071 Granada, Spain
7. Maternal and Child Health Network, Carlos III Health Institute, 28029 Madrid, Spain
8. Pediatric Clinical Management Unit. "Virgen de las Nieves" University Hospital, 18071 Granada, Spain
* Correspondence: nestares@ugr.es; Tel.: +34-696989989

Received: 28 February 2020; Accepted: 19 March 2020; Published: 21 March 2020

Abstract: The current study assesses whether the use of a gluten-free diet (GFD) is sufficient for maintaining correct iron status in children with celiac disease (CD). The study included 101 children. The celiac group ($n = 68$) included children with CD, with long (> 6 months) ($n = 47$) or recent (< 6 months) ($n = 21$) adherence to a GFD. The control group ($n = 43$) included healthy children. Dietary assessment was performed by a food frequency questionnaire and a 3-day food record. Celiac children had lower iron intake than controls, especially at the beginning of GFD ($p < 0.01$). The group CD-GFD >6 months showed a higher intake of cobalamin, meat derivatives and fish compared to that of CD-GFD <6 months (all, $p < 0.05$). The control group showed a higher consumption of folate, iron, magnesium, selenium and meat derivatives than that of children CD-GFD >6 months (all, $p < 0.05$). Control children also showed a higher consumption of folate and iron compared to that of children CD-GFD <6 months (both, $p < 0.05$). The diet of celiac children was nutritionally less balanced than that of the control. Participation of dietitians is necessary in the management of CD to guide the GFD as well as assess the inclusion of iron supplementation and other micronutrients that may be deficient.

Keywords: celiac disease; gluten-free diet; nutritional adequacy; iron deficiency anemia; children

1. Introduction

Celiac disease (CD) occurs in about 1% of people in most populations [1,2]. Diagnosis rates are increasing, which seems to be due to a true rise in incidence that requires greater awareness and early detection. In response to unknown environmental factors, it is believed that ingestion of gluten promotes an immunologically mediated small intestinal enteropathy in genetically susceptible individuals [3]. The disease primarily affects the small intestine; however, the clinical manifestations are large, with both intestinal and extra-intestinal symptoms. Patients with CD might also present with various deficiency states, including anemia, osteopenia or osteoporosis. Upon diagnosis, patients should be tested, since between 20%–38% of CD patients show nutritional deficiencies. Specifically,

12%–69% display iron deficiency, more frequent in adults than in children [4], and 8%–41% display Vitamin B12 deficiency, and about 31% of patients with CD present low ferritin concentrations [5].

A lifelong strict gluten-free diet (GFD) is the only available treatment for CD. Improvement and resolution of symptoms typically occur within days or weeks, and often precede the normalization of serological markers and of duodenal villous atrophy [6]. About 20% of patients with CD have persistent or recurrent symptoms despite having a good adherence to a GFD [7], and the nutritional adequacy of the GFD remains controversial [8], although evidence suggests that GFD is nutritionally unbalanced [8]. In fact, wheat is a source of iron, folates and B vitamins (thiamin, riboflavin and niacin) and not only a major source of protein. Indeed, gluten-free products are low in these nutrients compared to their gluten-containing equivalents [9–11].

An essential micronutrient for adequate erythropoietic function is iron, which is implicated in oxidative metabolism, enzymatic activities and cellular immune responses [12]. Iron deficiency anemia (IDA) is a public health problem where children are one of the weaker groups [13]. CD leads to decreased absorption of many nutrients in duodenum-mucosal damage, including iron [14] (the site of maximal iron absorption). Therefore, iron malabsorption is usually observed in CD and may be the presenting clinical feature even in the absence of weight loss or diarrhea [15–17]. Although IDA is very common in CD, it could persist after the initiation of a GFD [18]. Unfortunately, the relationship between IDA and CD has been poorly explored.

Therefore, the purpose of the present study was to determine the importance of a GFD in the normalization of iron metabolism in patients with CD, as well as to test the influence of the time in a GFD on iron metabolism.

2. Materials and Methods

2.1. Subjects

The study was carried out according to the principles of the Declaration of Helsinki and its later amendments and approved by the Ethics Committee of the University of Granada (Ref. 201202400000697). The study included 101 children aged 7–18 years old, attending the Gastroenterology, Hepatology and Child Nutrition Service from the "Virgen de las Nieves" University Hospital in Granada, Spain.

The control group included 43 healthy children, whose serological screening was detected to be negative and who had no history of any chronic disease. These children attended this Service due to minor symptoms related to chronic functional constipation, according to the Rome IV criteria. After verifying that it was due to transitory gastrointestinal symptoms (functional constipation), they were included in the control group. The inclusion criteria for the control group were age between 7 and 18 years, absence of serum IgA and IgG anti-transglutaminase (tTG) antibodies, normal weight for the age, absence of gastrointestinal disorders in the previous year and normal appetite. Children with CD diagnosed in accordance with the European Society for Pediatric Gastroenterology Hepatology and Nutrition (ESPGHAN) [19] were included in the CD group ($n = 68$), which was divided into patients on a GFD longer than 6 months (GFD > 6, $n = 47$) and patients following a GFD less than 6 months (GFD < 6, $n = 21$). The exclusion criteria for both groups were liver or kidney diseases, acute and chronic inflammation, inflammatory bowel disease, diabetes, chronic asthma and consumption of dietary supplements containing substances with antioxidant activity. We also excluded obese patients (according to the criteria of the International Task Force) [20] and those who did not sign the informed consent. Written informed consent was obtained from all parents.

2.2. Clinical and Socio-Demographics

Participants' clinical and socio-demographic characteristics including age, household composition, parents' marital status, educational level and smoking habit were assessed by the same group of researchers.

When IDA was detected in CD children, elemental iron was administered at doses of 3 to 5 mg per kilogram of weight per day. When iron deficiency without anemia was detected, prophylactic doses of elemental iron were prescribed at a dose of 2 mg per kilogram per day in two daily doses for 2–3 months [21].

2.3. Anthropometric Measures

Anthropometric characteristics (weight, height) were assessed in the control and the celiac subjects. Height was measured to the nearest 5 mm using a stadiometer (Seca 22, Hamburg, Germany). Body weight was measured using the same mechanical balance (Seca 200, Hamburg, Germany).

2.4. Blood Haematological and Biochemical Anaemia-Related Markers

Venous blood samples were collected into anticoagulated tubes with sodium heparin during morning hours from fasting patients. In order to obtain plasma, blood samples were centrifuged at $2500\times g$ at 4 °C for 10 min. Plasma samples were frozen (−80 °C) until measurements. All hematological and biochemical parameters studied were measured using an automated hematology analyzer (K-1000D, Sysmex, Tokyo, Japan). The following biochemical parameters were determined: iron, ferritin, transferrin, thyroid-stimulating hormone (TSH) and thyroxine.

2.5. Dietary Assessment

Dietary intake was assessed through a semi-quantitative 78-item food frequency questionnaire (FFQ) previously validated in Spain by Mataix et al. [22] and a three-day food record, two on weekdays and one on the weekend. The diary was carefully explained, face to face, by the same trained dietitian to the children and their parents and was accompanied by detailed instructions for the compilation and a photographic atlas including different portion size pictures and a set of household measures [23]. The survey included a daily record of all foods consumed during the different meals (breakfast, morning snack, lunch, afternoon snack, dinner). For each meal, participants were requested to report an exhaustive description of the food and the recipes (including cooking methods and sugar or fats added during the meal preparation), food amount (according to the atlas) and the brands of packaged foods consumed.

All diaries were analyzed by the same trained dietitian using the Evalfinut software that includes the Spanish Food Composition Database [24]. The program estimated the energy intake (kilocalories) and macronutrients (proteins, total fats, saturated fats, carbohydrates, simple sugars and fiber, expressed in grams) and the percentage of energy provided by each macronutrient. Recommended Energy and Nutrient Intake Levels for Spanish population [24] were taken as reference values for energy and nutrient intake and for food group consumption. The composition of GF products was retrieved from product labels.

2.6. Data Analyses

We employed descriptive statistics (mean, standard deviation) for quantitative variables and percentage of participants (%) for categorical variables to describe the baseline characteristics of the study sample. We conducted Student's t-test to explore differences in the continuous variables. Furthermore, we assessed differences in categorical variables by using the chi-squared test.

A one-way analysis of covariance (ANCOVA) after adjustment for age, sex and body weight was employed to assess the differences in hematological and biochemical anemia-related markers between the celiac and control healthy groups. An ANCOVA after adjustment for age, sex and body weight was also performed to explore differences in hematological and biochemical anemia-related markers and dietary behavior between the healthy controls, the patients with a GFD in the last 6 months and the patients engaged in a GFD less than 6 months. Significant pairwise comparisons with Bonferroni adjustment were performed to keep the experiment error rate at $\alpha = 0.05$ and to identify between which groups the differences were significant (e.g., control healthy group vs. less than 6 months in a GFD).

The data analyses were conducted with the Statistical Package for Social Sciences (IBM SPSS Statistics for Windows, Version 20, IBM Corp, Armonk, NY, USA), and statistical significance was set at $p \leq 0.05$.

3. Results

The baseline sociodemographic and anthropometric characteristics of the study sample are shown in Table 1. A total of 68 children with CD participated in the study (mean age 8.5 ± 4.1 years). More than half of the participants with CD followed a GFD for more than 6 months and met physical activity recommendations. The control group included 43 healthy children (mean age 10.3 ± 4.5 years). There were differences in height ($p = 0.006$) and weight ($p = 0.002$) between groups. Regarding the hematological results, the CD group showed lower levels of hemoglobin, erythrocyte and hematocrit compared to healthy children ($p < 0.05$).

Table 1. Anthropometric, clinical and sociodemographic characteristics of the study participants.

Variable	Celiac Group ($n = 68$)	Healthy Group ($n = 43$)	p
Sex (female, n (%))	52 (76.5)	20 (46.5)	0.014
Age (years)	8.5 (4.1)	10.3 (4.5)	0.025
Anthropometry			
Height (cm)	129.2 (23.5)	142.2 (25.2)	0.006
Weight (kg)	30.5 (12.9)	39.6 (16.4)	0.002
Passive smoker (yes, %)	8.9	25.7	0.031
Time in gluten-free diet (%)			
Not started or less than 6 months	32.9	-	
More than 6 months	67.1	-	
Strictly following gluten-free diet (n, (%))	55 (85.9)	1 (1.8)	
Any other celiac family member (%)			
No (or unknown)	35.9	-	
Siblings or parents	46.9	-	
Cousins or uncles	6.3	-	
Various degrees of consanguinity	10.9	-	
Meet physical activity recommendations	75.5	88.9	0.161

Values shown as mean (standard deviation) unless otherwise indicated.

Differences in serum hematological and biochemical anemia-related markers between healthy control children, patients with a GFD in the last 6 months and patients with a GFD less than 6 months are shown in Table 2. Serum erythrocytes differed between groups ($p = 0.016$), with pairwise comparisons showing lower erythrocyte counts in both groups of CD patients compared to the healthy control group ($p < 0.05$). Hematocrit also differed between groups ($p = 0.031$), with pairwise comparisons showing lower hematocrit concentration in the CD group following the GFD for less than 6 months compared to the control group (38.6 ± 0.7 versus 41.0 ± 0.4, respectively, $p < 0.05$). Finally, hemoglobin levels differed between groups ($p < 0.05$), being lower in CD groups but without pairwise significant difference.

Table 2. Differences between healthy control children, patients with a gluten-free diet in the last 6 months and patients with a gluten-free diet less than 6 months on serum hematological and biochemical anemia-related markers.

Variable	Less than 6 Months on Gluten-Free Diet (n = 21)	More than 6 Months on Gluten-Free Diet (n = 47)	Healthy Control Group (n = 43)	p
Erythrocytes (millions)	4.74 (0.08) [a]	4.80 (0.05) [b]	4.99 (0.05) [ab]	0.016
Hematocrit (%)	38.6 (0.70) [a]	40.0 (0.44)	41.0 (0.49) [a]	0.031
Hemoglobin (mg/dL)	13.2 (0.21)	13.4 (0.14)	13.9 (0.15)	0.046
Erythrocyte corpuscular volume (fL)	82.6 (1.28)	83.2 (0.80)	81.8 (0.89)	0.521
Hemoglobin corpuscular volume (fL)	28.3 (0.47)	28.0 (0.29)	27.9 (0.33)	0.744
RDW	13.3 (0.20)	13.7 (0.13)	13.5 (0.14)	0.130
Iron (µg/dL)	75.7 (8.0)	77.3 (4.5)	89.1 (5.4)	0.226
Ferritin (µg/dL)	44.3 (10.1)	41.9 (5.3)	50.3 (6.5)	0.618
Transferrin (mg/dL)	319.6 (13.3)	292.3 (8.4)	285.5 (11.6)	0.161
TSH (UI/L)	2.42 (0.25)	2.71 (0.17)	2.23 (0.18)	0.150
Thyroxine (µg/dL)	0.97 (0.03)	0.93 (0.02)	0.95 (0.02)	0.588

Values shown as mean (standard error); TSH: thyroid-stimulating hormone; RDW: red blood cell distribution width. Model adjusted for sex, age and body weight. [a,b] Common superscript in a same row indicates a significant difference ($p < 0.05$) between the groups. Pairwise comparisons were performed with Bonferroni's adjustment.

Tables 3 and 4 show the total daily energy and the macronutrient and micronutrient intakes in the three study groups, and the results from daily food group consumption, as collected by the FFQ. Total energy daily intake did not differ between groups. There were no significant differences for macronutrient intake. There were some differences for micronutrients involved in iron metabolism; iron intake was lower for CD groups vs controls ($p < 0.006$). Selenium and magnesium intake was lower for GFD > 6 months vs the control group ($p < 0.001$).

Table 3. Differences between healthy control children, patients with a gluten-free diet in the last 6 months and patients with a gluten-free diet less than 6 months on dietary intake outcomes.

Variable	Less than 6 Months on Gluten-Free Diet (n = 21)	More than 6 Months on Gluten-Free Diet (n = 47)	Healthy Control Group (n = 43)	p
Dietary intake				
Energy intake (Kcal/day)	1790 (150.5)	1814 (75.1)	1870 (88.9)	0.861
Fat (g/day)	60.3 (8.4)	78.1 (4.2)	75.9 (5.0)	0.171
Protein (g/day)	68.8 (7.5)	70.0 (3.5)	77.0 (4.2)	0.409
Fiber (g/day)	18.8 (1.7)	14.2 (0.8)	15.7 (1.0)	0.056
Carbohydrates (g/day)	179.3 (19.3)	200.1 (9.94)	212.6 (11.7)	0.376
Folate (µg)	159.8 (17.6) [a]	159.0 (9.0) [b]	191.4 (10.6) [ab]	0.075
Cobalamin (µg)	4.04 (1.99) [a]	7.50 (1.00) [a]	6.50 (1.18)	0.289
Calcium (mg)	741.8 (99.7)	732.1 (49.7)	798.1 (58.9)	0.701
Iron (mg)	7.32 (0.99) [a]	7.61 (0.49) [b]	10.1 (0.58) [ab]	0.006
Iodine (µg)	74.4 (9.4)	75.7 (6.3)	88.8 (6.8)	0.313
Magnesium (mg)	174.8 (18.4)	165.6 (9.23) [a]	206.9 (10.9) [a]	0.022
Selenium (µg)	52.3 (7.0)	45.5 (3.5) [a]	68.9 (4.2) [a]	<0.001
Zinc (mg)	6.50 (0.70)	5.81 (0.35)	7.11 (0.42)	0.070

Values shown as mean (standard error); s, servings; m, month; wk, week. Model adjusted for sex, age and body weight. Upper case [a,b] letters in the same row indicate a significant pairwise difference ($p < 0.05$) between groups with the same letter. Bonferroni's correction for multiple comparisons was applied to analyze pairwise differences.

Table 4. Differences between healthy control children, patients with a gluten-free diet in the last 6 months versus less than 6 months on food frequency outcomes.

Variable	Less than 6 Months on Gluten-Free Diet (n = 17)	More than 6 Months on Gluten-Free Diet (n = 35)	Healthy Control Group (n = 36)	p
Food frequency				
Chicken (s/m)	9.6 (3.3)	10.9 (2.2)	15.8 (2.3)	0.221
Beef (s/m)	3.7 (0.71) [a]	3.2 (0.47) [a]	3.5 (0.47)	0.802
Pork (s/m)	4.9 (1.40)	7.7 (0.94)	6.5 (0.96)	0.256
Cured ham (s/m)	7.1 (2.09) [ab]	13.7 (1.40) [a]	13.0 (1.40) [b]	0.034
Ham (s/m)	7.1 (2.68) [a]	13.6 (1.79) [ab]	7.3 (1.81) [b]	0.030
Tukey(s/m)	10.4 (3.27)	10.3 (2.19)	8.59 (2.21)	0.843
Meat derivatives (s/m)	5.5 (2.81) [a]	13.5 (1.88) [ab]	7.0 (1.90) [b]	0.020
Viscera (s/m)	0.13 (0.19)	0.34 (0.13)	0.11 (0.13)	0.440
White fish (s/m)	3.8 (0.9) [a]	5.9 (0.7)	7.3 (0.7) [a]	0.025
Blue fish (s/m)	3.1 (0.7)	4.0 (0.5)	5.1 (0.5)	0.104
Lentils (s/m)	3.5 (0.87)	4.3 (0.59)	3.7 (0.59)	0.661
Grouped fish and seafood (s/m)	14.1 (2.86) [a]	22.8 (1.89) [a]	21.4 (1.88)	0.044
Grouped red meat and subproducts (s/m)	28.5 (5.13) [a]	52.1 (3.43) [a]	37.4 (3.47)	<0.001
Olive oil (s/m)	50.1 (10.9)	61.7 (7.35)	68.7 (7.43)	0.407
Nuts (s/m)	6.46 (6.73)	9.33 (4.24)	18.4 (4.33)	0.232

Values shown as mean (standard error); s, servings; m, month; wk, week. Model adjusted for sex, age and body weight. Upper case [a,b] letters in the same row indicate a significant pairwise difference ($p < 0.05$) between groups with the same letter. Bonferroni's correction for multiple comparisons was applied to analyze pairwise differences.

The differences in dietary habits of the study participants between the control group, the celiac children following a GFD for at least 6 months and the celiac children following a GFD for less than 6 months are shown in Table 3. The children with CD who followed a GFD for at least 6 months showed a higher intake of cobalamin, meat derivatives and fish when compared with those patients who followed a GFD for less than 6 months (all, $p < 0.05$). The children in the healthy control group showed a higher consumption of folate, iron, magnesium, selenium and meat derivatives than those children with CD following a GFD for at least 6 months (all, $p < 0.05$). The children in the control group showed a higher consumption of folate and iron compared with the children with CD following a GFD for less than 6 months (both, $p < 0.05$).

4. Discussion

The main findings of the present study indicate that patients with CD showed lower levels of hemoglobin, erythrocyte and hematocrit compared to healthy children, although neither group presented average values compatible with anemia, nor microcytosis. Regardless of the GFD tracking time, those patients following a GFD for more than 6 months showed a lower hematocrit than healthy controls. Moreover, both CD groups had lower iron and folate intake than the healthy controls. In addition, a lower intake of magnesium and selenium was also observed in patients with CD who had followed a GFD for more than 6 months compared to the control group. Finally, the children with CD who had followed a GFD for less than 6 months showed a lower cobalamin intake compared to those with a greater period of adherence.

In our study, there were 52 (76.5%) celiac females vs 20 (46.5%) healthy females, a sample that is representative of the real incidence of CD by sex [25] and consistent with other similar ones [26]. Moreover, the groups differed in age and weight, but we controlled all the analyses for such covariates.

It is well known that CD is a cause of anemia as a result of malabsorption of iron, folic acid and cobalamin [5]. IDA is a frequent finding in patients with CD and adherence to a GFD may be sufficient to reverse IDA and iron deficiency, although both may persist despite a good adherence to a GFD [7,23]. In fact, in the present study, erythrocyte count, hemoglobin and hematocrit were lower in CD patients compared to healthy controls. However, these patients cannot be considered anemic (despite hemoglobin was lower in CD groups, these values were within the normal range for its age). It is possible that the non-presence of IDA in our patients with CD may be due to the fact that, in addition to the GFD, all children who presented IDA at the time of the diagnosis of CD were prescribed oral iron supplements (ferrous sulfate). This fact could induce a normalization of both the IDA and ID indicators in the first months of treatment, despite the fact that dietary iron intake was lower than recommended [22]. A strict monitoring of the GFD leads to the remission of clinical symptoms, the normalization of serological markers of CD and the recovery of the histological lesion in the small intestine, but the IDA and/or the ID may take a long time in recovering, between 6 months and a year or even longer [17,23]. In addition, it should be taken into account that anemia is present in 22%–63% of patients with CD at the time of diagnosis [15]; the more severe the villus lesion of the intestine, the higher the incidence of anemia [27].

In addition to ID, it is known that in CD there are other micronutrient deficiencies (copper, zinc, folic acid and vitamins A, D, E, K, B6 and B12) as a consequence of the malabsorption [28]. Gluten is found in cereals rich in the referred micronutrients, so a GFD may predispose to its deficiency [29]. In our study, children with CD who followed a GFD for more than 6 months had a lower intake of folic acid, magnesium and selenium than the control group. These data are consistent with those reported in other studies [30–32] that described a lower intake of folic acid, magnesium and selenium, among other micronutrients. Folate intake in children with CD has been poorly investigated, and there are data that indicate lower folate intake with a GFD [33]. One of the factors that could also explain the differences found in the study in relation to micronutrient intake is the pattern of the diet. However, when we evaluate the frequency of consumption of the different food groups, we only found differences in the intake of meat derivatives that was higher in patients with CD who had followed the GFD for at least 6 months, compared with the control group ($p < 0.020$); these results that have also been described previously [26].

Daily energy intake does not meet Recommended Daily Intake for Spanish population [24] since these are around 2000 kcal for children aged 6 to 9 years and 2400 kcal for children aged 10 to 12 years. With respect to food group consumption, as collected by FFQ, CD > 6 consumed more red meat and subproducts, which has been described in CD by other authors [26]. The daily intake of carbohydrates and the energy intake provided by carbohydrates were lower in the CD < 6 group, although not significantly, and in all groups the percentage of energy supplied by carbohydrates reached the recommendations [24]. Several studies have shown that children have a high risk of consuming excess fats, and that this problem may be increased in patients with CD, because GF bakery products have a higher total fat content and saturated fat [34]. This higher fat intake may predispose to suffer from overweight and obesity, although there are no consistent data to support this fact [35]. In our study no increase in total fat intake was observed.

Previous studies [36] revealed, through a skin model derived from fibroblasts, the importance of nutrient restriction in early stages of life, being one of the earliest determining factors that mark accelerated aging. Fibroblasts have been associated with resistance to multiple forms of cellular stress and with DNA repair mechanisms, increased proteastasis, and resistance to cellular senescence. In CD, it is known that there is an uncontrolled activation of the proinflammatory pathway [37] that maintains the production of free radicals that causes oxidative stress through the increase of reactive oxygen species and consequent damage to cellular DNA [38], and it has been documented that chronic inflammation may be involved in at least a third of cancer cases worldwide [39], so it is essential to ensure a correct balance of micronutrients from childhood.

Another problem that is usually described in children with CD is a low fiber intake due to the lower content of it in the flours used for the manufacture of GF products [40]. In the present study, all children covered the recommended daily intakes due to the consumption of GF vegetables and grains with a fiber content similar to wheat [35]. Data from a study conducted in Spanish children with CD also showed that fiber intake was adequate [41].

In general, patients with CD who participated in the present study were well controlled from a nutritional point of view, and the majority (86%) was aware of the dietary recommendations to be followed (strict GFD) and the performance of physical activity. It has been described that higher levels of adherence to a GFD are positively associated with the perceived adoption of healthy behaviors [42]. In fact, among our patients, it seems that low compliance could be related to a lack of nutritional knowledge and that over time they would acquire more information and there would be greater adherence to the GFD. This is achieved through medical visits during the follow-up of the disease and the participation and dedication of the dietitian, essential for the acquisition of knowledge and obtaining positive reinforcement [43,44].

5. Strengths and Limitations

The present study sample size was relatively small, and, consequently, the present results must be interpreted with caution. Based on the present findings, it is advisable to recruit a higher number of participants to render the obtained results with more statistical relevance. Moreover, the groups differed in age, weight and sex, but we controlled all the analyses for such covariates. On the other hand, this is the first study exploring the effect of nutritional adequacy of the GFD and the influence of the time following this GFD on iron status.

6. Conclusions

In conclusion, CD may be associated with iron deficiency, due to malabsorption, but also as a result of a poor adherence to a balanced GFD; it is not clear what percentage each factor influences. We believe that the participation of dietitians in the management of the disease is necessary to guide the GFD, to make the diet more balanced, as well as to fortify it in iron and other micronutrients such as folate that may be deficient.

Author Contributions: Conceptualization, T.N. and R.M.-M.; Methodology; T.N., R.M.-M and J.M.; Validation, T.N.; V.A.A.; R.M.-M.; M.L.-F.; A.L.; M.F.-A. and J.M.; Formal Analysis, V.A.A. and M.F.-A.; Investigation, T.N.; R.M.-M. and J.M.; Resources, T.N. and M.L.-F.; Data Curation, R.M.-M.; J.M. and A.L.; Writing—original Draft preparation, T.N.; V.A.A.; J.M. and R.M.-M.; Writing—Review & Editing: T.N.; V.A.A.; and R.M.-M.; Project Administration, T.N.; Funding Acquisition, T.N. and M.L-F. All authors have read and agreed to the published version of the manuscript.

Funding: This study was partially funded by the Regional Government of Andalusia, Excellence Research Project No P12-AGR-2581. This study was also supported by the University of Granada Research and Knowledge Transfer Fund (PPIT)2016, Excellence Actions Programme: Scientific Units of Excellence (UCEES), and the Regional Ministry of Economy, Knowledge, Enterprises and University, European Regional Development Funds (ref. SOMM17/6107/UGR). MFA was additionally funded by the Spanish Ministry of Education, Culture and Sports (Grant number FPU17/03715).

Acknowledgments: The authors thank the patients for their participation in the current study. We are grateful to Ana Yara Postigo Fuentes for her assistance with the English language.

Conflicts of Interest: The authors declare no conflicts of interest.

References

1. Choung, R.S.; Larson, S.A.; Khaleghi, S.; Rubio-Tapia, A.; Ovsyannikova, I.G.; King, K.S.; Larson, J.J.; Lahr, B.D.; Poland, G.A.; Camilleri, M.J.; et al. Prevalence and Morbidity of Undiagnosed CD Froma Community-Based Study. *Gastroenterology* **2017**, *152*, 830–839.e5. [CrossRef]
2. Rubio-Tapia, A.; Ludvigsson, J.F.; Brantner, T.L.; Murray, J.A.; Everhart, J.E. The Prevalence of CDin the United States. *Am. J. Gastroenterol.* **2012**, *107*, 1538–1544. [CrossRef]
3. Mahadev, S.; Laszkowska, M.; Sundström, J.; Björkholm, M.; Lebwohl, B.; Green, P.H.R.; Ludvigsson, J.F. Prevalence of CDin Patients with Iron Deficiency Anemia—A Systematic Review With Meta-analysis. *Gastroenterology* **2018**, *155*, 374–382.e1. [CrossRef]
4. Bottaro, G.; Cataldo, F.; Rotolo, N.; Spina, M.; Corazza, G.R. The clinical pattern of subclinical/silent celiac disease: An analysis on 1026 consecutive cases 1. *Am. J. Gastroenterol.* **1999**, *94*, 691–696. [CrossRef]

5. Martin-Masot, R.; Nestares, M.T.; Diaz-Castro, J.; López-Aliaga, I.; Muñoz Alférez, M.J.; Moreno-Fernández, J.; Maldonado, J. Multifactorial Etiology of Anemia in CDand Effect of Gluten-Free Diet: A Comprehensive Review. *Nutrients* **2019**, *11*, 2557. [CrossRef]
6. Murray, J.A.; Watson, T.; Clearman, B.; Mitros, F. Effect of a GFD on gastrointestinal symptoms in celiac disease. *Am. J. Clin. Nutr.* **2004**, *79*, 669–673. [CrossRef]
7. Leffler, D.A.; Dennis, M.; Hyett, B.; Kelly, E.; Schuppan, D.; Kelly, C.P. Etiologies and Predictors of Diagnosis in Nonresponsive Celiac Disease. *Clin. Gastroenterol. Hepatol.* **2007**, *5*, 445–450. [CrossRef]
8. Penagini, F.; Dilillo, D.; Meneghin, F.; Mameli, C.; Fabiano, V.; Zuccotti, G.V. GFD in children: An approach to a nutritionally adequate and balanced diet. *Nutrients* **2013**, *5*, 4553–4565. [CrossRef]
9. Thompson, T. Folate, Iron, and Dietary Fiber Contents of the Gluten-free Diet. *J. Am. Diet. Assoc.* **2000**, *100*, 1389–1396. [CrossRef]
10. Thompson, T. Thiamin, riboflavin, and niacin contents of the gluten-free diet: Is there cause for concern? *J. Am. Diet. Assoc.* **1999**, *99*, 858–862. [CrossRef]
11. Hallert, C.; Grant, C.; Grehn, S.; Grännö, C.; Hultén, S.; Midhagen, G.; Ström, M.; Svensson, H.; Valdimarsson, T. Evidence of poor vitamin status in coeliac patients on a GFDfor 10 years. *Aliment. Pharmacol. Ther.* **2002**, *16*, 1333–1339. [CrossRef]
12. Muñoz, M.; Villar, I.; García-Erce, J.A. An update on iron physiology. *World J. Gastroenterol.* **2009**, *15*, 4617. [CrossRef]
13. Leung, A.K.; Chan, K.W. Iron deficiency anemia. *Adv. Pediatr.* **2001**, *48*, 385–408.
14. Repo, M.; Lindfors, K.; Mäki, M.; Huhtala, H.; Laurila, K.; Lähdeaho, M.L.; Saavalainen, P.; Kaukinen, K.; Kurppa, K. Anemia and iron deficiency in children with potential celiac disease. *J. Pediatr. Gastroenterol. Nutr.* **2017**, *64*, 56–62. [CrossRef]
15. Harper, J.W.; Holleran, S.F.; Ramakrishnan, R.; Bhagat, G.; Green, P.H.R. Anemia in CD is multifactorial in etiology. *Am. J. Hematol.* **2007**, *82*, 996–1000. [CrossRef]
16. Kalayci, A.G.; Kanber, Y.; Birinci, A.; Yildiz, L.; Albayrak, D. The prevalence of coeliac disease as detected by screening in children with iron deficiency anaemia. *Acta Paediatr.* **2005**, *94*, 678–681. [CrossRef]
17. Freeman, H.J. Iron deficiency anemia in celiac disease. *World J. Gastroenterol.* **2015**, *21*, 9233–9238. [CrossRef]
18. Annibale, B.; Severi, C.; Chistolini, A.; Antonelli, G.; Lahner, E.; Marcheggiano, A.; Iannoni, C.; Monarca, B.; DelleFave, G. Efficacy of GFDalone on recovery from iron deficiency anemia in adult celiac patients. *Am. J. Gastroenterol.* **2001**, *96*, 132–137. [CrossRef]
19. Husby, S.; Koletzko, S.; Korponay-Szabo, I.R.; Mearin, M.L.; Phillips, A.; Shamir, R.; Troncone, R.; Giersiepen, K.; Branski, D.; Catassi, C.; et al. European Society for Pediatric Gastroenterology, Hepatology, and Nutrition guidelines for the diagnosis of coeliac disease. *J. Pediatr. Gastroenterol. Nutr.* **2012**, *54*, 136–160. [CrossRef]
20. Cole, T.J.; Bellizzi, M.C.; Flegal, K.M.; Dietz, W.H. Establishing a standard definition for child overweight and obesity worldwide: International survey. *BMJ* **2000**, *320*, 1240–1243. [CrossRef]
21. Kapur, G.; Patwari, A.K.; Narayan, S.; Anand, V.K. Iron Supplementation in Children with Celiac Disease. *Indian J. Pediatr.* **2003**, *70*, 955–958. [CrossRef]
22. Mataix, J.L.; Martinez de Victoria, E.; Montellano, M.A.; Lopez, M.; Aranda, P.L. *Valoración del Estado Nutricional de la ComunidadAutónoma de Andalucía*; Consejería de Salud de la Junta de Andalucía: Sevilla, Spain, 2000.
23. Ruiz, M.D.; Artacho, R. *Guía Para EstudiosDietéticos: ÁlbumFotográfico de Alimentos*; Universidad de Granada: Granada, Spain, 2011.
24. Moreiras, O.; Carbajal, A.; Cabrera, L.; Cuadrado, C. Ingestasdiariasrecomendadas de energía y nutrientespara la poblaciónespañola. In *Tablas de Composición de Alimentos*, 18th ed.; Ediciones Pirámide: Madrid, Spain, 2016.
25. King, J.A.; Jeong, J.; Underwood, F.E.; Quan, J.; Panaccione, N.; Windsor, J.W.; Coward, S.; de Bruyn, J.; Ronksley, P.E.; Shaheen, A.A.; et al. Incidence of Celiac Disease Is Increasing Over Time: A Systematic Review and Meta-analysis. *Am. J. Gastroenterol.* **2020**. [CrossRef]
26. Lionetti, E.; Antonucci, N.; Marinelli, M.; Bartolomei, B.; Franceschini, E.; Gatti, S.; Catassi, G.N.; Verma, A.K.; Monachesi, C.; Catassi, C. Nutritional status, dietary intake, and adherence to the mediterranean diet of children with CD on a gluten-free diet: A case-control prospective study. *Nutrients* **2020**, *12*, 143. [CrossRef] [PubMed]

27. Rajalahti, T.; Repo, M.; Kivelä, L.; Huhtala, H.; Mäki, M.; Kaukinen, K.; Kurpaa, K. Anemia in pediatric celiac disease: Association with clinical and histogical features and response to gluten-free diet. *J. Pediatr. Gastroenterol. Nutr.* **2017**, *64*, e1–e6. [CrossRef] [PubMed]
28. Di Nardo, G.; Villa, M.P.; Conti, L.; Ranucci, G.; Pacchiarotti, C.; Principessa, L.; Rauci, U.; Parisei, P. Nutritional deficiencies in children with celiac disease resulting from a gluten-free diet: A systematic review. *Nutrients* **2019**, *11*, 1588. [CrossRef] [PubMed]
29. Melini, V.; Melini, F. Gluten-free diet: Gaps and needs for a healthier diet. *Nutrients* **2019**, *11*, 170. [CrossRef]
30. Kautto, E.; Ivarsson, A.; Norström, F.; Högberg, L.; Carlsson, A.; Hörnell, A. Nutrient intake in adolescent girls and boys diagnosed with coeliac disease at an early age is mostly comparable to their non-coeliac contemporaries. *J. Hum. Nutr. Diet.* **2014**, *27*, 41–53. [CrossRef]
31. Balamtekin, N.; Aksoy, Ç.; Baysoy, G.; Uslu, N.; Demir, H.; Köksal, G.; Saltık-Temizel, İ.N.; Özen, H.; Gürakan, F.; Yüce, A. Is compliance with GFDsufficient? Diet composition of celiac patients. *Turk. J. Pediatr.* **2015**, *57*, 374–379.
32. Alzaben, A.; Turner, J.; Shirton, L.; Samuel, T.M.; Persad, R.; Mager, D. Assessing Nutritional Quality and Adherence to the GFDin Children and Adolescents with Celiac Disease. *Can. J. Diet. Pract. Res.* **2015**, *76*, 56–63. [CrossRef]
33. Babio, N.; Alcázar, M.; Castillejo, G.; Recasens, M.; Martínez-Cerezo, F.; Gutiérrez-Pensado, V.; Masip, G.; Vaqué, C.; Vila-Martí, A.; Torres-Moreno, M.; et al. Patients With Celiac Disease Reported Higher Consumption of Added Sugar and Total Fat Than Healthy Individuals. *J. Pediatr. Gastroenterol. Nutr.* **2017**, *64*, 63–69. [CrossRef]
34. Miranda, J.; Lasa, A.; Bustamante, M.A.; Churruca, I.; Simón, E. Nutritional differences between a gluten-free diet and a diet containing equivalent products with gluten. *Plant Foods Hum. Nutr.* **2014**, *69*, 182–187. [CrossRef] [PubMed]
35. Sue, A.; Dehlsen, K.; Ooi, C.Y. Paediatric Patients with Coeliac Disease on a Gluten-Free Diet: Nutritional Adequacy and Macro- and Micronutrient Imbalances. *Curr. Gastroenterol. Rep.* **2018**, *20*, 2. [CrossRef] [PubMed]
36. Salmon, A.B.; Dorigatti, J.; Huber, H.F.; Li, C.; Nathanielsz, P.W. Maternal nutrient restriction in baboon programs later-life cellular growth and respiration of cultured skin fibroblasts: A potential model for the study of aging-programming interactions. *GeroScience* **2018**, *40*, 269–278. [CrossRef]
37. Diaz-Castro, J.; Muriel-Neyra, C.; Martin-Masot, R.; Moreno-Fernandez, J.; Maldonado, J.; Nestares, T. Oxidative stress, DNA stability and evoked inflammatory signaling in young celiac patients consuming a gluten-free diet. *Eur. J. Nutr.* **2019**. [CrossRef]
38. Nilsen, E.M.; Lundin, K.E.; Krajci, P.; Scott, H.; Sollid, L.M.; Brandtzaeg, P. Gluten specific, HLA-DQ restricted T cells from coeliac mucosa produce cytokines with Th1 or Th0 profile dominated by interferon gamma. *Gut* **1995**, *37*, 766–776. [CrossRef]
39. Coussens, L.M.; Werb, Z. Inflammation and cancer. *Nature* **2002**, *420*, 860–867. [CrossRef]
40. Martin, J.; Geisel, T.; Marech, C.; Krieger, K.; Stein, J. Inadequate nutrient intake in patient with celiac disease. Results from a German dietary survey. *Digestion* **2013**, *87*, 240–246. [CrossRef]
41. BallesteroFernández, C.; Varela-Moreiras, G.; Úbeda, N.; Alonso-Aperte, E. Nutritional status in spanish children and adolescents with celiac disease on a gluten free diet compared to non-celiac disease controls. *Nutrients* **2019**, *11*, 2329. [CrossRef]
42. Fueyo-Díaz, R.; Magallón-Botaya, R.; Gascón-Santos, S.; Asensio-Martínez, Á.; Palacios-Navarro, G.; Sebastián-Domingo, J.J. The effect of self-efficacy expectations in the adherence to a gluten free diet in celiac disease. *Psychol. Health.* **2019**, *13*, 1–16. [CrossRef]
43. Grupo de trabajo del Protocolopara el diagnósticoprecoz de la enfermedadcelíaca. *Protocolo Para el DiagnósticoPrecoz de la EnfermedadCelíaca*; Ministerio de Sanidad, ServiciosSociales e Igualdad. Servicio de Evaluación del ServicioCanario de la Salud (SESCS): Las Palmas de Gran Canaria, Spain, 2018.
44. Fok, C.Y.; Holland, K.S.; Gil-Zaragozano, E.; Paul, S.P. The role of nurses and dietitians in managing paediatric coeliac disease. *Br. J. Nurs.* **2016**, *25*, 449–455. [CrossRef]

© 2020 by the authors. Licensee MDPI, Basel, Switzerland. This article is an open access article distributed under the terms and conditions of the Creative Commons Attribution (CC BY) license (http://creativecommons.org/licenses/by/4.0/).

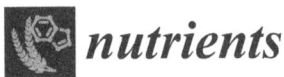

Article

Adjusting Haemoglobin Values for Altitude Maximizes Combined Sensitivity and Specificity to Detect Iron Deficiency among Women of Reproductive Age in Johannesburg, South Africa

Takana Mary Silubonde [1,2,*,†], Jeannine Baumgartner [1,3,†], Lisa Jayne Ware [2], Linda Malan [1], Cornelius Mattheus Smuts [1] and Shane Norris [2,4]

1. Centre of Excellence for Nutrition, Faculty of Health Sciences, North-West University, Potchefstroom 2531, South Africa; jeannine.baumgartner@hest.ethz.ch (J.B.); Linda.Malan@nwu.ac.za (L.M.); Marius.Smuts@nwu.ac.za (C.M.S.)
2. SAMRC/Wits Developmental Pathways for Health Research Unit, Faculty of Health Sciences, University of the Witwatersrand, Johannesburg 2000, South Africa; lisa.ware@wits.ac.za (L.J.W.); Shane.Norris@wits.ac.za (S.N.)
3. Laboratory of Human Nutrition, Department of Health Sciences and Technology, ETH Zurich, 8092 Zurich, Switzerland
4. School of Health and Human Development, University of Southampton, Southampton S016 6YD, UK
* Correspondence: 31260632@student.g.nwu.ac.za
† These authors contributed equally to this work.

Received: 31 January 2020; Accepted: 16 February 2020; Published: 27 February 2020

Abstract: In South Africa, haemoglobin (Hb) is measured to screen for iron deficiency (ID). However, low levels of Hb are only a late stage indicator of ID. Furthermore, Hb values are generally not adjusted for altitude even though recommended by WHO. We determined the Hb threshold with the highest combined sensitivity and specificity for detecting ID among South African women living at 1700 m above sea level. In a cross-sectional study of 492 18–25-year-old women, we measured Hb and iron status biomarkers. Using receiver operating characteristic curves, we determined the Hb threshold with maximum Youden Index for detecting ID. This threshold of <12.35 g/dL resulted in a 37.2% anaemia prevalence (20.9% IDA), and sensitivity and specificity of 55.7% and 73.9%, respectively. The WHO altitude-adjusted threshold of <12.5 g/dL resulted in a 39% anaemia prevalence (21.3% IDA), and sensitivity and specificity of 56.8% and 70.8%, respectively. In contrast, using the unadjusted Hb cut-off of <12 g/dL resulted in a 18.5% anaemia prevalence (12.6% IDA), and sensitivity and specificity of 35.1% and 88.6%, respectively. In this sample of South African women of reproductive age an Hb threshold <12.35 g/dL had the highest combined sensitivity and specificity for detecting ID. The diagnostic performance of this Receiver operating characteristic curve-determined threshold was comparable to the altitude-adjusted threshold proposed by WHO. Thus, clinical and public health practice in South Africa should adopt adjustment of Hb for altitude to avoid underestimation of ID and missing women in need for intervention.

Keywords: anaemia; altitude adjustment; haemoglobin; iron; South Africa; women of reproductive age

1. Introduction

Iron deficiency (ID) is the most common micronutrient deficiency worldwide and the major cause of anaemia. Women of reproductive age (WRA) have high iron requirements because of iron loss through menstruation. An estimated half a billion WRA are affected by anaemia, with ID being responsible for approximately half the cases [1]. During pregnancy, physiological iron requirements increase even further to ensure adequate blood volume expansion and optimal placental and foetal development [2]. However, in low-and middle-income countries, iron intake and/or absorption are often inadequate to meet demands, resulting in ID and ID anaemia (IDA) [3].

Maternal ID and IDA are associated with serious consequences for the mother and her offspring, including an increased risk of morbidity and mortality, adverse birth outcomes, and impaired physical and neurological development in the offspring [4]. In an effort to prevent the adverse health effects of ID and IDA, the World Health Organization (WHO) recommends intermittent iron-folic acid supplementation in menstruating women living in settings where the prevalence of anaemia is 20% or higher [5], and daily oral iron-folic acid supplementation in all pregnant women as part of routine antenatal care [6]. To identify populations at risk for ID and individuals in need for treatment, accurate diagnosis is imperative.

In primary health care settings, the measurement of haemoglobin (Hb) concentration is commonly used to screen individuals who require iron supplementation, e.g., by using inexpensive and easy to use point-of-care haemoglobinometers [7]. Hb is an iron-containing protein found within red blood cells (RBCs). Mature human RBCs have a life span of ~120 days, after which they become senescent and are phagocytosed by macrophages, with iron being recycled [8]. Thus, Hb concentrations only drop when iron stores are depleted (the late stages of ID) or when iron cannot be mobilized from storage in hepatocytes or macrophages, e.g., in the presence of inflammation [9,10]. Furthermore, anaemia has a multifactorial aetiology and can exist without ID [11]. Therefore, measuring Hb concentrations has generally low sensitivity (ability of a test to correctly identify those with the condition) and specificity (ability of the test to correctly identify those without the condition) for the detection of ID [12,13]. Nonetheless, due to the lack of a single, inexpensive, and simple measure of iron status, measuring Hb concentration remains the method of choice for ID screening in primary healthcare, particularly in low-resource settings.

However, the interpretation of Hb values is not free of challenges. Hb cut-off points to diagnose anaemia remained relatively unchanged since 1968, and have been defined for different age categories of children, men, non-pregnant and pregnant women [12]. Since 2001, the WHO further recommended adjusting Hb concentrations downwards (or correcting cut-off point upwards) in individuals residing at altitudes higher than 1000 m above sea level [12]. Erythropoiesis (production of RBCs) increases as a result of chronic hypoxia [14]. Partial pressure of oxygen decreases as altitude increases, resulting in a lower oxygen saturation of RBCs and an increase in erythropoiesis as an adaptive response [15]. Thus, failure to adjust Hb values for altitude may lead to an underestimation of the anaemia and IDA prevalence at population level, and missed diagnosis and subsequent treatment at an individual level.

Despite these risks, the adjustment of Hb values for altitude is not a standard practice, neither by researchers nor by health care professionals in clinical settings, and remains a matter of debate [16,17]. Sharma and colleagues recently re-examined associations of Hb with altitude in a dataset including 68,193 observations among preschool-aged children and WRA from all WHO regions (except South-East Asia) [18]. The authors confirmed that Hb should be adjusted for altitude, but indicated that current recommendations may underestimate anaemia for those residing at lower altitudes (<2000 m) and overestimate anaemia for those residing at higher altitudes (<3000 m). Furthermore, small differences in Hb concentrations may exist between different ethnic groups. Thus, Karakochuk et al. recently stated that the validity of adjusting Hb cut-offs in individuals of African origin warrants further research [7].

South Africa occupies the southern tip of Africa, and consists of a high-lying inland plateau separated from the narrow, low-lying coastal plain by mountainous escarpment. The country's mean altitude is approximately 1200 m, and at least 40% of the surface is at a higher elevation [19]. Nonetheless, South African clinical guidelines do not advise adjusting Hb values [20–22], which is therefore not a general practice in the public healthcare sector. However, in the most recent South African Demographic and Health Survey (SADHS) conducted in 2016 [23], anaemia prevalence rates were reported based on altitude-adjusted Hb values, while previous national surveys, such as the

2012 South African National Health and Nutrition Examination Survey (SANHANES) [24], reported unadjusted values. It can be speculated that this may explain the increase in anaemia prevalence in WRA from 23.1% to 31.5% in the 2012 and 2016 surveys, respectively. Consensus is needed on whether to adjust Hb values for altitude or not in South African population surveys and in the primary health care sector.

Therefore, the aim of this study was to establish an Hb threshold ($\approx$adjustment value) that would maximize the combined sensitivity and specificity for the detection of ID among WRA residing in Soweto, South Africa, situated at 1700 m above sea level. Our objectives were three-fold: (i) to determine the Hb cut-off point with the highest combined sensitivity and specificity (maximum Youden Index) for detecting ID based on ferritin [adjusted and non-adjusted for inflammation] and iron deficient erythropoiesis (IDE) based on soluble transferrin receptor (sTfR); (ii) to assess and compare the sensitivity and specificity of the Hb cut-off points adjusted for altitude (as recommended by WHO) and without adjustment for the detection of ID; and (iii) to determine and compare the prevalence of anaemia, IDA and ID without anaemia using these different cut-off points.

2. Materials and Methods

2.1. Study Setting and Population

For this study, we used data collected between 2018 and 2019 from the *Soweto Young Women's Survey*, a prospective study conducted in Gauteng, South Africa's most populous province (home to approximately 26% of the South African population). Data collection took place at the South African Medical Research Medical Council (SAMRC) Developmental Pathways to Health Research Unit (DPHRU), located within the Chris Hani Baragwanath Academic Hospital (CHBAH), a tertiary hospital in Soweto (South Western Township). Generally healthy, 18–25-year-old, non-pregnant WRA were recruited from Soweto, a historically disadvantaged urban area of 200 km^2 in the city of Johannesburg, Gauteng province. Over 1.3 million people reside in Soweto (6400/km^2) with 98.5% of the population being of black African descent. Women were eligible for inclusion if they were aged 18–25 years; proficient in local languages; born in South Africa or neighbouring countries; and if they had been residing in their home in Soweto for at least 3 months. Women were excluded if they had a previous diagnosis of type-1 diabetes; cancer or epilepsy; or not able or willing to provide written informed consent. Due to South Africa's high prevalence of HIV infection (23.2% of women aged 15–49 years [25]), women who were HIV positive were included in the study for the sample to be a better representation of the general population. As a result, HIV was self-reported and CD4 and viral load were not assessed.

A cluster design was employed for recruitment, where each Soweto community centre was a cluster. Thirty clusters with a radius of 1 km^2 each were identified around Soweto using churches as the midpoint of each cluster. An online search was performed using the Google search engine to locate the information of all churches in Soweto. Using street address information, geolocations of each church structure were obtained, and each church was visited by fieldworkers and verified. The latitude and longitude of the 104 churches identified and verified were then classified using k-means clustering. The church with the shortest straight line distance to the cluster centroid was selected for inclusion in the study as it was at the centre of a cluster of churches that was maximally distant from the other churches in Soweto. An equal number of participants were recruited from two randomly selected clusters.

During the recruitment process, all households in the selected community clusters were approached to identify those where young women lived. Once identified, potential participants were visited in their homes and were informed in their home language about: (i) the objectives of the study; (ii) the use of the results; and (iii) the risks and benefits of the study. An informed consent form was supplied to potentially eligible women who were interested in being part of the study. The interested women were then invited to the study site for the signing of informed consent and data collection.

2.2. Ethical Considerations

This study was conducted in accordance with the ethical principles laid down in the Declaration of Helsinki, and all procedures involving human participants were approved by the Human Research Ethics Committees of the North-West University, Potchefstroom (NWU-0042919-S1), and the University of the Witwatersrand, Johannesburg (M171137).

2.3. Measurement of Anthropometric Indicators and Socio-Demographic Information

Weight (kg) and height (cm) of participants were measured in order to calculate body mass index: BMI = weight (kg)/(height [m])^2. Weight was measured using the Seca 877 Scale (Seca, Hamburg, Germany) and recorded to the nearest 100 g. Women wore light clothing and removed shoes and heavy outerwear (e.g., sweaters) before obtaining weight. Height was measured to the nearest 0.1 cm using a single calibrated Holtain Stadiometer (Holtain Limited, Crymych, UK). Participants were measured either barefoot or wearing thin socks. Mid upper arm circumference (MUAC) was measured to the nearest 0.1 cm using a plastic measuring tape. Measurement was taken at the mid-point of the upper arm, between the acromion process and the tip of the olecranon. A MUAC ≤24 cm was used to define undernutrition [26]. A questionnaire was administered by a trained research assistant to assess socio-economic and demographic characteristics of the women. Food insecurity (hunger) was assessed by a shortened version of the Community Childhood Hunger Identification Project (CCHIP) Index [27].

2.4. Biomarker Analysis

Hb concentrations were measured at the health research unit in capillary blood collected by an experienced nurse using a calibrated Hb 201+ HemoCue® system (HemoCue Johannesburg, South Africa). The HemoCue® system is an easy-to-use haemoglobinometer that is commonly used for determining haemoglobin concentrations in health research and for point-of-care testing in primary health care settings [7,28]. The South African point-of-care cut-off to diagnose anaemia and ID in WRA is a finger-prick Hb <12 g/dL [20,22]. Participants diagnosed with anaemia, according to these national guidelines, were given a referral letter to visit their nearest clinic.

Venous blood samples were drawn into lithium heparin tubes (BD, Plymouth, UK). Plasma was separated within 1 h after blood collection, and aliquots stored at −20 °C for a maximum of 14 days until transportation (on dry ice) for storage at −80 °C until analysis. For the analysis of iron status indices and the inflammation/infection markers C-reactive protein (CRP) and alpha-1-acid glycoprotein (AGP), the Q-Plex™ Human Micronutrient Array (7-plex, Quansys Bioscience, Logan, UT, USA) was used [29].

As plasma ferritin concentrations are elevated in the presence of inflammation, ferritin concentrations were adjusted for inflammation using the correction factors proposed by Thurnham et al. [30]. For participants in the incubation phase (CRP > 5 mg/L and AGP ≤ 1 g/L), ferritin values were adjusted using a correction factor of 0.77. For the early convalescence phase (CRP > 5 mg/L and AGP > 1 g/L), a correction factor of 0.53 was used, while in the late convalescence phase (CRP ≤ 5 mg/L and AGP > 1 g/L), a correction factor of 0.75 was applied.

Participants were classified as being iron deficient if their inflammation-adjusted plasma ferritin concentration was <15 µg/L or, if their unadjusted plasma ferritin concentration was <30 µg/L as recommended by WHO in settings where infection or inflammation is prevalent [31]. However, since the ferritin cut-off of <15 µg/L is still commonly used for unadjusted ferritin values in the diagnosis of ID in the public health sector in South Africa (e.g., population surveys), we also reported the ID prevalence based on unadjusted ferritin values using a cut-off of <15 µg/L. IDA was defined as ferritin <15 µg/L (adjusted) or <30 µg/L (unadjusted) plus haemoglobin <12 g/dL. Iron deficient erythropoiesis (IDE) was defined as sTfR ≥8.3 mg/L.

2.5. Data and Statistical Analysis

Study data were collected and managed using REDCap electronic data capture tools hosted at the University of Witwatersrand [32]. Data processing and statistical analysis of data were performed using Microsoft Office Excel 2010 (Microsoft, Redmond, WA, USA) and SPSS version 25 (SPSS Inc., Chicago, IL, USA).

Data were tested for normality by means of visual inspection using Q-Q plots and histograms, and the Shapiro–Wilk test. Normally distributed data are expressed as means ± SD; non-normally distributed data are expressed as medians (IQR).

Receiver operating characteristic (ROC) curves were created for the use of Hb in the detection of ID defined by ferritin (inflammation-adjusted <15 µg/L; unadjusted <30 µg/L) and sTfR (≥8.3 mg/L). The diagnostic threshold of Hb indicative of ID was selected based on the Youden Index, which is defined by the formula: sensitivity + specificity − 1. The maximal Youden Index identifies the optimal threshold when sensitivity and specificity are considered of equal importance, and this maximal value is the "knee" of the ROC curve [33]. For each ROC curve, the area under the curve (AUC) is reported. An AUC value of 0.50 indicates completely random predictions while a value of 1 indicates perfect predictions.

Furthermore, we determined the sensitivity, specificity, and Youden Index for the diagnostic thresholds indicative of ID (based on inflammation-adjusted and unadjusted ferritin or cut-off values) when Hb values were adjusted for altitude (Hb value—0.5 g/dL at 1700 m above sea level), which is equivalent to the use of an Hb cut-off of <12.5 g/dL, as recommended by WHO [12].

3. Results

3.1. Sample Characteristics

The characteristics of the 492 WRA participating in this study are shown in Table 1. All women were of African descent with a median age of 21 years (IQR 19–23). The majority of the women (61%) had obtained a high school leaving certificate. The median household size was six residents (IQR 4–8) and 47% of women reported food insecurity. Half of the women (51%) were nulliparous. The median BMI was 24.4 (21.2–29.6) kg/m^2, with 22% of women overweight and 24% obese.

3.2. Hematological Indicators

Table 2 presents the inflammatory and iron status indicators in the sample of WRA. Thirty-four percent of the women had inflammation/infection (CRP > 5 mg/L and/or AGP > 1 g/L) with 14% of the women in the late convalescence stage. The median adjusted ferritin concentration was 25.9 (8.0–55.1) µg/L, and the median unadjusted ferritin 28.2 (9.3–62.9) µg/L. The prevalence of ID based on the adjusted and unadjusted ferritin values was 38% and 36%, respectively, when using the cut-off point of <15 µg/L, but 52% for unadjusted ferritin values with the cut-off point of <30 µg/L. The prevalence of IDE (sTfR > 8.3 mg/L) was 42%.

Figure 1 shows receiver operating characteristic (ROC) curves for the use of Hb to diagnose ID (Figure 1a–c) and IDE (Figure 1d). ROC curve analysis resulted in an Hb threshold of 12.35 g/dL with maximum sensitivity and specificity (Youden Index = 0.30) and an AUC of 0.681 to detect ID based on an inflammation-adjusted ferritin <15 µg/L (Figure 1a). To detect ID based on an unadjusted ferritin <30 µg/L (WHO recommendation) or <15 µg/L (current clinical and public health practice), ROC curve analysis resulted in an Hb threshold of 12.45 g/dL (Figure 1b,c) and an AUC of 0.651 and 0.675, respectively. When using sTfR to define IDE, ROC curve analysis resulted in an Hb threshold of 12.35 g/dL and AUC of 0.633.

Table 1. Characteristics of 18–25 year-old women of reproductive age (WRA) residing in Soweto, South Africa ($n = 492$).

Characteristics	Median (IQR) or n (%)
Age	21 (19–23)
BMI (kg/m^2)	24.4 (21.2–29.6)
Underweight (<18.5 kg/m^2)	41 (8)
Normal weight (18.5–24.9 kg/m^2)	224 (46)
Overweight (25–29.9 kg/m^2)	110 (22)
Obese (>30 kg/m^2)	117 (24)
MUAC (cm)	27.6 (24.8–31.5)
Undernutrition (≤24 cm)	94 (19)
HIV positive (self-reported) Yes	22 (4)
Food insecurity	
Yes	230 (47)
Household asset score	9 (7–10)
Low (1–5)	38 (8)
Medium (6–9)	308 (63)
High (10–13)	146 (30)
Highest level of education	195 (40)
Primary school or less	297 (61)
High school leaving certificate	
Household size (number of people)	6 (4–8)
1–4	154 (32)
5–10	269 (56)
>10	57 (12)
Parity	
Nulliparous	253 (51)
Primiparous	192 (39)
Multiparous	47 (10)

BMI = body mass index, MUAC = mid upper arm circumference.

Table 2. Inflammatory and iron status indicators in 18–25 year-old women of reproductive age residing in Soweto, South Africa ($n = 492$).

Biomarker	Median (IQR) or n (%)
CRP (mg/L)	1.41 (0.44–3.84)
AGP (g/L)	0.86 (0.72–1.02)
Inflammatory status	
No inflammation (CRP ≤ 5 mg/L and AGP ≤ 1 g/L)	327 (67)
Incubation (CRP >5 mg/L and AGP ≤ 1 g/L)	57 (12)
Early convalescence (CRP > 5 mg/L and AGP > 1 g/L)	41 (8)
Late convalescence (CRP ≤ 5 mg/L and AGP > 1 g/L)	67 (14)
Inflammation-adjusted ferritin (μg/L) [1]	25.9 (8.0–55.1)
Non-ID (ferritin ≥ 15 μg/L)	307 (63)
ID (ferritin < 15 μg/L)	185 (38)
Unadjusted ferritin (μg/L)	28.2 (9.3–62.9)
Non-ID (ferritin ≥ 30 μg/L)	238 (48)
ID (ferritin < 30 μg/L)	254 (52)
Non-ID (ferritin ≥ 15 μg/L)	314 (64)
ID (ferritin < 15 μg/L)	178 (36)
sTfR (mg/L)	7.5 (5.7–10.5)
Non-IDE (sTfR ≤ 8.3 mg/L)	288 (59)
IDE (sTfR > 8.3 mg/L)	204 (42)

AGP, α-1-acid glycoprotein; CRP, C-reactive protein; ID, iron deficiency; IDA, iron deficiency anaemia; sTfR, serum transferrin receptor; IDE, iron deficient erythropoiesis. [1] Ferritin values were adjusted for inflammation using the correction factors suggested by Thurnham et al. [30].

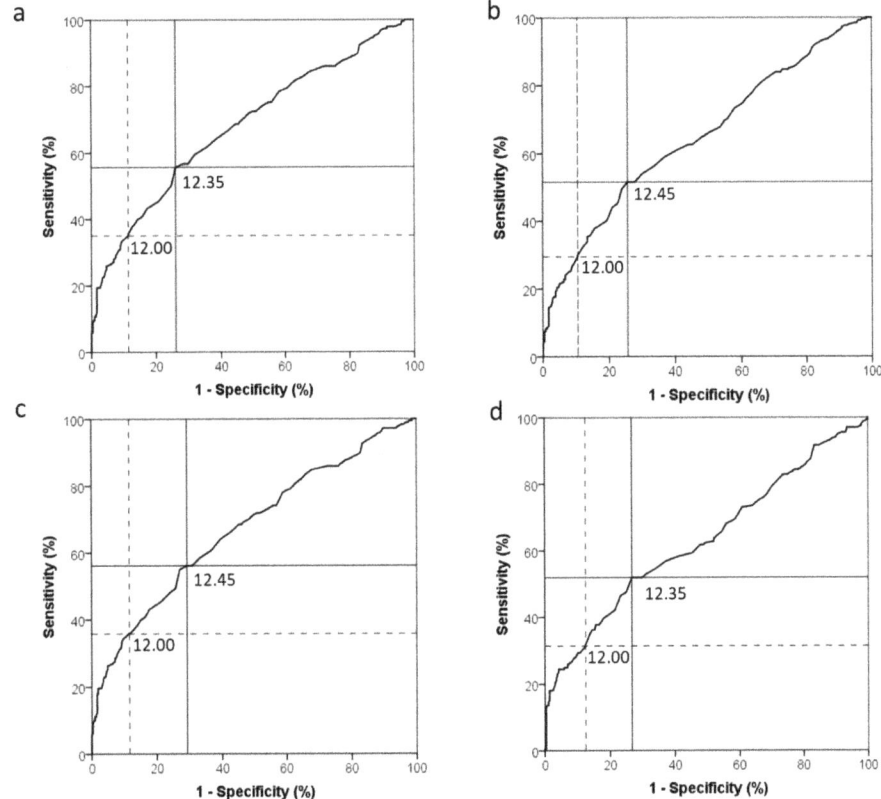

Figure 1. Receiver operating characteristic curves for the use of haemoglobin to diagnose iron deficiency in 18–25 year-old non-pregnant women of reproductive age (n = 492) based on: (**a**) Inflammation-adjusted ferritin (<15 µg/L), area under the curve (AUC) = 0.681; (**b**) unadjusted ferritin (<30 µg/L), AUC = 0.651; (**c**) unadjusted ferritin (<15 µg/L), AUC = 0.675; and (**d**) soluble transferrin receptor (sTfR > 8.3 mg/L), AUC = 0.633. The solid line indicates the haemoglobin cut-off point with the highest combined sensitivity and specificity (maximum Youden Index), while the dotted line indicates the unadjusted haemoglobin cut-off point, typically used in the public healthcare sector.

Table 3 shows the diagnostic accuracy of the Hb cut-off points to detect ID based on inflammation-adjusted and unadjusted ferritin values, and presents the iron and anaemia status of the participating WRA based on the different Hb cut-off points and ferritin criteria to define ID. The unadjusted Hb cut-off point of <12.00 g/dL, that is currently used in primary health care, had a sensitivity of 35.1% and specificity of 88.6% to diagnose ID based on an inflammation-adjusted ferritin <15 µg/L. It resulted in an anaemia, IDA and ID without anaemia prevalence of 18.5% and 12.6% and 25.0%, respectively. The ROC-curve-determined Hb cut-off point of 12.35 g/dL optimized to diagnose ID based on an inflammation-adjusted ferritin <15 µg/L had a sensitivity of 55.7% and specificity of 73.9%. It resulted in an anaemia, IDA and ID without anaemia prevalence of 37.2% and 20.9% and 16.7%, respectively. The ROC-curve-determined Hb cut-off point of 12.45 g/dL to determine ID based on an unadjusted ferritin <30 µg/L had a sensitivity of 51.6% and a specificity of 74.4%. It resulted in an anaemia, IDA and ID without anaemia prevalence of 39.0% and 26.6% and 25.0%, respectively. The ROC-curve-determined Hb cut-off point of 12.45 g/dL to determine ID based on an unadjusted ferritin <15 µg/L had a sensitivity of 56.2% and a specificity of 70.7%, and resulted in an anaemia, IDA and ID without anaemia prevalence of 39.0% and 20.3% and 14.6%, respectively. The altitude-adjusted

Hb cut-off point of <12.5 g/dL, as recommended by WHO, had a sensitivity of 56.8% and a specificity of 70.8%. It resulted in an anaemia, IDA and ID without anaemia prevalence of 39.0% and 21.3% and 16.3%, respectively.

Table 3. Diagnostic accuracy of the different Hb cut-off points to detect ID based on inflammation-adjusted and unadjusted ferritin, and iron and anaemia status in 18–25 year-old non-pregnant women of reproductive age residing in Soweto, South Africa (n = 492).

	Total Anaemia (n [%])	IDA (n [%])	Anaemia without ID (n [%])	ID without Anaemia (n [%])	Non-ID & Non-Anaemic (n [%])	Diagnostic Performance of Hb Cut-off Points to Detect ID		
						Sensitivity (%)	Specificity (%)	Youden Index
Hb <12.00 g/dL (As currently used in SA primary health care clinics to diagnose ID [inflammation-adjusted ferritin <15 µg/L])	91 (18.5)	62 (12.6)	29 (5.9)	123 (25.0)	278 (56.5)	35.1	88.6	0.24
Hb <12.35 g/dL (ROC-curve-determined to diagnose ID [inflammation-adjusted ferritin <15 µg/L])	183 (37.2)	103 (20.9)	80 (16.3)	82 (16.7)	227 (46.1)	55.7	73.9	0.30
Hb <12.45 g/dL (ROC-curve-determined to diagnose ID [unadjusted ferritin <30 µg/L])	192 (39.0)	131 (26.6)	61 (12.4)	132 (25.0)	177 (36.0)	51.6	74.4	0.26
Hb <12.45 g/dL (ROC-curve-determined to diagnose ID [unadjusted ferritin <15 µg/L])	192 (39.0)	100 (20.3)	92 (18.7)	72 (14.6)	228 (46.3)	56.2	70.7	0.27
Hb <12.50 g/dL (Altitude-adjusted based on WHO recommendations to diagnose ID [inflammation-adjusted ferritin <15 µg/L])	192 (39.0)	105 (21.3)	87 (17.7)	80 (16.3)	220 (44.7)	56.8	70.8	0.27

Hb, haemoglobin; ID, iron deficiency; ROC, receiver operation characteristics; SA, South Africa; WHO, World Health Organization.

4. Discussion

The results of this analysis among 18–25 year-old South African WRA living at 1700 m above sea level showed that the Hb threshold with the highest combined sensitivity and specificity for detecting both ID (based on inflammation-adjusted ferritin <15 µg/L) and IDE (based on sTfR > 8.3 mg/L) is <12.35 g/dL. The diagnostic performance of this ROC-curve-determined cut-off value was comparable to the altitude-adjusted Hb cut-off of <12.5 g/dL proposed by WHO for this altitude. In contrast, the Hb cut-off of <12.00 g/dL, which is currently used in the South African primary health care setting without adjusting Hb values for altitude, had a lower sensitivity for the detection of ID than the ROC-curve-determined and altitude-adjusted cut-offs (35% versus ~56%). According to our analysis, the current Hb threshold used in primary health care for the detection of anaemia missed more than half of the anaemia cases detected when using an altitude adjusted Hb threshold (18.5% versus 39%), and resulted in a markedly lower prevalence of IDA (12.6% versus 21%), and a higher prevalence of ID without anaemia (25% versus ~16%). The latter indicates the proportion of women with depleted iron stores who would be missed if measuring Hb to screen for ID.

According to the 2018 Standard Treatment Guidelines and Essential Medicines List for South Africa, the first step in the diagnosis of ID at primary healthcare level is measuring Hb [22]. Thereby, a Hb <12 g/dL is considered indicative of anaemia in non-pregnant WRA, which requests a full blood count to determine the likely aetiology of anaemia based on measured mean corpuscular volume (MCV; average size and volume of red blood cells). If MCV is normal, systemic disease or haemolysis are considered likely causes, and if MCV is low then ID is the most likely cause, while high MCV is indicative of a folate and/or vitamin B_{12} deficiency [22]. Only an estimated 50% of anaemia cases are attributable to ID [28], and therefore proper identification of the anaemia cause is necessary to ensure cause-specific treatment [34]. However, follow-up assessments to confirm the cause of anaemia and the presence of IDA, including the one described above, are rarely done in primary healthcare clinics in South Africa.

Furthermore, clinical guidelines do not specify how to interpret Hb values from individuals residing in higher altitude settings [20–22], which makes up a substantial proportion of South Africa's population [35]. The results of this study indicate that the current point-of-care threshold to detect anaemia (<12 g/dL) has poor sensitivity (35.1%) for the detection of ID (88.6% specificity) in women residing at an altitude of 1700 m above sea level. In our sample, the ROC curve was optimized at an Hb threshold of <12.35 (AUC = 0.681) using the Youden Index, which defines the maximum potential effectiveness of Hb to detect ID when equal weight is given to sensitivity and specificity. Thereby, the ROC curve-determined threshold increased sensitivity to 55.7%, while reducing specificity to 73.9%. The diagnostic performance of this threshold was comparable to the performance of the altitude-adjusted Hb threshold (<12.5 g/dL) proposed by WHO, which slightly improved sensitivity (56.8%) while maintaining a favourable specificity (70.8%). This confirms the findings by Sharma et al., who recently re-examined haemoglobin adjustments to define anaemia among WRA residing at different altitudes and concluded that Hb values (or thresholds) should be adjusted for altitude [18].

Not only can the lack of altitude-adjustment lead to missed diagnosis and treatment of ID in primary health care clinics, it can also result in an underestimation of the anaemia burden in the population. At the public health level, WHO recommends intermittent (once, twice, or three times per week on non-consecutive days) iron and folic acid supplementation of adult women and adolescent girls in populations where the prevalence of anaemia among WRA is 20% or higher [5]. The recommendation for blanket iron supplementation emphasizes that sensitivity of Hb as a screening tool to detect ID is more important than specificity in the public health context. Nonetheless, sensitivity alone does not provide the basis for informed decisions following positive screening test results because those positive results could contain many false positive outcomes [36], hence the use of the Youden Index to define a cut-off with maximum combined sensitivity and specificity. The anaemia prevalence of 18.5% obtained in our sample when using the non-adjusted Hb cut-off of <12.00 g/dL would indicate that no intervention at the public health level is needed. In contrast, the 39% anaemia prevalence obtained when using the ROC-curve-determined and the altitude-adjusted cut-offs would indicate a moderate to borderline severe public health problem that requires intervention. Recent national surveys have reported discrepant anaemia prevalence rates among South African WRA. The (South African Demographic Health Survey) SADHS conducted in 2016 reported an anaemia prevalence in WRA of 31.5% [23], while the South African National Health and Nutrition Examination Survey (SANHANES) 2012 reported an anaemia prevalence of 23.1% [24]. The latter survey did not adjust Hb values for altitude and used the HemoCue 201+ system to measure Hb while SANHANES 2012 used an automated haematology analyser. These and other factors make it impossible to conclude whether the situation truly got worse or whether the 2012 survey potentially underestimated the anaemia prevalence [37].

Another challenge lays in the interpretation of ferritin in settings with a high prevalence of inflammation. Ferritin is not only a marker of iron stores but also an acute-phase protein that increases during inflammation independently of iron status [38,39]. In this study, 34% of women had inflammation, highlighting the importance of considering inflammation when interpreting ferritin values and determining ID prevalence. Possible strategies to interpret ferritin values in settings with a high inflammatory burden are to raise the cut-off that defines deficiency [31], or to adjust ferritin values of individuals with inflammation [30,39]. The latter requires the measurement of inflammatory markers, which is not always feasible. Furthermore, there is currently no consensus on the most appropriate adjustment method. For the determination of an optimized Hb threshold to detect ID, we defined ID using different ferritin interpretation approaches. ROC analysis using unadjusted ferritin cut-off values of either <30 or <15 μg/L to define ID resulted in an optimized Hb cut-off of <12.45 g/dL. However, the highest Youden Index and AUC for Hb to detect ID was obtained when ferritin was adjusted for inflammation using the correction factors proposed by Thurnham et al. In the current study, we used the correction factors proposed by Thurnham et al. [30]. However, for interest sake we also adjusted ferritin values using the Biomarkers Reflecting Inflammation and Nutritional Determinants of Anaemia (BRINDA) approach and repeated the ROC curve analysis for Hb to detect ID based on BRINDA-adjusted ferritin <15 μg/L [40]. This resulted in an even lower median ferritin concentration of 19.8 (6.2–41.2) μg/L and ID prevalence of 55.3%. Nonetheless, the Hb threshold with optimized combined sensitivity and specificity to detect ID remained at <12.35 g/dL (Youden Index = 0.281), with a sensitivity and specificity of 52.7% and 74.4%, respectively. Thus, overall, the different approaches to interpret ferritin did not relevantly affect the diagnostic performance of Hb to detect ID, but the use of the higher ferritin cut-off of <30 µg/L likely resulted in an overestimation of ID and IDA.

When interpreting the results of this study, the following limitations must be considered. Firstly, since we only included data from women residing at one particular altitude, we cannot draw a definite conclusion on whether the lack in sensitivity of the current point-of-care cut-off is driven by altitude or by other factors. Thus, future studies should repeat these analyses in South African women residing at different altitudes. Secondly, we did not perform a full blood count using an automated haematology analzyer to validate the accuracy of the HemoCue 201+ system and to determine the likely causes of anaemia using MCV. The HemoCue 201+ system has been used in the most recent SADHS survey (versus automated haematology analyser in SANHANES) and is being used in most primary healthcare settings in South Africa to screen for anaemia and IDA. Nonetheless, studies that compared the HemoCue 201+ system with automated haematology analyzers showed that Hb concentrations measured by the HemoCue 201+ system were on average 0.1 to 0.4 g/dL higher than when measured with the haematology analyser [7,37]. This would suggest that if measured with an automated haematology analyser, the ROC-curve-determined Hb threshold for detecting ID would have been slightly higher, and therefore getting even closer to the altitude-adjusted threshold recommended by WHO. Lastly, we did not consider the potential effects of smoking on Hb concentrations in our analysis, since information on smoking was incomplete. Similar to altitude-exposure, the reduced oxygen-carrying capacity in smokers caused by exposure to carbon monoxide results in a compensatory increase in Hb concentrations in individuals smoking ≥1/2 packet per day [40]. Therefore, WHO recommends adjustment of Hb for smoking, and Sharma et al. showed that adjustments for smoking and altitude are additive [12]. Thus, we cannot rule out that Hb concentrations of smoking WRA would have needed even further adjustment, again potentially closing the gap between the ROC-determined and the altitude-adjusted Hb threshold.

The strength of this study was the assessment of iron status by measuring two different biomarkers (ferritin and sTfR) using a validated method [29]. However, we do acknowledge that a recent study comparing the Quansys multiplex immunoassay with reference-type assays found poor precision for sTfR in comparison with the Roche cobas 6000 clinical analyser [41]. Nonetheless, the Hb threshold that we obtained by ROC curve analysis for the detection of ID (based on ferritin) was identical to the one for the detection of IDE (based on sTfR), although the latter mainly served as sensitivity analysis. In addition, the analysis of both CRP and AGP enabled us to adjust ferritin for inflammation and perform a sensitivity analysis.

5. Conclusions

In conclusion, the sensitivity and specificity of the optimized Hb cut-off point of 12.35 g/dL determined by ROC curve analysis for the detection of ID was comparable to the Hb cut-off point adjusted for altitude (<12.5 g/dL) as recommended by WHO. It further resulted in comparable anaemia, IDA, and ID without anaemia prevalence rates. In contrast, the use of an unadjusted Hb cut-off point (or lack of adjusting single Hb values) resulted in an underestimation of the anaemia and IDA prevalence, and missed detection of ID in 25% of women (versus 16% for altitude-adjusted cut-off) when analysis of additional iron status indicators is not possible or standard practice. Thus, this study confirms that clinical and public health practice should adopt the adjustment of Hb values for altitude according to WHO guidelines to avoid underestimation of the anaemia and IDA burden in the population and missing individuals in need for intervention. The lack of addressing a large anaemia burden in WRA may not only compromise their own health, but also the health of their baby if they become pregnant.

Author Contributions: Conceptualization, J.B., L.J.W., C.M.S. and S.N.; methodology, T.M.S., J.B., L.J.W., L.M., C.M.S. and S.N.; investigation, T.M.S. and L.J.W.; data curation, L.J.W. and L.M.; formal analysis, T.M.S. and J.B.; supervision, L.J.W., L.M., C.M.S. and S.N.; resources, C.M.S. and S.N.; project administration, T.M.S. and L.J.W.; funding acquisition, C.M.S. and S.N.; writing—original draft preparation, T.M.S. and J.B.; writing—review and editing, T.M.S., J.B., L.J.W., L.M., C.M.S. and S.N. All authors have read and agreed to the published version of the manuscript.

Funding: The HeLTI study is supported by the South African Medical Research Council, and the Canadian Institutes of Health Research. Additional funding for this study was provided by the North-West University in Potchefstroom, South Africa.

Acknowledgments: The authors thank the women who participated in this study, and Cecile Cooke (Centre of Excellence for Nutrition, North-West University, South Africa) for her assistance with sample management and laboratory analysis.

Conflicts of Interest: The authors declare no conflict of interest.

References

1. WHO. *The Global Prevalence of Anaemia in 2011*; World Health Organization: Geneva, Switzerland, 2011.
2. Fisher, A.L.; Nemeth, E. Iron homeostasis during pregnancy. *Am. J. Clin. Nutr.* **2017**, *106*, 1567S–1574S. [CrossRef]
3. Chaparro, C.M.; Suchdev, P.S. Anemia epidemiology, pathophysiology, and etiology in low- and middle-income countries. *Ann. N. Y. Acad. Sci.* **2019**, *1450*, 15–31. [CrossRef] [PubMed]
4. WHO. *Essential Nutrition Actions: Improving Maternal, Newborn, Infant and Young Child Health and Nutrition*; WHO: Geneva, Switzerland, 2013.
5. WHO. *Guideline: Intermittent Iron and Folic Acid Supplementation in Menstruating Women*; WHO: Geneva, Switzerland, 2011.
6. WHO. *WHO Recommendations on Antenatal Care for a Positive Pregnancy Experience*; WHO: Geneva, Switzerland, 2016.
7. Karakochuk, C.D.; Hess, S.Y.; Moorthy, D.; Namaste, S.; Parker, M.E.; Rappaport, A.I.; Wegmuller, R.; Dary, O. Measurement and interpretation of hemoglobin concentration in clinical and field settings: A narrative review. *Ann. N. Y. Acad. Sci.* **2019**, *1450*, 126–146. [CrossRef] [PubMed]
8. Korolnek, T.; Hamza, I. Macrophages and iron trafficking at the birth and death of red cells. *Blood* **2015**, *125*, 2893–2897. [CrossRef]
9. Muñoz, M.; Villar, I.; García-Erce, J.A. An update on iron physiology. *World J. Gastroenterol.* **2009**, *15*, 4617–4626. [CrossRef]
10. Muckenthaler, M.U.; Rivella, S.; Hentze, M.W.; Galy, B. A Red Carpet for Iron Metabolism. *Cell* **2017**, *168*, 344–361. [CrossRef] [PubMed]
11. Petry, N.; Olofin, I.; Hurrell, R.F.; Boy, E.; Wirth, J.P.; Moursi, M.; Donahue Angel, M.; Rohner, F. The Proportion of Anemia Associated with Iron Deficiency in Low, Medium, and High Human Development Index Countries: A Systematic Analysis of National Surveys. *Nutrients* **2016**, *8*, 693. [CrossRef]
12. WHO. *Haemoglobin Concentrations for the Diagnosis of Anaemia and Assessment of Severity*; World Health Organization: Geneva, Switzerland, 2011.
13. Lynch, S. *The Rationale for Selecting and Standardizing Iron Status Indicators*; World Health Organization: Geneva, Switzerland, 2012.
14. Haase, V.H. Hypoxic regulation of erythropoiesis and iron metabolism. *Am. J. Physiol. Ren. Physiol.* **2010**, *299*, F1–F13. [CrossRef]
15. Gassmann, M.; Muckenthaler, M.U. Adaptation of iron requirement to hypoxic conditions at high altitude. *J. Appl. Physiol.* **2015**, *119*, 1432–1440. [CrossRef]
16. Gonzales, G.F.; Rubín de Celis, V.; Begazo, J.; Del Rosario Hinojosa, M.; Yucra, S.; Zevallos-Concha, A.; Tapia, V. Correcting the cut-off point of hemoglobin at high altitude favors misclassification of anemia, erythrocytosis and excessive erythrocytosis. *Am. J. Hematol.* **2018**, *93*, E12–E16. [CrossRef]
17. Robalino, X.; Balladares-Saltos, M.; Miño, P.; Guerendiain, M. Comparison of Hemoglobin Concentration Adjusted for Altitude and Serum Iron and Ferritin to Diagnose Anemia in Childhood in Highlands. *Blood* **2016**, *128*, 2459. [CrossRef]

18. Sharma, A.J.; Addo, O.Y.; Mei, Z.; Suchdev, P.S. Reexamination of hemoglobin adjustments to define anemia: Altitude and smoking. *Ann. N. Y. Acad. Sci.* **2019**, *1450*, 190–203. [CrossRef] [PubMed]
19. Lowe, C.C.; Gordon, D.F.; Hall, M.; Bundy, C.J.; Thompson, L.M.; Cobbing, J.R.D.; Mabin, A.S.; Vigne, R. South Africa. Available online: https://www.britannica.com/place/South-Africa (accessed on 15 January 2019).
20. NDOH. *Adult Primary Care (APC) Guide*; National Department of Health: Pretoria, South Africa, 2016.
21. NDOH. *Guidelines for Maternity Care in South Africa*, 4th ed.; National Department of Health: Pretoria, South Africa, 2015.
22. NDOH. *Essential Drugs Programme*; Primary Healthcare Standard Treatment Guideline and Essential Medicine List; National Department of Health: Pretoria, South Africa, 2018.
23. Naitonal Department of Health (NDOH); Statistics South Africa (Stats SA); South African Medical Research Council (SAMRC); ICF. *South African Demographic and Health Survey 2016: Key Indicators*; National Department of Health: Pretoria, South Africa; Rockville, MD, USA, 2017.
24. Shisana, O.; Labadarios, D.; Rehle, T.; Simbayi, L.; Zuma, K.; Dhansay, A.; Reddy, P.; Parker, W.A.; Hoosain, E.; Naidoo, P.; et al. *South African National Health and Nutrition Examination Survey (SANHANES-1)*; HSRC Press: Cape Town, South Africa, 2013.
25. Shisana, O.; Rehle, T.; Simbayi, L.C.; Zuma, K.; Jooste, S.; Zungu, N.; Labadarios, D.; Onoya, D. *South African National HIV Prevalence, Incidence and Behaviour Survey, 2012*; HSRC Press: Cape Town, South Africa, 2015.
26. Tang, A.M.; Chung, M.; Dong, K.; Wanke, C.; Charlton, K.; Hong, S.; Nguyen, P.H.; Patsche, C.B.; Deitchler, M.; Maalouf-Manasseh, Z. *Determining a Global Mid-Upper Arm Circumference Cutoff to Assess Underweight in Adults (Men and Nonpregnant Women)*; USAID: Washington, DC, USA, 2017.
27. Wehler, C.A.; Scott, R.I.; Anderson, J.J. The Community Childhood Hunger Identification Project: A model of domestic hunger—Demonstration project in Seattle, Washington. *J. Nutr. Educ.* **1992**, *24*, 29S–35S. [CrossRef]
28. WHO; UN. *Iron Deficiency Anaemia: Assessment, Prevention, and Control*; WHO: Geneva, Switzerland, 2001.
29. Brindle, E.; Lillis, L.; Barney, R.; Hess, S.Y.; Wessells, K.R.; Ouédraogo, C.T.; Stinca, S.; Kalnoky, M.; Peck, R.; Tyler, A.; et al. Simultaneous assessment of iodine, iron, vitamin A, malarial antigenemia, and inflammation status biomarkers via a multiplex immunoassay method on a population of pregnant women from Niger. *PLoS ONE* **2017**, *12*, e0185868. [CrossRef] [PubMed]
30. Thurnham, D.I.; Northrop-Clewes, C.A.; Knowles, J. The use of adjustment factors to address the impact of inflammation on vitamin a and iron status in humans. *J. Nutr.* **2015**, *145*, 1137S–1143S. [CrossRef] [PubMed]
31. WHO. *Serum Ferritin Concentrations for the Assessment of Iron Status and Iron Deficiency in Populations*; World Health Organization: Geneva, Switzerland, 2011.
32. Harris, P.A.; Taylor, R.; Minor, B.L.; Elliott, V.; Fernandez, M.; O'Neal, L.; McLeod, L.; Delacqua, G.; Delacqua, F.; Kirby, J. The REDCap consortium: Building an international community of software platform partners. *J. Biomed. Inform.* **2019**, *95*, 103208. [CrossRef]
33. Youden, W.J. Index for rating diagnostic tests. *Cancer* **1950**, *3*, 32–35. [CrossRef]
34. Moodley, V.; Alant, J. The straight and marrow—A primary care approach to anaemia. *S. Afr. Fam. Pract.* **2018**. [CrossRef]
35. Hofmeyr, R.; Tölken, G.; De Decker, R. Acute high-altitude illness. *S. Afr. Med. J.* **2017**, *107*, 556–561. [CrossRef]
36. Trevethan, R. Sensitivity, Specificity, and Predictive Values: Foundations, Pliabilities, and Pitfalls in Research and Practice. *Front. Public Health* **2017**, *5*, 307. [CrossRef]
37. Chen, P.; Short, T.; Leung, D.H.; Oh, T. A clinical evaluation of the Hemocue haemoglobinometer using capillary, venous and arterial samples. *Anaesth. Intensive Care* **1992**, *20*, 497–500. [CrossRef] [PubMed]
38. Kernan, K.F.; Carcillo, J.A. Hyperferritinemia and inflammation. *Int. Immunol.* **2017**, *29*, 401–409. [CrossRef] [PubMed]
39. Namaste, S.M.; Rohner, F.; Huang, J.; Bhushan, N.L.; Flores-Ayala, R.; Kupka, R.; Mei, Z.; Rawat, R.; Williams, A.M.; Raiten, D.J.; et al. Adjusting ferritin concentrations for inflammation: Biomarkers Reflecting Inflammation and Nutritional Determinants of Anemia (BRINDA) project. *Am. J. Clin. Nutr.* **2017**, *106*, 359S–371S. [CrossRef] [PubMed]

40. Nordenberg, D.; Yip, R.; Binkin, N.J. The effect of cigarette smoking on hemoglobin levels and anemia screening. *JAMA* **1990**, *264*, 1556–1559. [CrossRef]
41. Esmaeili, R.; Zhang, M.; Sternberg, M.R.; Mapango, C.; Pfeiffer, C.M. The Quansys multiplex immunoassay for serum ferritin, C-reactive protein, and α-1-acid glycoprotein showed good comparability with reference-type assays but not for soluble transferrin receptor and retinol-binding protein. *PLoS ONE* **2019**, *14*, e0215782. [CrossRef]

© 2020 by the authors. Licensee MDPI, Basel, Switzerland. This article is an open access article distributed under the terms and conditions of the Creative Commons Attribution (CC BY) license (http://creativecommons.org/licenses/by/4.0/).

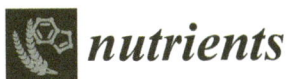

Article

Acai Extract Transiently Upregulates Erythropoietin by Inducing a Renal Hypoxic Condition in Mice

Shuichi Shibuya [1,2], Toshihiko Toda [2], Yusuke Ozawa [2], Mario Jose Villegas Yata [3] and Takahiko Shimizu [1,2,*]

1. Aging Stress Response Research Project Team, National Center for Geriatrics and Gerontology, 7-430 Morioka-cho, Obu, Aichi 474-8511, Japan; s-shibuya@ncgg.go.jp
2. Department of Endocrinology, Hematology and Gerontology, Chiba University Graduate School of Medicine, 1-8-1 Inohana, Chuo-ku, Chiba 260-8670, Japan; hik_toda-jac@proteome.jp (T.T.); ozawayusuke3@gmail.com (Y.O.)
3. FRUTA FRUTA, Inc., 3-3 Kandajimbo-cho, Chiyoda-ku, Tokyo 101-0051, Japan; mario@frutafruta.com
* Correspondence: shimizut@ncgg.go.jp; Tel.: +81-562-44-5651; Fax: +81-562-48-2373

Received: 18 January 2020; Accepted: 17 February 2020; Published: 19 February 2020

Abstract: Acai (*Euterpe oleracea* Mart. Palmae, Arecaceae) is a palm plant native to the Brazilian Amazon. It contains many nutrients, such as polyphenols, iron, vitamin E, and unsaturated fatty acids, so in recent years, many of the antioxidant and anti-inflammatory effects of acai have been reported. However, the effects of acai on hematopoiesis have not been investigated yet. In the present study, we administered acai extract to mice and evaluated its hematopoietic effects. Acai treatment significantly increased the erythrocytes, hemoglobin, and hematocrit contents compared to controls for four days. Then, we examined the hematopoietic-related markers following a single injection. Acai administration significantly increased the levels of the hematopoietic-related hormone erythropoietin in blood compared to controls and also transiently upregulated the gene expression of *Epo* in the kidney. Furthermore, in the mice treated with acai extract, the kidneys were positively stained with the hypoxic probe pimonidazole in comparison to the controls. These results demonstrated that acai increases the erythropoietin expression via hypoxic action in the kidney. Acai can be expected to improve motility through hematopoiesis.

Keywords: acai; erythropoiesis; erythropoietin

1. Introduction

To maintain oxygen homeostasis, mammals have hematopoietic regulatory mechanisms, including erythropoiesis. Erythropoietin (EPO) is a hematological factor mainly expressed in the kidney in adults [1]. EPO is induced under conditions of reduced oxygen levels, as well as blood loss [2]. The *Epo* transcription is regulated by hypoxia-inducible transcription factors (HIFs), which have two oxygen-responsive sites associated with prolyl hydroxylase and lead to degradation by ubiquitination under normoxia [3]. This evidence demonstrates that the redox states on renal proteins containing HIF are potential indicators of erythropoiesis in adult mammals.

Acai (*Euterpe oleracea* Mart. Palmae, Arecaceae) is a large palm plant found in the northern region of South America, called the "Amazon", in Brazil. Acai berries have a high polyphenol content, including anthocyanins, such as cyanidine-3-glucoside (C3Glc), cyanidine-3-diglucoside, and cyanidin-3-rutinoside, which contribute to antioxidant activity [4]. In several rodent studies, the benefits of acai intervention have been reported to include improving cardiac dysfunction following myocardial infarction [5], protection from diet-induced obesity [6] and hepatic steatosis [7], prevention of brain oxidative damage [8], and modulation of age-related hippocampal inflammation [9]. Acai intake is also expected to be a useful therapeutic strategy for chronic kidney disease with oxidative stress, inflammation, and dysbiosis [10]. However, no studies have determined the erythropoietic effect of acai on renal redox alteration.

In the present study, in order to clarify the erythropoietic action of acai, we administered acai extract to mice and examined the relationship between the erythropoietic factors and the redox change in the kidney.

2. Materials and Methods

2.1. Animals

C57BL/6NCrSlc mice were purchased from Japan SLC (Shizuoka, Japan) and inbred in our own cohorts. The animals were housed under a 12-h light/dark cycle and fed an MF diet (Oriental Yeast Co., Ltd., Tokyo, Japan) ad libitum. The mice were maintained and studied according to the protocols approved by the Animal Care Committee of the Chiba University.

2.2. Administration

Acai extract (Table 1, Lot. 171115 and 180622) provided by FRUTA FRUTA, Inc. (Tokyo, Japan) was made by finely grinding whole fruit and filtrating with a #30 strainer. The extract was orally administered at 10 mL/kg/day via gavage to mice 1 time ($n = 8$) and for four days ($n = 4$) at 12–16 weeks of age. C3Glc (NS380102) was purchased from Nagara Science (Gifu, Japan). ASP1517 (roxadustat, #15294) was purchased from Cayman Chemical (Ann Arbor, MI, USA). The water-dissolved C3Glc (50 mg/kg, $n = 6$) and 0.5% carboxymethyl cellulose-suspended ASP1517 (80 mg/kg, $n = 7$) were administered orally once to littermate mice of the acai-treated cohort. The study was performed using the blood and kidney tissue of animals collected under anesthesia 2–3 h after the final administration.

Table 1. Contents in 100 g of acai extract.

Contents		Fatty Acids	(%)
Energy intake	82.0 kcal	Palmitic acid (C16:0)	22.5
Protein	1.4 g	Palmitoleic acid (C16:1)	3.3
Total lipids	6.9 g	Stearic acid (C18:0)	1.9
Carbohydrates	2.0 g	Oleic acid (C18:1)	61.2
Dietary fiber	3.3 g	Linoleic acid (C18:2)	10.6
Total polyphenols	390 mg	Linolenic acid (C18:3)	0.5
Iron	1.0 mg		

2.3. Histology

To evaluate the tissue hypoxic area, Hypoxyprobe™-1 Omni (Hypoxyprobe, Inc., Burlington, MA, USA) was used [11]. Mice were sacrificed 15 min after being intraperitoneally injected with anesthetic and 60 mg/kg of pimonidazole. The kidney was fixed in a 4% paraformaldehyde phosphate buffered saline (PBS) (Nacalai Tesque, Inc., Kyoto, Japan) and embedded in paraffin. The rehydrated sections were antigen retrieved with 10 mM citrate buffer (pH 6.0, with 0.05% Tween 20) at 95 °C for 30 min, washed with PBS containing 0.1% Tween 20 three times, and intrinsic peroxidases were quenched with 3% H_2O_2 for 30 min. We performed blocking with 3% goat serum or Blocking One Histo (Nacalai Tesque) and then treated samples with 1:200 or 1:20 diluted anti-pimonidazole antibody (Hypoxyprobe, Inc.). The pimonidazole-positive area was evaluated by the QWin V3 imaging software program (Leica, Wetzlar, Germany) or a BZ-X710 analyzer (Olympus Co., Tokyo, Japan) using the ABC staining kit (Vector Labs., Inc., Burlingame, CA, USA) or the FITC-fluorescence method (goat anti-rabbit antibody #AP307F, Sigma (St. Louis, MO, USA) and Fluoro-KEEPER Antifade Reagent with DAPI #12745-74; Nacalai Tesque), respectively.

2.4. Measurement of EPO

The plasma EPO level was measured using the Mouse Erythropoietin Quantikine ELISA kit (#MEP00B; R&D Systems, Inc., Minneapolis, MN, USA) according to the manufacturer's instructions. In brief, thawed plasma was diluted 2-fold by calibrator diluents and then incubated on an antibody-coated microplate with each volume of assay diluents for 2 h using an orbital shaker. Washed wells were treated with antiserum conjugate for 2 h and with a substrate mixture for 30 min. The optical density measured at 450 and 540 nm was analyzed with the standards curve using the 4-parameter logistic curve-fit.

2.5. Quantitative Polymerase Chain Reaction (PCR)

Total RNA was extracted from the kidney using the RNAlater (Thermo Fisher Scientific, Waltham, MA, USA) and the Sepasol-RNA I Super G reagent (Nacalai Tesque) according to the manufacturer's instructions. The cDNA was synthesized from 1 mg total RNA using ReverTra Ace qPCR RT Master Mix (Toyobo, Osaka, Japan). Real-time PCR was performed with the SsoAdvanced SYBR Green Supermix (Bio-Rad, Hercules, CA, USA) on a Mini-Opticon (Bio-Rad) according to the manufacturer's protocols. All data were normalized to the level of the housekeeping gene β-Actin/*Actb*. The following primers were used for the analysis: *Actb*, forward, 5′-GCC CTA GGC ACC AGG GTG TGA-3′, and reverse, 5′-TCC TCA GGG GCC ACA CGC A-3′; *Epo*, forward, 5′-TCA TCT GCG ACA GTC GAG TTC TG-3′, and reverse, 5′-GGT ATC TGG AGG CGA CAT CAA TTC-3′; and *Vegfa*, forward, 5′-GCA GCT TGA GTT AAA CGA ACG-3′, and reverse, 5′-GGT TCC CGA AAC CCT GAG-3′.

2.6. Hematological Cytometry

The number of red blood cells and leukocytes, hemoglobin levels, and hematocrit levels were measured by the Oriental Yeast hematology analyzing service (Tokyo, Japan).

2.7. Statistical Analyses

The statistical analyses were performed using the Student's *t*-test for comparisons between two groups and a one-way analysis of variance/Tukey's test for comparisons of three or more groups. Differences between the data were considered significant when the p-values were less than 0.05. All data are expressed as the mean ± standard deviation (SD).

3. Results

3.1. Acai Extract Alters Hematological Parameters

First, to investigate the hematological effects, we administered acai extract and measured the hematological parameters in mice. Treatment with acai extract significantly increased the erythrocyte content (RBC), hemoglobin level (HGB), and hematocrit level (HCT) but not the leukocyte content (WBC) or reticulocyte count (RET) in blood for four days (Table 2). Acai extract also induced no significant change in the erythrocyte mean cell volume (MCV), mean cell hemoglobin (MCH), mean cell hemoglobin concentration (MCHC), or platelet content (PLT) (Table 2). These results suggest that acai induced a hemopoietic effect or suppressed red blood cell degradation.

Table 2. Effect of acai extract on the hematological parameters in mice ($n = 4$).

	Control	10 g/kg of Acai for Four Days
WBC (/μL)	2500 ± 804	2275 ± 660
RBC (×10^4/μL)	876 ± 11	931 ± 12 *
HGB (g/dL)	14.1 ± 0.5	14.9 ± 0.4 *
HCT (%)	47.6 ± 0.6	51.1 ± 1.4 *
MCV (fL)	54.4 ± 0.7	54.9 ± 0.8
MCH (pg)	16.0 ± 0.5	16.0 ± 0.4
MCHC (%)	29.5 ± 0.8	29.3 ± 0.9
PLT (×10^4/μL)	95 ± 5	97 ± 13
RET (‰)	27.8 ± 4.8	23.0 ± 1.2

Hematological parameters in blood treated with acai extract (10 g/kg) daily for four days orally. WBC: Leukocyte content; RBC: Erythrocyte content; HGB: Hemoglobin; HCT: Hematocrit; MCV: Mean cell volume; MCH: Mean cell hemoglobin; MCHC: Mean cell hemoglobin concentration; PLT: Platelet content; RET: Reticulocytes. * $P < 0.05$ by t-test.

3.2. Acai Extract Acutely Upregulates the EPO Contents in Blood

EPO is the principle regulator of red blood cell production [12]. In general, the *Epo* expression is transiently stimulated by a hypoxic condition [2]. After four days of administration of acai, the renal *Epo* expression showed a slight increase (Figure 1A). In this context, we performed a transient experiment, administering acai extract to mice and measuring the EPO contents in plasma 2–3 h after treatment. The acai treatment caused a significant increase in the plasma EPO level compared with vehicle control (Figure 1B). Furthermore, acai upregulated the *Epo* transcript level in the kidney compared with the control (Figure 1C). The erythropoiesis inducer roxadustat (ASP1517), which is also used to treat renal anemia, also upregulated both the EPO contents in plasma and the *Epo* transcript level in kidney (Figure 1B,C). In contrast to acai, the administration of C3Glc caused no significant change in either the EPO contents or the *Epo* level (Figure 1B,C). Furthermore, the relationship between the plasma EPO concentration and the kidney *Epo* transcript level was positive (Figure 1D). These results suggest that acai extract transcriptionally induced EPO production in the kidney.

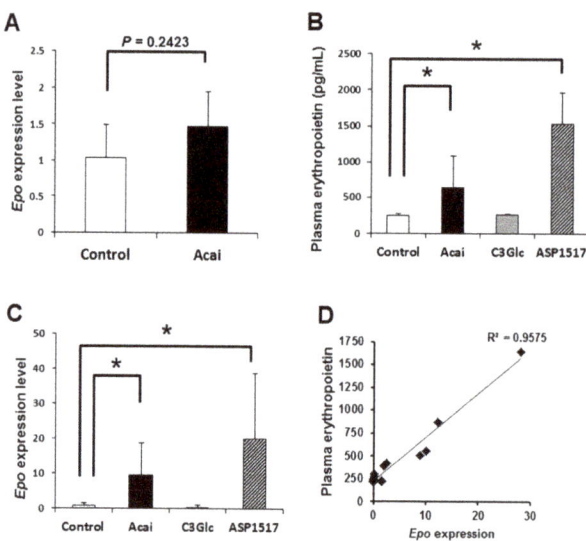

Figure 1. Acai extract upregulates both the plasma erythropoietin (EPO) concentration and kidney *Epo* expression. (**A**). The relative *Epo* transcript level in the kidney after the oral administration of acai extract

(10 g/kg) dairy for four days. * $P < 0.05$ by *t*-test. (**B**) The plasma EPO concentration in mice 2–3 h after the oral administration of acai extract (10 g/kg), C3Glc (50 mg/kg), and ASP1517 (80 mg/kg). (**C**) Relative *Epo* transcript levels in kidney 2–3 h after the oral administration of acai extract (10 g/kg), C3Glc (50 mg/kg), and ASP1517 (80 mg/kg). (**D**) Relationship between the plasma EPO concentration and *Epo* transcription in kidney. Error bars indicate the standard deviation. * $P < 0.05$ by an ANOVA/Tukey's test.

3.3. Acai Extract Induces a Renal Hypoxic Condition

Finally, to investigate the relationship between EPO induction and renal hypoxia under acai administration, we administered the hypoxic probe pimonidazole to mice and histologically detected renal hypoxia. By immunostaining with pimonidazole, which accumulates in hypoxic areas, acai extract was shown to induce renal hypoxia (Figure 2A). A quantitative analysis with the fluorescence intensity of pimonidazole staining showed that acai created a significantly larger hypoxic area than was seen in the controls (Figure 2B,C). Furthermore, acai induced renal hypoxia mainly at the corticomedullary junction where erythropoietin is produced (Figure 2A,B). Along with hypoxia induction, acai also increased the expression of *Vegfa*, which located downstream of HIF, in the kidney (Figure 2D). These results suggest that renal erythropoietin production caused by acai depends on the hypoxic reaction in the kidney.

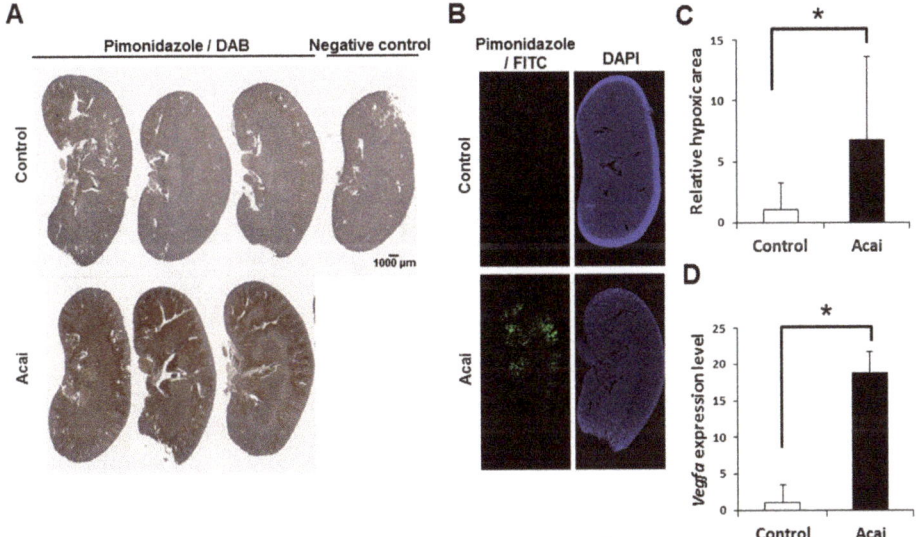

Figure 2. Acai extract induces a hypoxic reaction in kidney. (**A–C**) The pimonidazole-positive hypoxic area in kidney sections 2–3 h after the oral administration of acai extract (10 g/kg) was detected by 3,3′-diaminobenzidine (**A**) and fluorescein isothiocyanate (**B,C**). (**D**) Relative *Vegfa* transcript level in the kidney 2–3 h after acai extract. Scale bar denotes 1 mm. Error bar indicates the standard deviation. * $P < 0.05$ by *t*-test.

4. Discussion

Since EPO, a hematopoietic hormone that controls erythropoiesis, is produced in response to tissue hypoxia, athletes often incorporate high-altitude training. The induction of EPO expression mainly involves the transcription factor HIF induced by hypoxia [3]. Under hypoxic conditions, degradation of HIF is inhibited by ubiquitination due to the suppression of proline hydroxylase, thereby promoting hematopoiesis [3]. ASP1517 induces the production of erythrocytes via the prevention of HIF degradation by inhibiting the proline hydroxylase [13]. Actually, the remarkable induction of renal hypoxia by acai suggests the HIF-mediated *Epo* and *Vegfa* upregulation (Figures 1 and 2).

In our study, acai administration did not increase RET, which is in contrast to the increases it induced in erythropoietin and HCT (Table 2). Testosterone supplementation improved anemia in aged mice without increasing the number of reticulocytes, suggesting the contributions of an increase in erythrocyte-related genes in spleen and the normalization of iron homeostasis [14]. Since acai contains a large amount of iron, it can also increase the ferritin and iron contents, leading to iron-related hematopoiesis. As EPO is transiently induced by hypoxic conditions [2], the upregulation of EPO by acai may affect acute erythropoiesis. These findings suggest that, in contrast to the HIF-mediated erythropoiesis mechanism of ASP1517, acai may exert multiple hematopoietic mechanisms. Since the combination of EPO-stimulating and iron agents is an important anemia management strategy for patients undergoing hemodialysis [15], acai has potential applications in therapy for various types of anemia. We need to analyze the mechanisms underlying the hematopoietic effect of acai more strictly in future studies.

Acai contains large amounts of iron, various polyphenols, and long-chain fatty acids, such as oleate, palmitate and linoleate (Table 1), suggesting various beneficial effects for anemia. The monounsaturated oleic acid depresses the cytokine expression in vitro [16]. Stoner et al. reported that acai reduced the serum IL-5 and IL-8 levels in rats [17]. Anemia in the elderly population is caused by the increased expression of proinflammatory cytokines [18]. Acai may protect against anemia by reducing the levels of inflammatory cytokines increased by aging and various stressors. Furthermore, acai treatment attenuated renal ischemia/reperfusion injury via protection against renal oxidative stress in diabetic and spontaneously hypertensive rats [19,20]. In a rat study, acai treatment significantly decreased the 8-isoprostane immunostaining level and thiobarbituric acid reactive substances level in the kidney [20], suggesting the transition from an oxidative to a reductive condition in the kidney. These findings show that acai induces erythropoietic action via an altered redox status in the kidney. Mitochondrial angiotensin II receptors regulate oxygen consumption in kidney mitochondria [21], suggesting a deep association with the renal status and oxygen consumption. Hernandez-Vargas et al. reported that the suppressors of cytokine signaling (SOCS) family negatively regulated the angiotensin II-activated signal pathway, including JNK, resulting in a decreased renal oxygen consumption [22]. AICAR, an AMPK activator, decreased the renal oxygen consumption via the modulation of SOCS1 [23]. In this context, acai may inhibit the SOCS family, leading to the activation of the angiotensin II-mediated pathway associated with increased oxygen consumption and hypoxia in the kidney.

Polyphenols protect against reactive oxygen species-induced hemolysis via increased red blood cell integrity associated with the inhibition of lipid peroxidation [24–27]. Similarly, red cabbage extracts rich in anthocyanins rescue oxidative hemolysis in streptozotocin-induced diabetes [28]. Anthocyanins also exert antisickling activity by stabilizing red blood cells and their membranes and inhibiting polymerization on hemoglobin S [29,30]. However, C3Glc alone did not alter the erythropoietin or *Epo* levels (Figure 2), suggesting that not only polyphenols but also iron and fatty acids of acai contribute to erythropoiesis.

Acai showed no toxicity in experimental models [31–36] nor any significant differences in the body weight or food consumption [17,31,32,36], suggesting potential applications in the prevention of various disease. Conversely, Mn, which is abundant in acai, suppresses Fe absorption, suggesting a risk for anemia [37]. The kidneys are prone to hypoxia because of their high energy consumption [38]. Chronic renal hypoxia is a final common pathway to end-stage renal failure, resulting in an irreversible decline in the renal function [39,40]. In a study of hypertensive rats, acai treatment for 45 days decreased the creatinine contents in the serum and urine, suggesting a protective effect on the kidney [20]. Since we only performed the acai trials for up to four days, a more detailed evaluation of the effects of longer-term treatment on the hematopoietic activity and renal function is needed. EPO formulations are presently banned as a doping substance. The erythropoietic mechanism of acai via EPO must be further clarified, and its use in sports needs to be carefully discussed.

In summary, acai induces an erythropoietic effect associated with renal hypoxia. These findings provide valuable insight into the potential utility of acai for future research on hematopoiesis in humans.

Author Contributions: S.S., T.T., and T.S. designed the study; S.S. and T.S. wrote the manuscript; S.S., T.T., M.J.V.Y., and Y.O. performed the experiments; S.S. analyzed the data; T.S. edited the article; and T.S. coordinated and directed the project. All authors have read and agreed to the published version of the manuscript.

Funding: This research was funded by FRUTA FRUTA, Inc.

Conflicts of Interest: This does not alter the authors' adherence to all *Nutrients* policies on sharing data and materials.

References

1. Zanjani, E.D.; Ascensao, J.L.; McGlave, P.B.; Banisadre, M.; Ash, R.C. Studies on the liver to kidney switch of erythropoietin production. *J. Clin. Investig.* **1981**, *67*, 1183–1188. [CrossRef] [PubMed]
2. Fandrey, J. Oxygen-dependent and tissue-specific regulation of erythropoietin gene expression. *Am. J. Physiol. Regul. Integr. Comp. Physiol.* **2004**, *286*, R977–R988. [CrossRef] [PubMed]
3. Wenger, R.H.; Hoogewijs, D. Regulated oxygen sensing by protein hydroxylation in renal erythropoietin-producing cells. *Am. J. Physiol. Renal. Physiol.* **2010**, *298*, F1287–F1296. [CrossRef] [PubMed]
4. Schauss, A.G.; Wu, X.; Prior, R.L.; Ou, B.; Huang, D.; Owens, J.; Agarwal, A.; Jensen, G.S.; Hart, A.N.; Shanbrom, E. Antioxidant capacity and other bioactivities of the freeze-dried Amazonian palm berry, *Euterpe oleraceae* mart. (acai). *J. Agric. Food Chem.* **2006**, *54*, 8604–8610. [CrossRef] [PubMed]
5. Zapata-Sudo, G.; da Silva, J.S.; Pereira, S.L.; Souza, P.J.; de Moura, R.S.; Sudo, R.T. Oral treatment with *Euterpe oleracea* Mart. (acai) extract improves cardiac dysfunction and exercise intolerance in rats subjected to myocardial infarction. *BMC Complement. Altern. Med.* **2014**, *14*, 227. [CrossRef]
6. de Oliveira, P.R.; da Costa, C.A.; de Bem, G.F.; Cordeiro, V.S.; Santos, I.B.; de Carvalho, L.C.; da Conceicao, E.P.; Lisboa, P.C.; Ognibene, D.T.; Sousa, P.J.; et al. *Euterpe oleracea* Mart.-Derived Polyphenols Protect Mice from Diet-Induced Obesity and Fatty Liver by Regulating Hepatic Lipogenesis and Cholesterol Excretion. *PLoS ONE* **2015**, *10*, e0143721. [CrossRef]
7. Pereira, R.R.; de Abreu, I.C.; Guerra, J.F.; Lage, N.N.; Lopes, J.M.; Silva, M.; de Lima, W.G.; Silva, M.E.; Pedrosa, M.L. Acai (*Euterpe oleracea* Mart.) Upregulates Paraoxonase 1 Gene Expression and Activity with Concomitant Reduction of Hepatic Steatosis in High-Fat Diet-Fed Rats. *Oxid Med. Cell Longev.* **2016**, *2016*, 8379105. [CrossRef]
8. de Souza Machado, F.; Kuo, J.; Wohlenberg, M.F.; da Rocha Frusciante, M.; Freitas, M.; Oliveira, A.S.; Andrade, R.B.; Wannmacher, C.M.; Dani, C.; Funchal, C. Subchronic treatment with acai frozen pulp prevents the brain oxidative damage in rats with acute liver failure. *Metab. Brain Dis.* **2016**, *31*, 1427–1434. [CrossRef]
9. Poulose, S.M.; Bielinski, D.F.; Carey, A.; Schauss, A.G.; Shukitt-Hale, B. Modulation of oxidative stress, inflammation, autophagy and expression of Nrf2 in hippocampus and frontal cortex of rats fed with acai-enriched diets. *Nutr. Neurosci.* **2017**, *20*, 305–315. [CrossRef]
10. Martins, I.; Borges, N.A.; Stenvinkel, P.; Lindholm, B.; Rogez, H.; Pinheiro, M.C.N.; Nascimento, J.L.M.; Mafra, D. The value of the Brazilian acai fruit as a therapeutic nutritional strategy for chronic kidney disease patients. *Int. Urol. Nephrol.* **2018**, *50*, 2207–2220. [CrossRef]
11. Souma, T.; Nezu, M.; Nakano, D.; Yamazaki, S.; Hirano, I.; Sekine, H.; Dan, T.; Takeda, K.; Fong, G.H.; Nishiyama, A.; et al. Erythropoietin Synthesis in Renal Myofibroblasts Is Restored by Activation of Hypoxia Signaling. *J. Am. Soc. Nephrol.* **2016**, *27*, 428–438. [CrossRef] [PubMed]
12. Jelkmann, W. Erythropoietin: Structure, control of production, and function. *Physiol. Rev.* **1992**, *72*, 449–489. [CrossRef] [PubMed]
13. Provenzano, R.; Besarab, A.; Sun, C.H.; Diamond, S.A.; Durham, J.H.; Cangiano, J.L.; Aiello, J.R.; Novak, J.E.; Lee, T.; Leong, R.; et al. Oral Hypoxia-Inducible Factor Prolyl Hydroxylase Inhibitor Roxadustat (FG-4592) for the Treatment of Anemia in Patients with CKD. *Clin. J. Am. Soc. Nephrol.* **2016**, *11*, 982–991. [CrossRef] [PubMed]
14. Guo, W.; Li, M.; Bhasin, S. Testosterone supplementation improves anemia in aging male mice. *J. Gerontol. A Biol. Sci. Med. Sci.* **2014**, *69*, 505–513. [CrossRef] [PubMed]
15. Fishbane, S.; Shah, H.H. Ferric pyrophosphate citrate as an iron replacement agent for patients receiving hemodialysis. *Hemodial. Int.* **2017**, *21* (Suppl. 1), S104–S109. [CrossRef] [PubMed]

16. Verlengia, R.; Gorjao, R.; Kanunfre, C.C.; Bordin, S.; de Lima, T.M.; Curi, R. Effect of arachidonic acid on proliferation, cytokines production and pleiotropic genes expression in Jurkat cells—A comparison with oleic acid. *Life Sci.* **2003**, *73*, 2939–2951. [CrossRef]
17. Stoner, G.D.; Wang, L.S.; Seguin, C.; Rocha, C.; Stoner, K.; Chiu, S.; Kinghorn, A.D. Multiple berry types prevent N-nitrosomethylbenzylamine-induced esophageal cancer in rats. *Pharm. Res.* **2010**, *27*, 1138–1145. [CrossRef]
18. Balducci, L. Anemia, fatigue and aging. *Transfus. Clin. Biol.* **2010**, *17*, 375–381. [CrossRef]
19. El Morsy, E.M.; Ahmed, M.A.; Ahmed, A.A. Attenuation of renal ischemia/reperfusion injury by acai extract preconditioning in a rat model. *Life Sci.* **2015**, *123*, 35–42. [CrossRef]
20. da Silva Cristino Cordeiro, V.; de Bem, G.F.; da Costa, C.A.; Santos, I.B.; de Carvalho, L.; Ognibene, D.T.; da Rocha, A.P.M.; de Carvalho, J.J.; de Moura, R.S.; Resende, A.C. *Euterpe oleracea* Mart. seed extract protects against renal injury in diabetic and spontaneously hypertensive rats: Role of inflammation and oxidative stress. *Eur. J. Nutr.* **2018**, *57*, 817–832. [CrossRef]
21. Friederich-Persson, M.; Persson, P. Mitochondrial angiotensin II receptors regulate oxygen consumption in kidney mitochondria from healthy and type 1 diabetic rats. *Am. J. Physiol. Renal. Physiol.* **2020**. [CrossRef]
22. Hernandez-Vargas, P.; Lopez-Franco, O.; Sanjuan, G.; Ruperez, M.; Ortiz-Munoz, G.; Suzuki, Y.; Aguado-Roncero, P.; Perez-Tejerizo, G.; Blanco, J.; Egido, J.; et al. Suppressors of cytokine signaling regulate angiotensin II-activated Janus kinase-signal transducers and activators of transcription pathway in renal cells. *J. Am. Soc. Nephrol.* **2005**, *16*, 1673–1683. [CrossRef] [PubMed]
23. Tsogbadrakh, B.; Ryu, H.; Ju, K.D.; Lee, J.; Yun, S.; Yu, K.S.; Kim, H.J.; Ahn, C.; Oh, K.H. AICAR, an AMPK activator, protects against cisplatin-induced acute kidney injury through the JAK/STAT/SOCS pathway. *Biochem. Biophys. Res. Commun.* **2019**, *509*, 680–686. [CrossRef] [PubMed]
24. Youdim, K.A.; Shukitt-Hale, B.; MacKinnon, S.; Kalt, W.; Joseph, J.A. Polyphenolics enhance red blood cell resistance to oxidative stress: In vitro and in vivo. *Biochim. Biophys. Acta* **2000**, *1523*, 117–122. [CrossRef]
25. Nabavi, S.M.; Nabavi, S.F.; Setzer, W.N.; Alinezhad, H.; Zare, M.; Naqinezhad, A. Interaction of different extracts of Primula heterochroma Stapf. with red blood cell membrane lipids and proteins: Antioxidant and antihemolytic effects. *J. Diet Suppl.* **2012**, *9*, 285–292. [CrossRef] [PubMed]
26. Phrueksanan, W.; Yibchok-anun, S.; Adisakwattana, S. Protection of Clitoria ternatea flower petal extract against free radical-induced hemolysis and oxidative damage in canine erythrocytes. *Res. Vet. Sci.* **2014**, *97*, 357–363. [CrossRef] [PubMed]
27. Tedesco, I.; Moccia, S.; Volpe, S.; Alfieri, G.; Strollo, D.; Bilotto, S.; Spagnuolo, C.; Di Renzo, M.; Aquino, R.P.; Russo, G.L. Red wine activates plasma membrane redox system in human erythrocytes. *Free Radic. Res.* **2016**, *50*, 557–569. [CrossRef]
28. Buko, V.; Zavodnik, I.; Kanuka, O.; Belonovskaya, E.; Naruta, E.; Lukivskaya, O.; Kirko, S.; Budryn, G.; Zyzelewicz, D.; Oracz, J.; et al. Antidiabetic effects and erythrocyte stabilization by red cabbage extract in streptozotocin-treated rats. *Food Funct.* **2018**, *9*, 1850–1863. [CrossRef]
29. Mpiana, P.T.; Mudogo, V.; Tshibangu, D.S.; Kitwa, E.K.; Kanangila, A.B.; Lumbu, J.B.; Ngbolua, K.N.; Atibu, E.K.; Kakule, M.K. Antisickling activity of anthocyanins from Bombax pentadrum, Ficus capensis and Ziziphus mucronata: Photodegradation effect. *J. Ethnopharmacol* **2008**, *120*, 413–418. [CrossRef]
30. Mpiana, P.T.; Ngbolua, K.N.; Bokota, M.T.; Kasonga, T.K.; Atibu, E.K.; Tshibangu, D.S.; Mudogo, V. In vitro effects of anthocyanin extracts from Justicia secunda Vahl on the solubility of haemoglobin S and membrane stability of sickle erythrocytes. *Blood Transfus.* **2010**, *8*, 248–254.
31. Fragoso, M.F.; Prado, M.G.; Barbosa, L.; Rocha, N.S.; Barbisan, L.F. Inhibition of mouse urinary bladder carcinogenesis by acai fruit (*Euterpe oleraceae* Martius) intake. *Plant Foods Hum. Nutr.* **2012**, *67*, 235–241. [CrossRef] [PubMed]
32. Fragoso, M.F.; Romualdo, G.R.; Ribeiro, D.A.; Barbisan, L.F. Acai (*Euterpe oleracea* Mart.) feeding attenuates dimethylhydrazine-induced rat colon carcinogenesis. *Food Chem. Toxicol.* **2013**, *58*, 68–76. [CrossRef]
33. Monge-Fuentes, V.; Muehlmann, L.A.; Longo, J.P.; Silva, J.R.; Fascineli, M.L.; de Souza, P.; Faria, F.; Degterev, I.A.; Rodriguez, A.; Carneiro, F.P.; et al. Photodynamic therapy mediated by acai oil (*Euterpe oleracea* Martius) in nanoemulsion: A potential treatment for melanoma. *J. Photochem. Photobiol. B* **2017**, *166*, 301–310. [CrossRef] [PubMed]

34. Ribeiro, J.C.; Antunes, L.M.; Aissa, A.F.; Darin, J.D.; De Rosso, V.V.; Mercadante, A.Z.; de Bianchi, M.L. Evaluation of the genotoxic and antigenotoxic effects after acute and subacute treatments with acai pulp (*Euterpe oleracea* Mart.) on mice using the erythrocytes micronucleus test and the comet assay. *Mutat. Res.* **2010**, *695*, 22–28. [CrossRef] [PubMed]
35. Marques, E.S.; Froder, J.G.; Carvalho, J.C.; Rosa, P.C.; Perazzo, F.F.; Maistro, E.L. Evaluation of the genotoxicity of *Euterpe oleraceae* Mart. (Arecaceae) fruit oil (acai), in mammalian cells in vivo. *Food Chem. Toxicol.* **2016**, *93*, 13–19. [CrossRef] [PubMed]
36. Schauss, A.G.; Clewell, A.; Balogh, L.; Szakonyi, I.P.; Financsek, I.; Horvath, J.; Thuroczy, J.; Beres, E.; Vertesi, A.; Hirka, G. Safety evaluation of an acai-fortified fruit and berry functional juice beverage (MonaVie Active(R)). *Toxicology* **2010**, *278*, 46–54. [CrossRef] [PubMed]
37. da Silva Santos, V.; de Almeida Teixeira, G.H.; Barbosa, F., Jr. Acai (*Euterpe oleracea* Mart.): A tropical fruit with high levels of essential minerals-especially manganese-and its contribution as a source of natural mineral supplementation. *J. Toxicol. Environ. Health A* **2014**, *77*, 80–89. [CrossRef]
38. Gallagher, D.; Belmonte, D.; Deurenberg, P.; Wang, Z.; Krasnow, N.; Pi-Sunyer, F.X.; Heymsfield, S.B. Organ-tissue mass measurement allows modeling of REE and metabolically active tissue mass. *Am. J. Physiol.* **1998**, *275*, E249–E258. [CrossRef]
39. Mimura, I.; Nangaku, M. The suffocating kidney: Tubulointerstitial hypoxia in end-stage renal disease. *Nat. Rev. Nephrol.* **2010**, *6*, 667–678. [CrossRef]
40. Nangaku, M. Chronic hypoxia and tubulointerstitial injury: A final common pathway to end-stage renal failure. *J. Am. Soc. Nephrol.* **2006**, *17*, 17–25. [CrossRef]

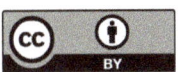

© 2020 by the authors. Licensee MDPI, Basel, Switzerland. This article is an open access article distributed under the terms and conditions of the Creative Commons Attribution (CC BY) license (http://creativecommons.org/licenses/by/4.0/).

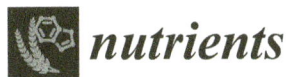

Article

Beneficial Effect of Ubiquinol on Hematological and Inflammatory Signaling during Exercise

Javier Diaz-Castro [1,2,*], Jorge Moreno-Fernandez [1,2], Ignacio Chirosa [3], Luis Javier Chirosa [3], Rafael Guisado [4] and Julio J. Ochoa [1,2]

[1] Institute of Nutrition and Food Technology "José Mataix", University of Granada, Biomedical Research Centre, Health-Sciences Technological Park, Avenida del Conocimiento s/n, Armilla, E-18071 Granada, Spain; jorgemf@ugr.es (J.M.-F.); jjoh@ugr.es (J.J.O.)
[2] Department of Physiology, University of Granada, E-18071 Granada, Spain
[3] Departament of Physical Education, University of Granada, E-18071 Granada, Spain; ichirosa@ugr.es (I.C.); lchirosa@ugr.es (L.J.C.)
[4] Faculty of Health Sciences, University of Granada, E-18071 Granada, Spain; rguisado@ugr.es
* Correspondence: javierdc@ugr.es; Tel.: +34-958-24-10-00 (ext. 20303)

Received: 13 January 2020; Accepted: 4 February 2020; Published: 6 February 2020

Abstract: Strenuous exercise (any activity that expends six metabolic equivalents per minute or more causing sensations of fatigue and exhaustion to occur, inducing deleterious effects, affecting negatively different cells), induces muscle damage and hematological changes associated with high production of pro-inflammatory mediators related to muscle damage and sports anemia. The objective of this study was to determine whether short-term oral ubiquinol supplementation can prevent accumulation of inflammatory mediators and hematological impairment associated to strenuous exercise. For this purpose, 100 healthy and well-trained firemen were classified in two groups: Ubiquinol (experimental group), and placebo group (control). The protocol was two identical strenuous exercise tests with rest period between tests of 24 h. Blood samples were collected before supplementation (basal value) (T1), after supplementation (T2), after first physical exercise test (T3), after 24 h of rest (T4), and after second physical exercise test (T5). Hematological parameters, pro- and anti-inflammatory cytokines and growth factors were measured. Red blood cells (RBC), hematocrit, hemoglobin, VEGF, NO, EGF, IL-1ra, and IL-10 increased in the ubiquinol group while IL-1, IL-8, and MCP-1 decreased. Ubiquinol supplementation during high intensity exercise could modulate inflammatory signaling, expression of pro-inflammatory, and increasing some anti-inflammatory cytokines. During exercise, RBC, hemoglobin, hematocrit, VEGF, and EGF increased in ubiquinol group, revealing a possible pro-angiogenic effect, improving oxygen supply and exerting a possible protective effect on other physiological alterations.

Keywords: high intensity exercise; ubiquinol; hematological parameters; inflammation; ergogenic effect

1. Introduction

There are multiple beneficial effects associated with regular and planned exercise [1,2], including the reduction in the age-related changes in nuclear pore complex proteins, protection of the neuromuscular junction, and the increase in the lives of susceptible motoneurons, preserving neuromuscular integrity and innervation status [3,4]. In addition, exercise increases blood flow and improves vascular integrity, enhancing angiogenesis, resulting in reversal of rarefaction and hypertension, and enhancement of cerebral blood flow and cognition [5].

On the other hand, strenuous exercise can induce a range of adverse effects including oxidative stress, hematological changes, and inflammatory response involved in activating catabolic pathways inducing muscle damage [6]. Strenuous exercise (defined as any activity that expends six metabolic equivalents (METS) per minute or more [7]) is harmful to health [8], because it causes structural damage to muscle cells indicated by muscle soreness and swelling, prolonged loss of muscle function, increased free radicals output, induction of the pro-inflammatory signaling, impairment of immune functions, including the immunoglobulin production or T-cell function, and leakage of muscle proteins into circulation, among other effects [9,10].

The aerobic energy metabolism during strenuous exercise (established when sensations of fatigue and exhaustion occur, inducing deleterious effects, affecting negatively different cells) plays a crucial role on the performance. Hematological changes such as decreases in the hemoglobin (Hb) concentrations and RBC counts are often found to result from participation in strenuous exercise [11]. In this sense, in athletes performing high intensity exercise, a high prevalence of "sports anemia" or iron deficiency anemia induced by strenuous exercise has been reported [12,13], which has been associated with hematological changes such as a decrease in RBC, hemoglobin, and hematocrit [14,15]. These changes are suggested to be mainly caused by iron deficiency and a negative iron balance caused by intense physical exercise [16].

Within the oxygen transport chain, RBC mass is crucial for oxygen supply to working muscles which could regulate the aerobic performance capacity [17]. However, although during the strenuous exercise there is a greater erythropoietic activity, an important loss of RBC is featured [14,18]. During exercise an inflammatory state is featured and a high production of free radicals, both factors affecting iron metabolism [18] and by a direct effect on the iron reduction due to its affinity for H_2O_2 [13]. In addition, skeletal muscle is a highly regenerative tissue, but muscle repair potential is limited, and inflammatory signaling contributes to muscle repair [19], however the pro-inflammatory cytokines can also be deleterious to health. Therefore, these cytokines are both cause and effect of inflammation [20]. Elevated levels of these inflammatory markers not only increase risk for chronic diseases, but also contribute to disease pathogenesis [21]. In addition, the composition of the serum microbiome is linked to indices of inflammation, altering immunity [22].

Athletes may be susceptible to a heightened anti-inflammatory state. These results can transiently suppress immune function and increase the risk of infection [23]. In this sense, reducing inflammation has been recognized as one of the ways to reduce the risk of chronic disease [24].

During regeneration, reconstitution of muscle fibers, RBC mass, and blood supply is imperative for full muscular recovery and prevention of muscle atrophy [25]. In this sense, vascular endothelial growth factor (VEGF) has a key role for angiogenesis and muscle fibers repair in skeletal muscle and has been shown to be upregulated by a single bout of dynamic exercise [26].

On the other hand, inflammation, angiogenesis, RBC mass, and oxygen supply have a key role on muscle damage associated to high intensity exercise and other physiological alterations that can affect physical performance. Therefore, it would be interesting to assess the effect of oral supplementation with a substance capable of improving hematological parameters and diminishing inflammatory signaling associated to this performance [27,28], however scarce studies are available about molecules with these characteristics to support the regeneration process of skeletal muscle after strenuous exercise. One of these substances could be coenzyme Q10 (CoQ10) [29].

The data available in the scientific literature have provided a direct link between physical performance and blood and muscle tissue CoQ10 levels [30]. However, most of these studies are focused mainly on the exercise performance and radical-scavenging activity of CoQ10 during low intensity exercise [30], with the studies about the influence of CoQ10 supplementation during the performance of high intensity (strenuous) exercise on the inflammatory signaling, hematology, and muscle recovery after strenuous exercise being scarce. CoQ10 exists in two forms: Ubiquinone (oxidized form), the most common form in CoQ10 supplements, and ubiquinol, the reduced and most active form, which has properties related to bioenergetic and antioxidant activity [31,32], but poorly studied. Therefore, we aimed to determine whether, a short term oral ubiquinol supplementation may be efficient ameliorating the pro-inflammatory effects, improving hematological parameters, effects that could promote skeletal muscles regeneration and oxygen supply after strenuous exercise.

2. Materials and Methods

2.1. Subjects and Supplementation Protocol

This study was a randomized, double-blind, and placebo-controlled trial. One hundred healthy and well trained, but not on an elite level, firemen of the Fire Department of the City of Granada were taking part in this study. Participants completed a medical and health history and physical activity questionnaire (IPAQ-SF) [33] prior to enrolment. All of them were nonsmokers, did not take any nutritional supplements and did not present febrile/inflammatory clinical symptoms, did not use immunosuppressive or nephrotoxic drugs, did not use energy, protein, and/or antioxidant supplements. The firemen were randomly divided into two groups: Ubiquinol group (ubiquinol) (n = 50), and placebo group (control) (n = 50). The ubiquinol group was supplemented with an oral dose of 200 mg/day of ubiquinol during two weeks, administrating two brown liquid filled hard gelatine capsules of 100 mg/day, and subjects assigned to the control group took placebo using the same scheme. The capsules Kaneka QH ubiquinol (Kaneka Corporation, Osaka, Japan) contained 100 mg of ubiquinol in a basis of canola oil, diglycerol monooleate, beeswax, and soy lecithin. The placebo capsules contained the same composition without ubiquinol and were also supplied by Kaneka (Kaneka Corporation, Osaka, Japan). The study was approved by the Commission of Ethics in Human Research of the University of Granada (ref. 804). The study has been registered in ClinicalTrials.gov, with number NCT01940627. Informed consent was obtained from all subjects with written consent to participate in this study.

2.2. Strenuous Exercise Performance Programme

Characteristics, intensity, and muscle damage (loss of skeletal muscle function and soreness) of this protocol was previously reported by measuring blood myoglobin and CK [32] and similar increases have been observed in other strenuous exercise tests [34]. After two-weeks period of ubiquinol or placebo supplementation, subjects performed the strenuous exercise protocol in order to induce muscle damage. Prior to the starting of each test, subjects performed a warm-up which was divided into two phases: General activation phase and specific phase. The protocol consisted of conducting two identical strenuous exercise tests, with a rest period between tests within 24 h. Circuit weight training (CWT), characterized by alternating exercises between upper- and lower-body segments performed at stations, has been widely used in practice settings. The main advantage of this method is that it allows faster training performance. Moreover, it is commonly used for persons interested in weight management, although a previous study showed similar effects on body composition and on muscular strength and size in trained men after CWT and multiple-set resistance training [35]. The rest time between sets was five minutes to allow recovery and complete the designed workout [35]. Both strenuous exercise tests consisted of performing a circuit composed of 10 bodybuilding exercises (1. athletic press; 2. chest press in Smith Machine; 3. seated oar; 4. shoulders press; 5. femoral biceps flexion; 6. chest press in Smith Machine; 7. step with weight; 8. surveyor's pole chest; 9. shove with weight; 10. quadriceps extension) [32]. In order to establish the minimum magnitude of the load to be displaced for each subject, one week before strenuous exercise protocol, a session of pre-training was held with the subjects to conform the load individually in terms of two parameters in each exercise: (a) Scale OMNI-RES [36] values of perceived exertion between 6–7, and (b) 10 repetitions.

2.3. Blood Sampling

Blood samples were collected from the participants by venous catheter into heparinized tubes before and immediately after the physical test. Five blood samples and urine were taken: Before supplementation (basal value) (T1), after supplementation (two weeks) (T2), after first physical exercise test (T3), after 24 h of rest (T4), after second physical exercise test (T5). One aliquot of blood was collected in tubes with an EDTA anticoagulant for hematological analysis. The remaining blood was immediately centrifuged at 1750 g for 10 min at 4 °C in a Beckman GS-6R refrigerated centrifuge

(Beckman, Fullerton, CA, USA) to separate plasma from red blood cell pellets. Plasma samples were immediately frozen and stored at −80 °C until analysis.

2.4. Inflammatory Parameters

Epidermal growth factor (EGF), interferon gamma (IFN-γ), vascular endothelial growth factor (VEGF), monocyte chemotactic protein 1 (MCP-1), tumor necrosis factor alpha (TNF-α), interleukin (IL)-1, IL-1ra (receptor agonist), IL-6, IL-10, and IL-15 were determined using the HCYTOMAG-60K Milliplex MAP Human Cytokine/Chemokine Magnetic Bead Panel (Millipore Corporation, Missouri, USA), based on immunoassays on the surface of fluorescent-coded beads (microspheres), following the specifications of the manufacturer (50 events per bead, 50 µL sample, gate settings: 8000–15,000, time out 60 s, melatonin bead set: 34). The plate was read on a LABScan 100 analyzer (Luminex Corporation, Austin, TX, USA) with xPONENT software for data acquisition. With these biomarkers we characterize mediators of adaptive immunity, mediators of innate immunity and inflammation, chemotaxis, haematopoietic mediators and growth factors, allowing us to have an overview of the various pathways of cytokines in the immune and inflammatory process. Average values for each set of duplicate samples or standards were within 15% of the mean. Cytokines concentrations in plasma samples were determined by comparing the mean of triplicate samples with the standard curve for each assay.

2.5. Hematological Parameters

Hemoglobin (Hb) concentration, red blood cells (RBC), hematocrit, mean corpuscular volume (MCV), mean corpuscular Hb (MCH), mean corpuscular Hb concentration (MCHC), red cell distribution width (RDW), platelets, mean platelets volume (MPV), leukocytes, neutrophils, lymphocytes, monocytes, eosinophils, basophils of fresh blood samples were measured using an automated hematology analyzer Mythic 22CT (C2 Diagnostics, Grabels, France).

2.6. Statistical Analysis

All data are presented as the mean ± standard error of the mean (SEM). All variables were tested to see if they followed the criteria of normality and homogeneity of variance using the Kolmogorov–Smirnoff's and Levene's tests, respectively. To compare general characteristics of the subjects in both experimental groups, unpaired Student's t-test was used. To assess the effect of the supplementation and the evolution in the time of each variable studied in each experimental group a general linear model of variance for repeated measures with an adjustment by means of Bonferroni's test has been performed. Bonferroni's test allowed us to know intra- and inter-subject differences (effect of time in each group and supplementation in each period, respectively) in a very robust way in terms of power. A value of $p < 0.05$ was considered significant. For data analysis we used the SPSS version 20.0 (SPSS Statistics for Windows, 20.0.0. SPSS INC. Chicago, IL, USA).

3. Results

No statistically significant differences between both groups were found for weight, age, height, and BMI (Table 1). In addition, no significant differences were recorded between groups for the short form of the International Physical Activity Questionnaire [32]. The subjects of both experimental groups were categorized as "Health Enhancing Physical Activity" (HEPA Active): Category 3, the highest measurement threshold of total physical activity of the questionnaire. In addition, as we have previously reported [32], the high intensity protocol induces muscle damage based on lactate output (increase of 290% (2.9 ± 0.1 vs. 8.5 ± 0.3 mmol/L) after the first exercise session and an increase of 355% (2.9 ± 0.1 vs. 10.5 ± 0.5 mmol/L) after the second training session, myoglobin increased 358% higher after the first session (25.7 ± 3.2 vs. 92.1 ± 7.9 ng/mL) and 387% after the second session (25.7 ± 3.2 vs. 99.3 ± 6.8 ng/mL) and creatine kinase (CK-MM) increased 158% after the first exercise test (2.01 ± 0.3 vs. 3.2 ± 0.4 ng/mL) and 196% after the second session (2.01 ± 0.3 vs. 4.0 ± 0.3 ng/mL). We have also reported that ubiquinol supplementation increased plasma CoQ10 levels 522% (1.00 ± 0.06 vs. 5.22 ± 0.41 mmol/L). The dropout percentage was similar in both groups (24% after finishing the first test and 32% after finishing the second exercise test) and neither differences were observed between dropout reasons in both groups [32].

Table 1. Subjects baseline characteristics.

	Age (Years)	Height (cm)	Weight (kg)	BMI (kg/m^2)	SBP (mmHg)	DBP (mmHg)	RHR (Beats/min)
Ubiquinol	38.9 ± 1.4	175.4 ± 0.8	76.8 ± 1.5	25.0 ± 0.4	137.0 ± 2.2	81.4 ± 1.5	57.4 ± 1.8
Control	38.2 ± 1.2	174.5 ± 1.2	76.3 ± 2.0	25.0 ± 0.5	134.1 ± 2.1	79.1 ± 1.9	57.1 ± 1.5

Data expressed as the mean ± SEM. BMI: Body mass index; SBP: Systolic blood pressure; DBP: Diastolic blood pressure; RHR: Resting heart rate.

IL-1 was lower in ubiquinol compared with the control group in T3. Regarding the evolution, IL-1 increased in the ubiquinol and control group in T5 compared with T1, T2, T3, and T4 (Figure 1A). No differences were observed in IL-1ra due to the supplementation. Regarding the evolution, IL-1ra increased in the ubiquinol group in T5 compared to T4, T2, and T1 (Figure 1B). No differences were observed in IL-6 due to the supplementation. Regarding the evolution, IL-6 increased in the ubiquinol group in T3 and T5 compared with T1, in T3 and T5 compared with T2, and also in T5 compared with T4, while decreased in T4 compared with T3 (Figure 1C). IL-8 was lower in the supplemented group in T3 compared with the control group. Regarding the evolution, in the ubiquinol group, IL-8 decreased in T4 with respect to T2, T3, and T5. In the control group, there was an increase in T3 with respect to T1, T2, and T4, and also increased in T5 with respect to T1 and T4 (Figure 1D). IL-10 was higher in ubiquinol compared with the control group in T5 (Figure 1E). Regarding the evolution, IL-10 increased in the ubiquinol group in T3 compared with T1 and T5, and also increased in T5 with respect to T1 and T4 while no differences by the evolution of time were observed in the control group. No differences were observed in IL-15 due to the supplementation. Regarding the evolution, IL-15 decreased in T4 compared with T3 in the control group (Figure 1F).

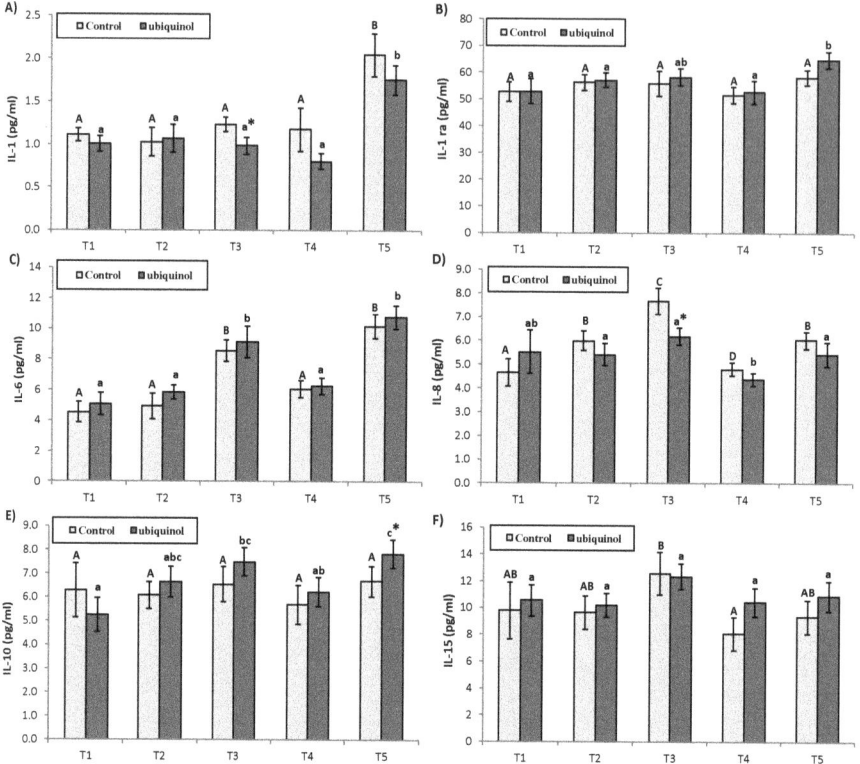

Figure 1. Effects of exercise and ubiquinol supplementation on plasma cytokines: interleukin (IL)-1 (**A**), IL-1ra (**B**), IL-6 (**C**), IL-8 (**D**), IL-10 (**E**), IL-15 (**F**). Results are expressed as the mean ± SEM. * means statistically significant differences between groups ($p < 0.05$). T1: Before supplementation (basal value); T2: After supplementation (two weeks) and before the first physical test; T3: After first physical exercise test; T4: After 24 h of rest and before the second physical test; T5: After second physical exercise test. Different letters in every group indicates significant differences due to the time (control (A, B, C, D, E); ubiquinol (a, b, c, d, e)) ($p < 0.05$).

No differences were observed in TNF-α due to the supplementation. Regarding the evolution, TNF-α increased in the ubiquinol group in T3 compared with T1 and T4. In the control group, TNF-α increased in T3 compared with the rest of the blood samples and also increased in T5 compared with T1 and T4 (Figure 2A). No differences were observed in IFN-γ due to the supplementation or evolution of time (Figure 2B). A higher level of EGF was observed in the ubiquinol compared with the control group in T2 and T3. Regarding the evolution, EGF increased in the ubiquinol group in T2 compared with T1 and in T3 compared with T1, T4, and T5. In the control group, EGF was higher in T1 with regard to T1, T2 and also increased in T4 with regard to T1 (Figure 2C). VEGF was higher in the ubiquinol compared with the control group in T3. VEGF increased in the ubiquinol group in T5 compared with T1 and T2, while no differences by the evolution of time were observed in the control group (Figure 2D). MCP-1 decreased in ubiquinol compared with the control group in T3 and T5. Regarding the evolution, MCP-1 increased in the ubiquinol group in T3 compared with T1, and in T5 compared with T4, while decreased in T4 compared with T2, and in T4 compared with T3. In the control group, MCP-1 increased in T2, T3, and T5 compared with T1, increased in T3 compared with T2, and in T5 compared with T4, while showed a decrease in T4 compared with T2, and in T4 and in T5 compared with T3 (Figure 2E).

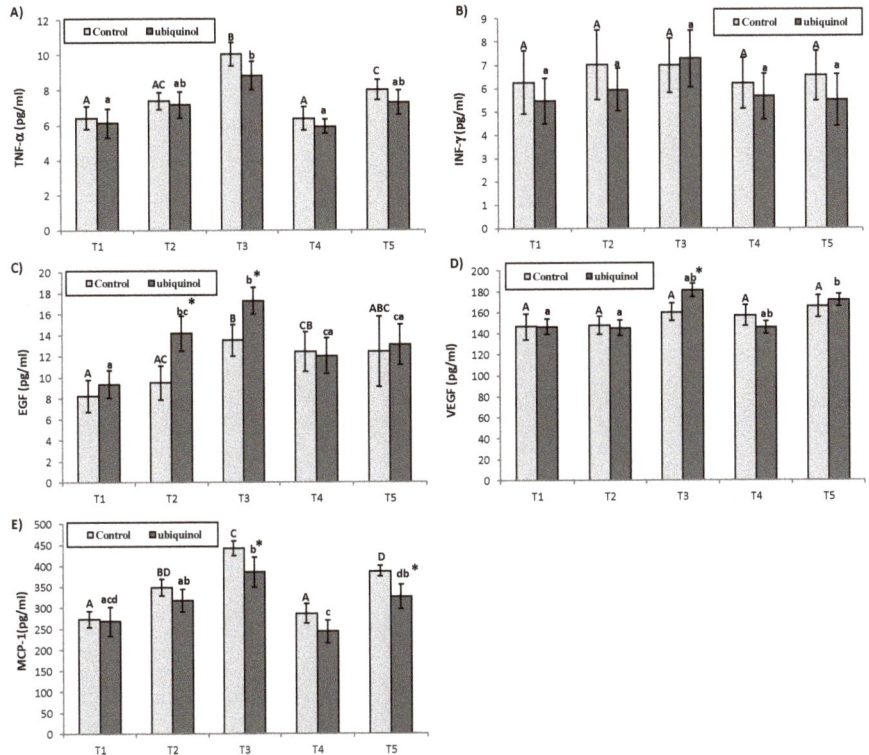

Figure 2. Effects of exercise and ubiquinol supplementation on plasma cytokines: tumor necrosis factor alpha (TNF-α) (**A**), interferon gamma (IFN-γ) (**B**), epidermal growth factor (EGF) (**C**), vascular endothelial growth factor (VEGF) (**D**), monocyte chemotactic protein 1 (MCP-1) (**E**). Results are expressed as mean ± SEM. * means statistically significant differences between groups ($p < 0.05$). T1: Before supplementation (basal value); T2: After supplementation (two weeks) and before the first physical test; T3: After first physical exercise test; T4: After 24 h of rest and before the second physical test; T5: After second physical exercise test. Different letters in every group indicates significant differences due to the time (control (A, B, C, D, E); ubiquinol (a, b, c, d, e)) ($p < 0.05$).

RBC increased in the ubiquinol compared with the control group in T3 and T4. Regarding the evolution, RBC increased in the ubiquinol group in T2 and T3 compared with T1 and T5, while decreased in the control group in T4 and T5 compared with T1 (Figure 3A). Hemoglobin levels were higher in ubiquinol compared with the control group in T3 and T4. In the control group, hemoglobin decreased in T4 compared with T1, T2, T3, and T5 (Figure 3B). Hematocrit increased in the ubiquinol compared with the control group in T3. Hematocrit decreased in T4 and T5 compared with T1 in the control group (Figure 3C).

Leukocytes increased in the ubiquinol group in T3 compared with T1 and T4. Neutrophils were higher in the ubiquinol compared with the control group in T4, also increased in the control group in T5 compared with T1, T2, and T4 and also in T3 and T5 in regard to T1, T2, and T4 in the ubiquinol group. Lymphocytes decreased in the ubiquinol group in T4, in T5 compared with T1 and T2 in the ubiquinol group and in T3, and also in T5 compared with T4 in the control group. Monocytes were lower in the ubiquinol compared with the control group in T4, also decreased in T2, T3, T4, and T5 compared with T1 in the control and ubiquinol group. Eosinophils decreased in T3 compared with T1 in the control and ubiquinol group. Basophils decreased in T4 and T5 compared with T1 in the ubiquinol group and increased in T5 compared with T1 and T4 in the control group. No changes were recorded in platelets during the study, MCV or MCH nor due to exercise and neither to ubiquinol. MCHC increased in the ubiquinol compared with the control group in T5 and also increased in T4 and T5 compared with T1 and T2 in the ubiquinol group, while decreased in T3, T4, and T5 compared with T1 in the control group. No significant changes were recorded in RDW and MPW due to exercise and neither to ubiquinol (Table 2).

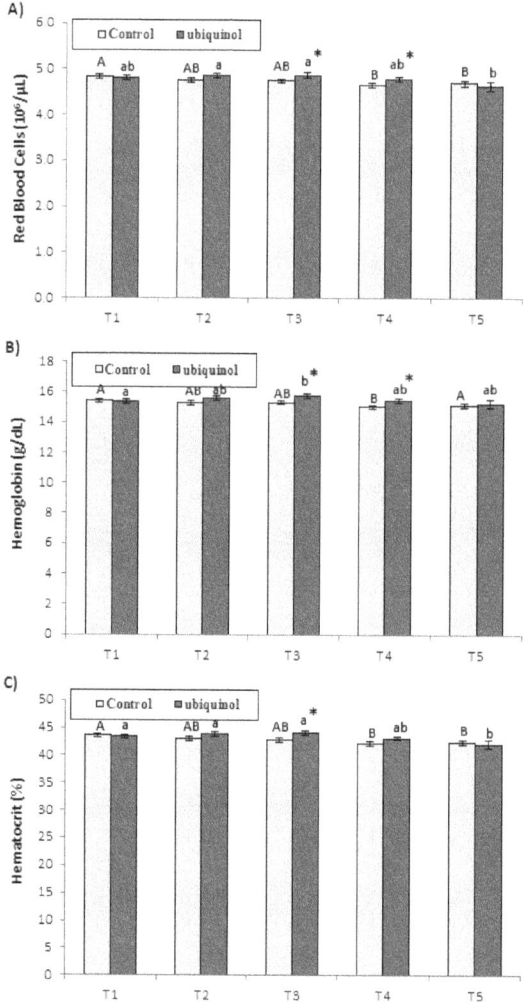

Figure 3. Effects of exercise and ubiquinol supplementation on hematological parameters: Red blood cells (**A**), hemoglobin (**B**), hematocrit (**C**). Results are expressed as mean ± SEM. * means statistically significant differences between groups ($p < 0.05$). T1: Before supplementation (basal value); T2: After supplementation (two weeks) and before the first physical test; T3: After first physical exercise test; T4: After 24 h of rest and before the second physical test; T5: After second physical exercise test. Different letters in every group indicates significant differences due to the time (control (A, B, C, D, E); ubiquinol (a, b, c, d, e)) ($p < 0.05$).

Table 2. Effects of exercise and ubiquinol supplementation on hematological parameters. Results are expressed as mean ± SEM. * means statistically significant differences between groups ($p < 0.05$). T1: Before supplementation (basal value); T2: After supplementation (two weeks) and before the first physical test; T3: After first physical exercise test; T4: After 24 h of rest and before the second physical test; T5: After second physical exercise test. Different letters in every group indicates significant differences due to the time (control (A, B, C, D, E); ubiquinol (a, b, c, d, e)) ($p < 0.05$).

		T1	T2	T3	T4	T5
Leukocytes ($10^3/\mu L$)						
	Control	5.9 ± 0.2 [A]	5.9 ± 0.2 [A]	6.2 ± 0.2 [A]	5.9 ± 0.2 [A]	6.2 ± 0.2 [A]
	Ubiquinol	5.8 ± 0.2 [a,c]	6.1 ± 0.2 [a,b,c]	6.8 ± 0.3 [b]	5.9 ± 0.2 [c]	6.4 ± 0.3 [a,b,c]
Neutrophils (%)						
	Control	52.0 ± 1.1 [A,C]	52.0 ± 1.1 [A,C]	57.1 ± 1.3 [B]	52.0 ± 1.1 [C]	56.0 ± 1.1 [B]
	Ubiquinol	59.9 ± 1.1 [a]	54.2 ± 1.0 [b]	57.9 ± 1.0 [c]	56.5 ± 1.5 [b,c,d,*]	60.1 ± 1.5 [d]
Lymphocytes (%)						
	Control	34.7 ± 1.1 [A,B,C,D]	35.4 ± 0.9 [A,C,D]	32.1 ± 1.3 [B,D]	36.8 ± 1.0 [C]	32.8 ± 1.3 [D]
	Ubiquinol	36.2 ± 1.1 [a]	34.5 ± 1.1 [a,b]	32.3 ± 1.0 [b,c]	33.6 ± 1.3 [a,b,c,*]	30.6 ± 1.3 [c]
Monocytes (%)						
	Control	8.1 ± 0.3 [A]	7.1 ± 0.3 [B]	6.6 ± 0.3 [B]	7.4 ± 0.3 [A,B]	6.7 ± 0.3 [B]
	Ubiquinol	8.5 ± 0.3 [a]	7.0 ± 0.3 [b]	6.5 ± 0.3 [b]	6.6 ± 0.3 [b,*]	6.4 ± 0.3 [b]
Eosinophils (%)						
	Control	4.8 ± 0.5 [A]	4.5 ± 0.6 [A,B]	3.5 ± 0.5 [B]	4.1 ± 0.5 [A,B]	3.8 ± 0.5 [A,B]
	Ubiquinol	4.1 ± 0.4 [a,c]	3.6 ± 0.3 [a,c]	2.7 ± 0.3 [b]	3.5 ± 0.3 [c]	3.2 ± 0.3 [a,b,c]
Basophils (%)						
	Control	0.4 ± 0.04 [A,C]	0.6 ± 0.05 [B,C,D]	0.7 ± 0.04 [C,D]	0.5 ± 0.04 [A,B]	0.7 ± 0.07 [D]
	Ubiquinol	0.4 ± 0.03 [a]	0.7 ± 0.05 [b]	0.6 ± 0.04 [b]	0.5 ± 0.04 [c]	0.6 ± 0.06 [b,c]
Platelets ($10^3/\mu L$)						
	Control	240.0 ± 6.3 [A]	232.9 ± 6.1 [A]	248.9 ± 7.9 [A]	231.9 ± 6.6 [A]	251.6 ± 12.6 [A]
	Ubiquinol	239.9 ± 5.8 [a]	239.8 ± 7.0 [a]	250.3 ± 6.2 [a]	244.7 ± 6.6 [a]	244.1 ± 5.6 [a]
MCV (fL)						
	Control	90.4 ± 0.5 [A]	90.5 ± 0.6 [A]	90.5 ± 0.6 [A]	90.8 ± 0.7 [A]	90.5 ± 0.7 [A]
	Ubiquinol	90.4 ± 0.7 [a]	90.5 ± 0.7 [a]	90.7 ± 0.7 [a]	90.4 ± 0.8 [a]	90.8 ± 0.8 [a]
MCH (pg)						
	Control	31.9 ± 0.3 [A]	32.0 ± 0.3 [A]	32.3 ± 0.3 [A]	32.3 ± 0.3 [A]	32.3 ± 0.3 [A]
	Ubiquinol	32.0 ± 0.3 [a]	32.1 ± 0.3 [a]	32.3 ± 0.3 [a]	32.3 ± 0.3 [a]	32.7 ± 0.3 [a]
MCHC (g/dL)						
	Control	35.3 ± 0.1 [A]	35.4 ± 0.1 [A,B]	35.6 ± 0.1 [B]	35.6 ± 0.1 [B]	35.6 ± 0.1 [B]
	Ubiquinol	35.4 ± 0.1 [a]	35.4 ± 0.1 [a]	35.6 ± 0.1 [a,b]	35.7 ± 0.1 [b]	36.0 ± 0.1 [c,*]
RDW (%)						
	Control	13.2 ± 0.1 [A]	13.1 ± 0.1 [A]	13.1 ± 0.1 [A]	13.2 ± 0.1 [A]	13.2 ± 0.1 [A]
	Ubiquinol	13.3 ± 0.1 [a]	13.2 ± 0.1 [a,b]	13.0 ± 0.1 [b]	13.2 ± 0.1 [a,b]	13.1 ± 0.1 [a,b]
MPV (fL)						
	Control	8.6 ± 0.1 [A]	8.8 ± 0.1 [A]	8.7 ± 0.1 [A]	8.7 ± 0.1 [A]	8.7 ± 0.1 [A]
	Ubiquinol	8.4 ± 0.1 [a]	8.6 ± 0.2 [a]	8.4 ± 0.1 [a]	8.5 ± 0.1 [a]	8.5 ± 0.1 [a]

MCV: Mean corpuscular volume; MCH: Mean corpuscular hemoglobin; MCHC: Mean corpuscular hemoglobin concentration; RDW: Red cell distribution width; MPV: Mean platelet volume.

4. Discussion

Regular physical exercise is associated with numerous health benefits including a lower risk of all-cause mortality [37,38], nevertheless, strenuous exercise specially in amateur athletes, promotes the generation of oxidative stress and a pro-inflammatory state, which are one of the main reasons for the muscular aggression observed in high intensity exercise, together with other physiological alterations such as sports anemia [12], characterized by hematological changes including decrease in RBC, hemoglobin, and hematocrit [12,13,15]. These changes reduce oxygen supply and energy production which could regulate the aerobic performance capacity [17], which could lead to a reduction in the physical performance, incorrect adaptation to training protocols, and other possible physiological alterations [12]. Taking into account the importance of inflammation in most of these alterations, supplementation with effective molecules against these alterations could be beneficial. CoQ10 could be suitable for a muscle-protective supplementation because it has anti-inflammatory and antioxidant activity and it is intimately involved in energy production [39,40]. However, scarce studies of CoQ10 supplementation investigating its effects during strenuous physical exercise are available in the scientific literature, especially in the field of the inflammatory signaling and hematological parameters and virtually nonexistent when referring to supplementation with the reduced form of this molecule (ubiquinol) [29,39]. Both groups studied were homogeneous in terms of weight, height, blood pressure, and age. In addition, as commented above, we have previously reported that both groups showed similar physical nutritional status and characteristics, and that our protocol of exercise features a high intensity and induced muscle damage [32].

During intense exercise, muscles are damaged and reconstitution of muscle fibers is imperative for full muscular recovery and prevention of muscle atrophy, being pivotal factors in this process the inflammatory signaling and an adequate RBC mass and blood supply. The inflammatory response during high intensity exercise initiates a rapid and sequential invasion of muscle fibers, mediating the repairing process during recovery from strenuous exercise. Thus, the inflammatory response induced by muscle damage may be a functionally response to favor muscle regeneration [41].

In response to exercise, skeletal muscle releases pro-inflammatory cytokines exponentially according to the exercise intensity, duration, mass of muscle recruited, and endurance capacity [42]. Acute bouts of exercise cause transient damage to contracting skeletal muscles, triggering an inflammatory response that increases the levels of pro-inflammatory cytokines and acute-phase reactants in the blood [43], such as IL-6 and TNF-α which are pro-inflammatory cytokines primarily secreted by stimulated immune cells (e.g., monocytes and macrophages) [44], nevertheless, although IL-6 and TNF-α are pro-inflammatory agents, they can stimulate the production of an anti-inflammatory cytokine such as IL-10 [45]. In the ubiquinol group, the increase in IL-6 is not preceded by an increase in tumor necrosis factor alpha (TNF-α) and, most importantly, is followed by increased levels of anti-inflammatory cytokines, namely IL-1 receptor antagonist (IL-1ra) and IL-10 [45,46], together with a decrease in IL-8, as well as lower expression of Il-1, IL-15, and MCP-1. In turn, IL-10 inhibits the synthesis of some pro-inflammatory cytokines such as TNF-α [47], a fact that can be observed especially after the second physical test. TNF-α seems to have a biphasic effect on muscle: High levels of the cytokine promote muscle catabolism, probably by a nuclear factor kB (NF-kB) mediated effect, whereas low levels of TNF-α such as those recorded in the ubiquinol group do not induce NF-kB and stimulate myogenesis [48].

During strenuous exercise, there is a reduction in RBC, which could imply a decrease in the oxygen supply to the cells. On the other hand, previous investigations have reported that lower cardiorespiratory fitness, assessed by maximal oxygen consumption (VO$_2$max kg^{-1}), is associated with higher basal IL-8 and MCP-1 concentrations [49,50]. High VO$_2$max kg^{-1} is correlated with low IL-8 levels [51], suggesting that low IL-8 levels is an important inflammatory parameter that predicts the level of cardiorespiratory fitness. In the current study, ubiquinol also reduced MCP-1 (key chemokine that regulates migration and infiltration of monocytes/macrophages in response to inflammation) and IL-8. Interestingly, at physiological concentration, MCP-1 is the only adipocytokine able to impair insulin signaling and glucose uptake in skeletal muscle and in this sense, a decrease in this biomarker during physical exercise facilitates insulin-mediated glucose disposal [52]. Therefore, we can assume that rather than pro-inflammatory, the acute exercise-induced increase in pro-inflammatory cytokines such as IL-6, in the ubiquinol group, may actually lead to an anti-inflammatory environment [53] and also an improvement in physical performance due to a higher cardiorespiratory fitness and glucose consumption.

Regarding the hematological changes associated with strenuous exercise, it is asserted that exercise performed until exhaustion decreases the number of leukocytes, a fact that can be associated with metabolic changes such as ischemia that occur during exercise and increased muscle activity leads to a greater incidence of capillary swelling and leukocyte adherence to venules [54]. However, as explained below, ubiquinol features a vasodilator activity and pro-angiogenic effect which avoids capillary swelling and leukocyte adherence to blood vessels, reducing impairment of immune functions related to strenuous exercise [55], avoiding this reduction in the leukocytes. Moreover, as mentioned above, ubiquinol reduced MCP-1 that plays an important role in selectively recruiting monocytes and lymphocytes [56], the reason why we recorded a decrease of these white cells after 24 h of the first physical test.

As previously mentioned, in elite athletes, a decrease in the percentages of RBC, hemoglobin and hematocrit is recorded and, in this situation, inflammation is one of the main causes. Even if there is only a small decrease in RBC, it is important to highlight that during strenuous exercise a greater demand for oxygen is necessary and therefore even a small decrease in RBC could affect the performance. Thus, an adequate RBC mass and blood supply is imperative for full muscular recovery, energy requirements, and prevention of muscle atrophy [25]. In this regard, there are three aspects that have to be taken into account: The vasodilation, the angiogenesis or generation of new blood vessels, and the RBC mass circulating, physiological pathways that are closely related to increase blood supply. In the current study, ubiquinol prevented the decrease in RBC, hemoglobin, and hematocrit after the first physical test, a fact that would increase oxygen delivering to tissues, especially muscles. During exercise, oxidative stress induces deleterious structural and functional changes in RBC, however, ubiquinol prevents those changes in erythrocytes, due to its antioxidant properties [29], avoiding the impairment in hematological changes such as decreases in Hb and RBC caused by strenuous exercise [11]. In addition, ubiquinol supplementation also increases NO output [32], a fact that is beneficial during physical activity, featuring a vasodilator action that helps both exercise performance and nutrient supply in muscle recovery, as well as improvement in the supply of substrates such as glucose, together facilitate the regulatory role in the immune system [57]. This can be explained by the link between VEGF and nitric oxide (NO). VEGF is a critical cytokine involved in angiogenesis, and NO is a downstream effector. Importantly, recent studies suggest that NO is an essential mediator of endothelial cells migration and VEGF-induced angiogenesis [58]. Angiogenesis is a crucial process for effective regeneration not only by providing stable vessels for supporting the metabolic activity of the regenerated tissue, but also by generating a new population of endothelial and periendothelial cells that will supply a large array of molecules that sustain myogenesis [25]. In this sense, EGF promotes growth and migration of vascular smooth muscle cells through activation of EGF receptor, and VEGF promotes the generation of new blood vessels, essential processes during vascular remodeling and muscular fibers reconstitution [59,60]. In our study, VEGF increased in the ubiquinol group, revealing not only a vasodilator action of ubiquinol due to the NO, but also a pro-angiogenic effect, a fact that would improve nutrient and oxygen supply and muscle recovery after strenuous exercise, supporting and explaining the possible ergogenic effect of ubiquinol during intense exercise. On the other hand, ubiquinol also increased EGF, probably due to its antioxidant activity [61]. VEGF and EGF increase due to the ubiquinol supplementation can be directly linked with the muscle fibers regeneration after intense exercise.

5. Conclusions

In summary, the present study demonstrates a strong correlation between the high intensity exercise and inflammatory signaling as shown by the overexpression in the pro-inflammatory cytokines. In addition, the present findings provide evidence that oral supplementation of ubiquinol during high intensity exercise could modulate the inflammatory signaling associated to exercise by reducing the overexpression of pro-inflammatory cytokines, together with an increase in anti-inflammatory cytokines which limits the detrimental, pro-inflammatory actions of strenuous exercise. In addition, during exercise, RBC, hemoglobin, hematocrit, VEG, NO, and EGF did not decrease in the ubiquinol group, revealing a possible pro-angiogenic effect, a fact that could improve nutrients and oxygen supply and therefore muscle recovery after strenuous exercise. Therefore, the knowledge gained from these findings reveals the benefit of ubiquinol supplement in athletes prior to the performance of strenuous exercise in order to reduce the undesirable effects of the inflammation signaling during high intensity exercise, increasing blood supply, reducing the muscle damage and hematological impairment, and improving skeletal muscle fibers regeneration.

Author Contributions: J.J.O. designed the research proposal and provided funding. J.D.-C. and J.M.-F. conducted the research and wrote the manuscript. I.C., L.J.C., and R.G. revised the data and the manuscript. All persons designated as authors qualify for authorship, and all those who qualify for authorship are listed. All authors have read and agree to the published version of the manuscript.

Funding: This research received no external funding.

Acknowledgments: J.M.-F. was supported by a fellowship from the Ministry of Education, Culture and Sport (Spain), and is grateful to the Excellence PhD Program "Nutrición y Ciencias de los Alimentos" from the University of Granada. We would like to thank the Fire Department of Granada for their participation in the current study. Funding for this work, ubiquinol, and placebo capsules were provided by (Kaneka Corporation, Osaka, Japan). The authors are grateful to Susan Stevenson for her efficient support in the revision of the English language.

Conflicts of Interest: The investigators and the University of Granada have no direct or indirect interest in the tested product (Kaneka QH) or in Kaneka Corporation and therefore the authors declare no conflict of interest.

References

1. Powers, S.K.; Jackson, M.J. Exercise-Induced Oxidative Stress: Cellular Mechanisms and Impact on Muscle Force Production. *Physiol. Rev.* **2008**, *88*, 1243–1276. [CrossRef] [PubMed]
2. Matheson, G.O.; Klugl, M.; Dvorak, J.; Engebretsen, L.; Meeuwisse, W.H.; Schwellnus, M.; Blair, S.N.; van Mechelen, W.; Derman, W.; Borjesson, M.; et al. Responsibility of sport and exercise medicine in preventing and managing chronic disease: Applying our knowledge and skill is overdue. *Br. J. Sports Med.* **2011**, *45*, 1272–1282. [CrossRef] [PubMed]
3. Gillon, A.; Nielsen, K.; Steel, C.; Cornwall, J.; Sheard, P. Exercise attenuates age-associated changes in motoneuron number, nucleocytoplasmic transport proteins and neuromuscular health. *GeroScience* **2018**, *40*, 177–192. [CrossRef] [PubMed]
4. LaRoche, D.P.; Melanson, E.L.; Baumgartner, M.P.; Bozzuto, B.M.; Libby, V.M.; Marshall, B.N. Physiological determinants of walking effort in older adults: Should they be targets for physical activity intervention? *GeroScience* **2018**, *40*, 305–315. [CrossRef]
5. Norling, A.M.; Gerstenecker, A.T.; Buford, T.W.; Khan, B.; Oparil, S.; Lazar, R.M. The role of exercise in the reversal of IGF-1 deficiencies in microvascular rarefaction and hypertension. *GeroScience* **2019**. [CrossRef] [PubMed]
6. Abbasi, A.; Hauth, M.; Walter, M.; Hudemann, J.; Wank, V.; Niess, A.M.; Northoff, H. Exhaustive exercise modifies different gene expression profiles and pathways in LPS-stimulated and un-stimulated whole blood cultures. *Brain Behav. Immun.* **2014**, *39*, 130–141. [CrossRef] [PubMed]
7. Piercy, K.L.; Troiano, R.P.; Ballard, R.M.; Carlson, S.A.; Fulton, J.E.; Galuska, D.A.; George, S.M.; Olson, R.D. The Physical Activity Guidelines for Americans. *JAMA* **2018**, *320*, 2020–2028. [CrossRef]
8. Roitt, I.; Delves, P. *Roitts Immunology*, 12th ed.; Blackwell Science: London, UK, 2013.

9. Suzuki, K.; Yamada, M.; Kurakake, S.; Okamura, N.; Yamaya, K.; Liu, Q.; Kudoh, S.; Kowatari, K.; Nakaji, S.; Sugawara, K. Circulating cytokines and hormones with immunosuppressive but neutrophil-priming potentials rise after endurance exercise in humans. *Eur. J. Appl. Physiol.* **2000**, *81*, 281–287. [CrossRef]
10. Simon, H.B. Exercise and Health: Dose and Response, Considering Both Ends of the Curve. *Am. J. Med.* **2015**, *128*, 1171–1177. [CrossRef]
11. El-Sayed, M.S. Effects of exercise on blood coagulation, fibrinolysis and platelet aggregation. *Sports Med. Auckl. N. Z.* **1996**, *22*, 282–298. [CrossRef]
12. Kong, W.N.; Gao, G.; Chang, Y.Z. Hepcidin and sports anemia. *Cell Biosci.* **2014**, *4*, 19. [CrossRef] [PubMed]
13. Dominguez, R.; Sanchez-Oliver, A.J.; Mata-Ordonez, F.; Feria-Madueno, A.; Grimaldi-Puyana, M.; Lopez-Samanes, A.; Perez-Lopez, A. Effects of an Acute Exercise Bout on Serum Hepcidin Levels. *Nutrients* **2018**, *10*, 209. [CrossRef]
14. Chang, C.W.; Chen, Y.M.; Hsu, Y.J.; Huang, C.C.; Wu, Y.T.; Hsu, M.C. Protective effects of the roots of Angelica sinensis on strenuous exercise-induced sports anemia in rats. *J. Ethnopharmacol.* **2016**, *193*, 169–178. [CrossRef] [PubMed]
15. Tang, Y.; Qi, R.; Wu, H.; Shi, W.; Xu, Y.; Li, M. Reduction of hemoglobin, not iron, inhibited maturation of red blood cells in male rats exposed to high intensity endurance exercises. *J. Trace Elem. Med. Biol. Organ Soc. Miner. Trace Elem. GMS* **2019**, *52*, 263–269. [CrossRef] [PubMed]
16. Beard, J.; Tobin, B. Iron status and exercise. *Am. J. Clin. Nutr.* **2000**, *72*, 594–597. [CrossRef] [PubMed]
17. Saris, W.H.; Senden, J.M.; Brouns, F. What is a normal red-blood cell mass for professional cyclists? *Lancet Lond. Engl.* **1998**, *352*, 1758. [CrossRef]
18. Peeling, P.; Dawson, B.; Goodman, C.; Landers, G.; Wiegerinck, E.T.; Swinkels, D.W.; Trinder, D. Training surface and intensity: Inflammation, hemolysis, and hepcidin expression. *Med. Sci. Sports Exerc.* **2009**, *41*, 1138–1145. [CrossRef]
19. Oh, J.; Sinha, I.; Tan, K.Y.; Rosner, B.; Dreyfuss, J.M.; Gjata, O.; Tran, P.; Shoelson, S.E.; Wagers, A.J. Age-associated NF-kappaB signaling in myofibers alters the satellite cell niche and re-strains muscle stem cell function. *Aging* **2016**, *8*, 2871–2896. [CrossRef]
20. Grivennikov, S.I.; Greten, F.R.; Karin, M. Immunity, inflammation, and cancer. *Cell* **2010**, *140*, 883–899. [CrossRef]
21. Swiderski, K.; Thakur, S.S.; Naim, T.; Trieu, J.; Chee, A.; Stapleton, D.I.; Koopman, R.; Lynch, G.S. Muscle-specific deletion of SOCS3 increases the early inflammatory response but does not affect regeneration after myotoxic injury. *Skelet. Muscle* **2016**, *6*, 36. [CrossRef]
22. Buford, T.W.; Carter, C.S.; VanDerPol, W.J.; Chen, D.; Lefkowitz, E.J.; Eipers, P.; Morrow, C.D.; Bamman, M.M. Composition and richness of the serum microbiome differ by age and link to systemic inflammation. *GeroScience* **2018**, *40*, 257–268. [CrossRef] [PubMed]
23. Shaw, D.M.; Merien, F.; Braakhuis, A.; Dulson, D. T-cells and their cytokine production: The anti-inflammatory and immunosuppressive effects of strenuous exercise. *Cytokine* **2018**, *104*, 136–142. [CrossRef] [PubMed]
24. Fan, L.; Feng, Y.; Chen, G.C.; Qin, L.Q.; Fu, C.L.; Chen, L.H. Effects of coenzyme Q10 supplementation on inflammatory markers: A systematic review and meta-analysis of randomized controlled trials. *Pharmacol. Res.* **2017**, *119*, 128–136. [CrossRef] [PubMed]
25. Abou-Khalil, R.; Mounier, R.; Chazaud, B. Regulation of myogenic stem cell behavior by vessel cells: The "menage a trois" of satellite cells, periendothelial cells and endothelial cells. *Cell Cycle (Georget. Tex.)* **2010**, *9*, 892–896. [CrossRef] [PubMed]
26. Jensen, L.; Pilegaard, H.; Neufer, P.D.; Hellsten, Y. Effect of acute exercise and exercise training on VEGF splice variants in human skeletal muscle. *Am. J. Physiol. Regul. Integr. Comp. Physiol.* **2004**, *287*, 397–402. [CrossRef]
27. Vina, J.; Gomez-Cabrera, M.C.; Lloret, A.; Marquez, R.; Minana, J.B.; Pallardo, F.V.; Sastre, J. Free radicals in exhaustive physical exercise: Mechanism of production, and protection by antioxidants. *IUBMB Life* **2000**, *50*, 271–277. [CrossRef]
28. Slattery, K.; Bentley, D.; Coutts, A.J. The role of oxidative, inflammatory and neuroendocrinological systems during exercise stress in athletes: Implications of antioxidant supplementation on physiological adaptation during intensified physical training. *Sports Med. (Auckl. N. Z.)* **2015**, *45*, 453–471. [CrossRef]

29. Sarmiento, A.; Diaz-Castro, J.; Pulido-Moran, M.; Kajarabille, N.; Guisado, R.; Ochoa, J.J. Coenzyme Q10 Supplementation and Exercise in Healthy Humans: A Systematic Review. *Curr. Drug Metab.* **2016**, *17*, 345–358. [CrossRef]
30. Cooke, M.; Iosia, M.; Buford, T.; Shelmadine, B.; Hudson, G.; Kerksick, C.; Rasmussen, C.; Greenwood, M.; Leutholtz, B.; Willoughby, D.; et al. Effects of acute and 14-day coenzyme Q10 supplementation on exercise performance in both trained and untrained individuals. *J. Int. Soc. Sports Nutr.* **2008**, *5*, 8. [CrossRef]
31. Littarru, G.P.; Tiano, L. Bioenergetic and antioxidant properties of coenzyme Q10: Recent developments. *Mol. Biotechnol.* **2007**, *37*, 31–37. [CrossRef]
32. Sarmiento, A.; Diaz-Castro, J.; Pulido-Moran, M.; Moreno-Fernandez, J.; Kajarabille, N.; Chirosa, I.; Guisado, I.M.; Javier Chirosa, L.; Guisado, R.; Ochoa, J.J. Short-term ubiquinol supplementation reduces oxidative stress associated with strenuous exercise in healthy adults: A randomized trial. *BioFactors (Oxf. Engl.)* **2016**, *42*, 612–622. [CrossRef] [PubMed]
33. Papathanasiou, G.; Georgoudis, G.; Georgakopoulos, D.; Katsouras, C.; Kalfakakou, V.; Evangelou, A. Criterion-related validity of the short International Physical Activity Questionnaire against exercise capacity in young adults. *Eur. J. Cardiovasc. Prev. Rehabil. Off. J. Eur. Soc. Cardiol. Work. Groups Epidemiol. Prev. Card. Rehabil. Exerc. Physiol.* **2010**, *17*, 380–386. [CrossRef] [PubMed]
34. Aboodarda, S.J.; George, J.; Mokhtar, A.H.; Thompson, M. Muscle Strength and Damage Following Two Modes of Variable Resistance Training. *J. Sports Sci. Med.* **2011**, *10*, 635–642. [PubMed]
35. Aniceto, R.R.; Ritti-Dias, R.M.; Dos Prazeres, T.M.; Farah, B.Q.; de Lima, F.F.; do Prado, W.L. Rating of Perceived Exertion During Circuit Weight Training: A Concurrent Validation Study. *J. Strength Cond. Res.* **2015**, *29*, 3336–3342. [CrossRef]
36. Robertson, R.J.; Goss, F.L.; Rutkowski, J.; Lenz, B.; Dixon, C.; Timmer, J.; Frazee, K.; Dube, J.; Andreacci, J. Concurrent validation of the OMNI perceived exertion scale for resistance exercise. *Med. Sci. Sports Exerc.* **2003**, *35*, 333–341. [CrossRef]
37. Kraus, W.E.; Slentz, C.A. Exercise training, lipid regulation, and insulin action: A tangled web of cause and effect. *Obesity* **2009**, *17*, 21–26. [CrossRef]
38. Warburton, D.E.; Bredin, S.S. Reflections on Physical Activity and Health: What Should We Recommend? *Can. J. Cardiol.* **2016**, *32*, 495–504. [CrossRef]
39. Littarru, G.P.; Tiano, L. Clinical aspects of coenzyme Q10: An update. *Curr. Opin. Clin. Nutr. Metab. Care* **2005**, *8*, 641–646. [CrossRef]
40. Saha, S.P.; Whayne, T.F., Jr. Coenzyme Q-10 in Human Health: Supporting Evidence? *South. Med. J.* **2016**, *109*, 17–21. [CrossRef]
41. Tidball, J.G. Inflammatory processes in muscle injury and repair. *Am. J. Physiol. Regul. Integr. Comp. Physiol.* **2005**, *288*, 345–353. [CrossRef]
42. Ostrowski, K.; Schjerling, P.; Pedersen, B.K. Physical activity and plasma interleukin-6 in humans–effect of intensity of exercise. *Eur. J. Appl. Physiol.* **2000**, *83*, 512–515. [CrossRef] [PubMed]
43. Zaldivar, F.; Wang-Rodriguez, J.; Nemet, D.; Schwindt, C.; Galassetti, P.; Mills, P.J.; Wilson, L.D.; Cooper, D.M. Constitutive pro- and anti-inflammatory cytokine and growth factor response to exercise in leukocytes. *J. Appl. Physiol. (Bethesda Md. 1985)* **2006**, *100*, 1124–1133. [CrossRef] [PubMed]
44. Akira, S.; Taga, T.; Kishimoto, T. Interleukin-6 in biology and medicine. *Adv. Immunol.* **1993**, *54*, 1–78. [PubMed]
45. Stoner, L.; Lucero, A.A.; Palmer, B.R.; Jones, L.M.; Young, J.M.; Faulkner, J. Inflammatory biomarkers for predicting cardiovascular disease. *Clin. Biochem.* **2013**, *46*, 1353–1371. [CrossRef] [PubMed]
46. Steensberg, A.; Fischer, C.P.; Keller, C.; Moller, K.; Pedersen, B.K. IL-6 enhances plasma IL-1ra, IL-10, and cortisol in humans. *Am. J. Physiol. Endocrinol. Metab.* **2003**, *285*, E433–E437. [CrossRef] [PubMed]
47. Nielsen, A.R.; Mounier, R.; Plomgaard, P.; Mortensen, O.H.; Penkowa, M.; Speerschneider, T.; Pilegaard, H.; Pedersen, B.K. Expression of interleukin-15 in human skeletal muscle effect of exercise and muscle fibre type composition. *J. Physiol.* **2007**, *584*, 305–312. [CrossRef]
48. Diaz-Castro, J.; Guisado, R.; Kajarabille, N.; Garcia, C.; Guisado, I.M.; de Teresa, C.; Ochoa, J.J. Coenzyme Q(10) supplementation ameliorates inflammatory signaling and oxidative stress associated with strenuous exercise. *Eur. J. Nutr.* **2012**, *51*, 791–799. [CrossRef]
49. Kullo, I.J.; Khaleghi, M.; Hensrud, D.D. Markers of inflammation are inversely associated with VO2 max in asymptomatic men. *J. Appl. Physiol. (Bethesda Md. 1985)* **2007**, *102*, 1374–1379. [CrossRef]

50. Utsal, L.; Tillmann, V.; Zilmer, M.; Maestu, J.; Purge, P.; Saar, M.; Latt, E.; Maasalu, K.; Jurimae, T.; Jurimae, J. Negative correlation between serum IL-6 level and cardiorespiratory fitness in 10- to 11-year-old boys with increased BMI. *J. Pediatric Endocrinol. Metab.* **2013**, *26*, 503–508. [CrossRef]
51. Jurimae, J.; Tillmann, V.; Purge, P.; Jurimae, T. Body composition, maximal aerobic performance and inflammatory biomarkers in endurance-trained athletes. *Clin. Physiol. Funct. Imaging* **2015**. [CrossRef]
52. Accattato, F.; Greco, M.; Pullano, S.A.; Care, I.; Fiorillo, A.S.; Pujia, A.; Montalcini, T.; Foti, D.P.; Brunetti, A.; Gulletta, E. Effects of acute physical exercise on oxidative stress and inflammatory status in young, sedentary obese subjects. *PLoS ONE* **2017**, *12*, e0178900. [CrossRef] [PubMed]
53. Benatti, F.B.; Pedersen, B.K. Exercise as an anti-inflammatory therapy for rheumatic diseases-myokine regulation. *Nat. Rev. Rheumatol.* **2015**, *11*, 86–97. [CrossRef] [PubMed]
54. Haas, T.L.; Lloyd, P.G.; Yang, H.T.; Terjung, R.L. Exercise training and peripheral arterial disease. *Compr. Physiol.* **2012**, *2*, 2933–3017. [CrossRef] [PubMed]
55. Tossige-Gomes, R.; Ottone, V.O.; Oliveira, P.N.; Viana, D.J.S.; Araújo, T.L.; Gripp, F.J.; Rocha-Vieira, E. Leukocytosis, muscle damage and increased lymphocyte proliferative response after an adventure sprint race. *Braz. J. Med. Biol. Res.* **2014**, *47*, 492–498. [CrossRef]
56. Deshmane, S.L.; Kremlev, S.; Amini, S.; Sawaya, B.E. Monocyte chemoattractant protein-1 (MCP-1): An overview. *J. Interferon Cytokine Res. Off. J. Int. Soc. Interferon Cytokine Res.* **2009**, *29*, 313–326. [CrossRef]
57. Belardinelli, R.; Mucaj, A.; Lacalaprice, F.; Solenghi, M.; Seddaiu, G.; Principi, F.; Tiano, L.; Littarru, G.P. Coenzyme Q10 and exercise training in chronic heart failure. *Eur. Heart J.* **2006**, *27*, 2675–2681. [CrossRef]
58. Chavakis, E.; Dernbach, E.; Hermann, C.; Mondorf, U.F.; Zeiher, A.M.; Dimmeler, S. Oxidized LDL inhibits vascular endothelial growth factor-induced endothelial cell migration by an inhibitory effect on the Akt/endothelial nitric oxide synthase pathway. *Circulation* **2001**, *103*, 2102–2107. [CrossRef]
59. Shin, H.S.; Lee, H.J.; Nishida, M.; Lee, M.S.; Tamura, R.; Yamashita, S.; Matsuzawa, Y.; Lee, I.K.; Koh, G.Y. Betacellulin and amphiregulin induce upregulation of cyclin D1 and DNA synthesis activity through differential signaling pathways in vascular smooth muscle cells. *Circ. Res.* **2003**, *93*, 302–310. [CrossRef]
60. Mifune, M.; Ohtsu, H.; Suzuki, H.; Frank, G.D.; Inagami, T.; Utsunomiya, H.; Dempsey, P.J.; Eguchi, S. Signal transduction of betacellulin in growth and migration of vascular smooth muscle cells. *Am. J. Physiol. Cell Physiol.* **2004**, *287*, C807–C813. [CrossRef]
61. Ojalvo, A.G.; Acosta, J.B.; Mari, Y.M.; Mayola, M.F.; Perez, C.V.; Gutierrez, W.S.; Marichal, I.I.; Seijas, E.A.; Kautzman, A.M.; Pacheco, A.E.; et al. Healing enhancement of diabetic wounds by locally infiltrated epidermal growth factor is associated with systemic oxidative stress reduction. *Int. Wound J.* **2017**, *14*, 214–225. [CrossRef]

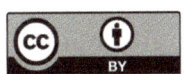

© 2020 by the authors. Licensee MDPI, Basel, Switzerland. This article is an open access article distributed under the terms and conditions of the Creative Commons Attribution (CC BY) license (http://creativecommons.org/licenses/by/4.0/).

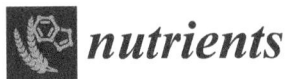

Article

Iron Status of Infants in the First Year of Life in Northern Taiwan

Chiao-Ming Chen [1,†], Shu-Ci Mu [2,3,†], Chun-Kuang Shih [4], Yi-Ling Chen [3,5], Li-Yi Tsai [3,6], Yung-Ting Kuo [7,8], In-Mei Cheong [1], Mei-Ling Chang [1], Yi-Chun Chen [4] and Sing-Chung Li [4,*]

[1] Department of Food Science, Nutrition, and Nutraceutical Biotechnology, Shih Chien University, Taipei 10462, Taiwan; charming@g2.usc.edu.tw (C.-M.C.); mei11792004@gmail.com (I.-M.C.); mlchang@g2.usc.edu.tw (M.-L.C.)
[2] School of Medicine, Fu-Jen Catholic University, New Taipei City 24205, Taiwan; musc1006@gmail.com
[3] Department of Pediatrics, Shin-Kong Wu Ho-Su Memorial Hospital, Taipei 11101, Taiwan; Ylchen1219@gmail.com (Y.-L.C.); Ly.tsai95@gmail.com (L.-Y.T.)
[4] School of Nutrition and Health Sciences, College of Nutrition, Taipei Medical University, 250 Wu-Hsing Street, Taipei 11031, Taiwan; ckshih@tmu.edu.tw (C.-K.S.); yichun@tmu.edu.tw (Y.-C.C.)
[5] School of Medicine, Taipei Medical University, Taipei 11031, Taiwan
[6] Institute of Environmental and Occupational Health Sciences, College of Public Health, National Taiwan University, Taipei 10617, Taiwan
[7] Department of Pediatrics, Shuang Ho Hospital, Ministry of Health and Welfare, Taipei Medical University, New Taipei 23561, Taiwan; pedkuoyt@tmu.edu.tw
[8] Department of Pediatrics, School of Medicine, College of Medicine, Taipei Medical University, Taipei 11031, Taiwan
* Correspondence: sinchung@tmu.edu.tw; Tel.: +886-2-27361661 (ext. 6560)
† These authors contributed equally to this work.

Received: 3 December 2019; Accepted: 31 December 2019; Published: 3 January 2020

Abstract: Iron deficiency (ID) and iron deficiency anemia (IDA) typically occur in developing countries. Notably, ID and IDA can affect an infant's emotion, cognition, and development. Breast milk is considered the best food for infants. However, recent studies have indicated that breastfeeding for more than six months increases the risk of ID. This study investigated the prevalence of ID and IDA, as well as the association between feeding type and iron nutritional status in northern Taiwan. A cross-sectional study was conducted on infants who returned to the well-baby clinic for routine examination from October 2012 to January 2014. Overall, 509 infants aged 1–12 months completed the iron nutritional status analysis, anthropometric measurement, and dietary intake assessment, including milk and complementary foods. The results revealed that 49 (10%) and 21 (4%) infants in their first year of life had ID and IDA, respectively, based on the World Health Organization criteria. Breastfed infants had a higher prevalence rate of ID and IDA than mixed-fed and formula-fed infants ($p < 0.001$). Regarding biomarkers of iron status, plasma hemoglobin (Hb), ferritin, and transferrin saturation (%) levels were significantly lower in ID and IDA groups. The prevalence of ID and IDA were 3.7% and 2.7%, respectively, in infants under six months of age, but increased to 20.4% and 6.6%, respectively, in infants above six months of age. The healthy group had a higher total iron intake than ID and IDA groups, mainly derived from infant formula. The total dietary iron intake was positively correlated with infants' Hb levels. Compared with formula-fed infants, the logistic regression revealed that the odds ratio for ID was 2.157 (95% confidence interval [CI]: 1.369–3.399) and that for IDA was 4.196 (95% CI: 1.780–9.887) among breastfed infants ($p < 0.001$) after adjusted for all confounding factors (including gestational week, birthweight, sex, body weight percentile, body length percentile, age of infants, mothers' BMI, gestational weight gain, education level, and hemoglobin level before delivery). In conclusion, our results determined that breastfeeding was associated with an increased the prevalence of ID and/or IDA, especially in infants above six months. This suggests that mothers who prolonged breastfeed after six months could provide high-quality iron-rich foods to reduce the prevalence of ID and IDA.

Keywords: infant; breast milk; formula milk; iron deficiency; iron deficiency anemia

1. Introduction

Breast milk is considered the optimal nutrition and healthy food for the first six months of life, and breastfeeding is typically complemented with other foods from six months of age until at least 12 months for nearly all infants [1]. A reappraisal of the evidence from a recent expert review for the European Food Safety Authority (EFSA) concluded that for infants across the EU, complementary foods might be introduced safely between the fourth and sixth month [2]. Studies have determined that the iron content in breast milk is low, infants fed with solid food before six months or received iron supplement will decrease the risk of IDA [3]. Anemia is defined as a reduced erythrocyte count or hemoglobin (Hb) value of 5 percentile below the normal hemoglobin value specified for that age in healthy individuals [4]. Therefore, the US Department of Agriculture and the Centers for Disease Control recommend the introduction of complementary food in infants aged between 4 and 6 months [5].

In addition to inadequate iron intake, reduced bioavailability of dietary iron, increased iron requirements, and chronic blood loss is common causes of iron deficiency (ID). ID is currently the most common micronutrient deficiencies worldwide, and a World Health Organization (WHO) survey in 2008 revealed that globally, approximately 293 million (47.4% prevalence) preschool-age children and approximately 56 million (41.8% prevalence) pregnant women suffer from anemia, among which approximately 50% cases are attributable to ID [6]. ID is undoubtedly the major cause of most anemia cases, although other minerals or vitamins can also be responsible for this pathology. Prolonged ID often leads to iron deficiency anemia (IDA) [7]. The American Academy of Pediatrics determined that IDA adversely affects an infant's social and emotional behavior development and cognitive performance [8]. Approximately 25% of infants in developing countries have IDA, and IDA during pregnancy increases the risk of preterm delivery and adverse perinatal outcomes, such as maternal hemorrhage, sepsis, low birth weight, and possibly poor neonatal health [9–11].

Recent studies have indicated that iron content in breast milk is low [12–14], and prolonged use of breast milk as the main food in infants might increase the risk of ID and IDA [15]. In Taiwan, the Ministry of Health and Welfare promotes the benefits of breastfeeding for a long period. Although Tsai et al. reported that IDA was associated with prolonged, predominant breastfeeding, the study sample size was small, and no relevant risk factors were evaluated [16]. The purpose of the present study was to investigate the iron status of infants in their first year of life and analyze the relevant influencing factors.

2. Participants and Methods

2.1. Study Subjects

A cross-sectional study was conducted in three hospitals, namely, Shin Kong Wu Ho-Su Memorial Hospital, Taipei Medical University Hospital, and Shuang Ho Hospital, from October 2012 to January 2014. Overall, 2804 healthy infants aged 1–12 months who came to the well-baby clinic for routine vaccination were screened for eligibility. The inclusion criteria for infants and mothers enrolled were as follows: No systemic diseases (toxemia, hypertension, diabetes mellitus, and heart disease) during pregnancy, age below one year, healthy and without any disease, as determined by a pediatrician. Infants with premature birth, congenital diseases (such as heart, lung, liver, and intestinal diseases), growth disorders, diagnosis of gastrointestinal disorders (nausea, vomiting, pain, flatulence, diarrhea, and malabsorption), and thalassemia were excluded.

The Ethics Committee of Shin Kong Wu Ho-Su Memorial Hospital and Taipei Medical University approved this study in accordance with the International Ethical Guidelines for Biomedical Research Involving Human Subjects and ethical principles of the Declaration of Helsinki (20120901R and

201308004). Written informed consent was obtained from all participants or legal representatives before the study procedures were performed.

2.2. Basic Characteristics and Dietary Iron Intake Assessment

The contents of the questionnaire were validated by experts, including the infant's basic information, such as gestational weeks, chronological age, birth weight, birth length; anthropometrics, such as body length, body weight, and head circumference; and dietary intake. Gestational weeks, chronological age, birth weight, and birth length were recorded per the medical chart. Body length and body weight were measured using an infantometer and weighing scales. The head circumference was measured by applying a plastic tape around the forehead (above the eyebrows) and the occipital protuberance. These measurements were converted to percentiles according to the growth charts for Taiwanese children released by the Ministry of Health and Welfare. The diet was assessed using a semi-quantitative frequency method, and the included food items were tofu, chicken, pork, beef, fish, egg yolk, viscera, vegetables, rice, wheat, baby rice cereal, baby wheat cereal, formula milk, juice, and puree. Complementary food and formula milk intakes were quantified based on standard bowls, spoons, and feeding bottles. Iron intake from the complementary food was calculated using the Nutritional Chamberlain Line, Nutritionist Edition, version 2002 (E-Kitchen Business Corp, Taiwan). Iron intake from formula milk and baby cereal was calculated according to their nutrient labels. Iron content in breast milk was obtained through actual measurement. Breast milk intake was obtained from mothers' reports. If the mothers were directly breastfeeding their infants, the total volume of breast milk intake was assessed according to the report of Lyu et al. [17]. Pre-pregnancy body weight (kg), gestational weight gain (kg), current weight, and education level were obtained from self-reported data. Current body weight (kg) and height (cm) were measured using an electronic health scale (Tanita corp., Tokyo, Japan). Complete blood count of the mothers, including Hb level, hematocrit (Hct) level, and mean corpuscular volume (MCV) before delivery at 37–40 weeks pregnancy were recorded according to the medical charts.

2.3. Breast Milk and Blood Collection

Breast milk from the mothers' unelated breast was collected using an electric milking machine (Lactina, Medela, Switzerland) for 20 min, which was then mixed, dispensed, and ice-cooled at −80 °C until analysis. Blood samples (4 mL) of infants were collected through an arterial puncture of one arm into vacutainers with and without anticoagulant ethylenediaminetetra-acetic acid (EDTA) by a trained technician. Serum was collected after centrifugation at 1400× g for 10 min at 4 °C and immediately sent to Central Laboratory, Shin-Kong Wu Ho-Su Memorial Hospital, for analysis.

2.4. Biochemical Analyses

Complete blood count was determined using an automatic blood cell analyzer (Biotecnica Instruments SpA, Roma, Italy). Ferritin was detected using a chemiluminescent immunoassay (Roche Diagnostics, Lewes, UK). Serum iron was analyzed using the ferrozine method (Siemens Healthcare, Marburg, Germany). Total iron binding capacity (TIBC) is the ability of transferrin to bind with iron that was measured by chemistry analyzer using dedicated reagents (Siemens Healthcare, Marburg, Germany). Transferrin saturation (TS, %) represents the percentage of transferrin bound to iron ions, calculated by dividing serum iron concentration by TIBC and multiplying the result by 100.

2.5. Breast Milk Iron Content Analysis

Aliquots of 0.5 mL of the mixed breast milk sample was added to 1.5 mL of 70% nitric acid and 0.5 mL of 30% hydrogen peroxide, separately. After mixing and allowing the samples resting for one night, the mixture was digested in a 50 mL polypropylene digestion bottle at 95 °C for 1 h. After cooling at room temperature, the digested sample was diluted using 50 mL of deionized water. Subsequently, 1 mL of the dilution was pipetted into a 15 mL centrifuge tube and diluted with 10 mL of 2% aqueous nitric acid solution to detect the iron content by using inductively coupled plasma mass spectrometry (ICP-MS) (ThermoFisher Scientific, Bremen, Germany) [18]. The iron content in breast milk was calculated using a standard curve constructed using pure iron standards for ICP-MS (Merck, Darmstadt, Germany); with an R value of ≥ 0.99, coefficient of variation (CV) at 2%, and a recovery rate of 80–120%.

2.6. Statistical Analysis

The WHO defines ID as a serum ferritin level less than 15.0 ng/mL and IDA as serum ferritin level less than 15.0 ng/mL and Hb less than 10.5 g/dL. We divided the subjects into three groups according to the WHO definitions: The normal, ID, and IDA groups. All data were confirmed to have a normal distribution by using the Kolmogorov–Smirnov test. Data are presented as means ± standard deviations (SDs), median (interquartile range), or percentage. Intergroup differences were determined using one-way ANOVA, followed by the Scheffé method for post hoc test or nonparametric statistics. Pearson's chi-squared test was used to assess categorical variables. The correlation between Hb and dietary iron intake was determined using the Pearson correlation test. The association between feeding types and anemia was determined using multivariable logistic regression. All data analyses were performed using SPSS (version 19; SPSS Inc., Chicago, IL, USA). Differences were considered significant at $p < 0.05$.

3. Results

3.1. Participant Characteristics and Infant Anemia Diagnosis

A total of 1368 infants were eligible for this study. However, 779 mothers did not provide consent to extract their infants' blood, and therefore, the 589 subjects were ultimately enrolled in this study. However, blood draws were unsuccessful in 39 infants. Thus, a total of 550 cases were included for data analysis. Because no introduction of complementary food to infants over six months of age was considered as abnormal feeding, four infants aged eight months and two aged 12 months were excluded accordingly. In addition, 35 infants with a WBC count of >0.000/mm^3, suspected of infection, were excluded. Data on the iron status analysis of 509 infants are presented in Figure 1.

Anemia was defined according to the WHO criteria, and 49 (10%) and 21 infants (4%) were diagnosed with ID and IDA, respectively, by the physician (Table 1). No statistically significant intergroup differences were noted in terms of sex gestational age, birthweight, body length, body weight, and head circumference of infants. The formula-fed type (52.8%) was the predominant population in the healthy group. The breastfed infants had a significantly higher prevalence of ID (65.3%) and IDA (85.7%) than the mixed-fed and formula-fed infants ($p < 0.001$). No significant intergroup differences were observed in terms of the mother's age, body mass index (BMI), gestational weight gain, and education.

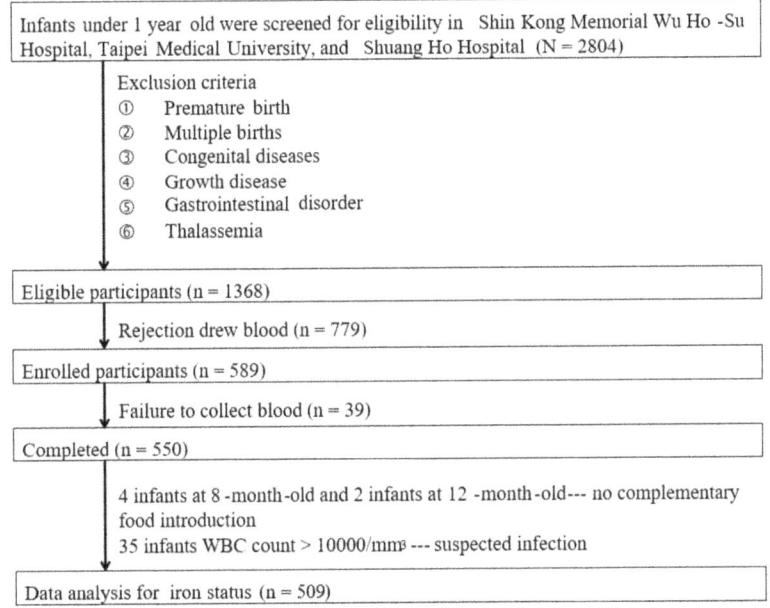

Figure 1. Flowchart of the enrolment of infants.

Table 1. Demographic characteristics of subjects diagnosed with iron deficiency (ID) or iron deficiency anemia (IDA) in the first year of life [a].

Characteristics	Normal N = 439	ID [b] N = 49	IDA N = 21	p Value
Infant				
Number (%)	439 (86)	49 (10)	21 (4)	
Male (%)	236 (53.8)	24 (49.0)	12 (57.1)	0.546
Gestational age	38.4 ± 1.5	38.2 ± 1.6	38.2 ± 1.4	0.673
Chronological age	5.9 ± 4.3	9.9 ± 3.6	9.6 ± 3.4	<0.001 *
Birth weight (kg)	3.0 ± 0.5	3.0 ± 0.6	3.0 ± 0.5	0.919
Body length (percentile)	52.9 ± 30.9	55.8 ± 31.4	37.9 ± 31.3	0.118
Body weight (percentile)	51.2 ± 28.3	51.3 ± 30.0	43.9 ± 30.4	0.568
Head circumference (percentile)	56.4 ± 30.2	50.1 ± 31.2	51.9 ± 20.3	0.424
Feeding type [c]				
Breast-fed (%)	127 (28.9)	32 (65.3)	18 (85.7)	<0.001 *
Mix-fed (%)	80 (18.2)	6 (12.2)	2 (9.5)	
Formula-fed (%)	232 (52.8)	11 (22.4)	1 (4.8)	
Mother				
Age (year)	32.6 ± 4.2	32.1 ± 3.6	32.4 ± 4.7	0.791
BMI (kg/m^2)	21.3 ± 3.7	20.8 ± 5.5	20.7 ± 3.8	0.654
Gestational weight gain (kg)	14.3 ± 7.9	16.3 ± 11.9	11.6 ± 5.5	0.125
Education (year)	14.6 ± 2.3	15.0 ± 2.3	15.2 ± 2.0	0.382

[a] Values are expressed as mean ± SD or n (%); [b] According to definitions by the World Health Organization, iron deficiency (ID): Serum ferritin < 15.0 ng/mL, iron deficiency anemia (IDA): Serum ferritin < 15.0 ng/mL and hemoglobin < 10.5 g/dL.; [c] Definition of feeding type: Breast-fed means that the dairy products in the infant's diet are all breast milk; Mix-fed means that the dairy products in the infant's diet include breast milk and formula milk; Formula-fed refers to the dairy products in the infant's diet only formula milk. * Differences between groups were tested using one-way ANOVA, followed by the Scheffé method for a post hoc or Chi-square test; $p < 0.05$ was considered statistically significant.

3.2. Analysis of Iron Status

The iron status of the infants and mothers before delivery are presented in Table 2. Biochemical parameters, ferritin, and TS were significantly low in ID and IDA groups. Although the mothers of infants with IDA had a slightly lower Hb level before delivery, no statistical difference was observed.

Table 2. Hematologic data of subjects [a].

Classification	Normal N = 439	ID [b] N = 49	IDA N = 21	p Value [c]
Infant				
Hb (g/L)	11.4 ± 1.3 [a]	11.6 ± 0.7 [a]	9.2 ± 1.4 [b]	<0.001
Ferritin (ng/mL)	55.0 (98.4) [a]	10.2 (5.7) [b]	5.2 (5.7) [b]	<0.001
TS (%)	22.5 ± 11.3 [a]	11.5 ± 5.5 [bc]	7.0 ± 4.5 [c]	<0.001
Maternal (before delivery)				
Hb (g/L)	12.0 ± 1.9	12.1 ± 1.4	11.3 ± 1.4	0.361
Hct (%)	36.2 ± 4.6	36.6 ± 3.2	34.5 ± 3.7	0.333
MCV (fl)	86.8 ± 8.2	87.1 ± 8.4	86.7 ± 8.1	0.584

[a] Data are presented as mean ± SD or median (interquartile range); [b] ID, iron deficiency; IDA, iron deficiency anemia; Hb, hemoglobin; TS, transferrin saturation; Hct, hematocrit; MCV, mean corpuscular volume; [c] Means in the column with different superscripts indicate a significant difference ($p < 0.05$), tested using one-way ANOVA, followed by the Scheffé method for post hoc test or the Kruskal–Wallis test.

3.3. Iron Intake of Infants

The total iron intake was calculated as the sum of the iron contents in milk and complementary food, as presented in Table 3. Because complementary food was introduced in only 17 infants, and most of the complementary foods were cereals and fruit purees for infants aged 4–6 months, data of the iron intake from complementary food are not shown. During ages 1–6 months, the daily iron intake from milk in the normal, ID, and IDA groups were 3.43, 0.13, and 0.13 mg, respectively. Moreover, the normal group had a higher total iron intake (3.49 mg daily) than the ID (0.13 mg daily) and IDA (0.13 mg daily) groups at ages 1–6 months. The low total iron intake in infants of the ID and IDA groups could be attributed to exclusive breastfeeding, and both ID and IDA were observed in infants aged 4–6 months.

Table 3. Iron intake of infants aged 1–6 months and 7–12 months [a].

Parameters	Normal	ID [b]	IDA	p Value
1–6 months				
Number (%)	307 (93.6)	12 (3.7)	9 (2.7)	
Chronological age	3.4 ± 1.8	5.0 ± 1.2	4.8 ± 1.1	0.007 *
Breastfeed (%)	174 (56.7)	12 (100)	9 (100)	0.001 *
Iron intake from milk (mg/day) [c]	3.43 (6.62)	0.13 (0.03)	0.13 (0.17)	0.003 *
Total iron intake (mg/day) [d]	3.49 (6.81)	0.13 (0.18)	0.13 (0.17)	0.007 *
7–12 months				
Number (%)	132 (73.0)	37 (20.4)	12 (6.6)	
Chronological age	11.3 ± 2.9	11.2 ± 2.9	11.3 ± 2.0	0.976
Breastfeed (%)	21 (15.9)	26 (70.3)	11 (91.7)	<0.001 *
Iron intake from milk (mg/day) [c]	5.04 (3.92)	0.14 (2.01)	0.14 (0.01)	<0.001 *
Iron intake from complementary food (mg/day)	1.04 (1.00)	1.29 (2.00)	1.20 (2.00)	0.840
Total iron intake (mg/day)	6.47 (4.35)	2.28 (3.02)	1.33 (0.98)	<0.001 *

[a] Data are presented as median (interquartile range); [b] ID, iron deficiency; IDA, iron deficiency anemia; [c] Iron intake from milk was the sum of iron intake from formula milk and breast milk.; [d] Total iron intake was the sum of iron intake from milk and complementary food; * Intergroup differences were tested using the Kruskal–Wallis test or chi square test; $p < 0.05$ was considered statistically significant.

The normal group had the highest iron intake from milk (5.04 mg daily), whereas, the ID and IDA groups had a low iron intake from milk. This could be attributed to the continuous breastfeeding of the infants in the ID and IDA groups. No intergroup differences were noted in terms of the iron intake from complementary food. Therefore, milk was the major source of iron intake in infants aged 7–12 months. Furthermore, we determined that the prevalence of ID and IDA in infants aged 7–12 months was 20.4% and 6.6%, respectively, which was significantly higher than 3.7% and 2.7%, respectively, in infants aged 1–6 months. Our results revealed that infants with ID or IDA before six months were all in aged 4–6 months and breastfed. The medium iron intake in infants aged 4–6 months in the normal, ID and IDA groups were 5.13 mg (6.54), 0.13 mg (0.18), and 0.13 mg (0.29), respectively. In aged 7–12 months, infants with IDA had the highest breastfeeding rate, followed by those with ID.

Iron is essential for hematopoiesis. We observed that the total dietary iron intake was positively correlated with Hb ($r = 0.292$, $p < 0.001$) (Figure 2A). We further divided the data into the following two subgroups: One to six months (Figure 2B) and 7–12 months (Figure 2C). The data revealed that the correlation between total dietary iron intake and Hb in infants aged 7–12 months was higher than in those aged 1–6 months ($r = 0.390$, $p < 0.001$ vs. $r = 0.130$, $p = 0.028$).

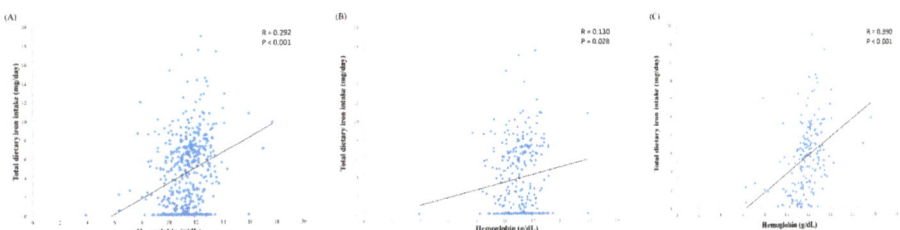

Figure 2. Correlations between total dietary iron intake and hemoglobin at 1–12 months (**A**), 1–6 months (**B**) and 7–12 months (**C**).

3.4. Association between Feeding Type and Iron Status

Logistic regression models were employed to identify predictors of ID and IDA. Our data revealed that feeding type was a major indicator in predicting anemia (Table 4). In model 1, no covariates were adjusted, and in model 2, gestational week, birthweight, sex, body weight percentile, body length percentile, and age of infants were adjusted. In model 3, in addition to the aforementioned variables for infants, mothers' BMI, gestational weight gain, education level, and Hb concentration before delivery were also adjusted. Compared with formula-fed infants, breastfed infants had a higher odds ratio (OR) for ID (OR: 2.715; 95% CI: 1.830–4.030) and IDA (OR: 4.338; 95% CI: 2.108–8.927) in model 1 ($p < 0.001$). Furthermore, ORs for ID and IDA significantly differed after adjustment for variables in models 2 and 3.

Table 4. Association between feeding type and iron status.

Variables	β	SE [a]	OR	95% CI	p Value
Model 1 [b]					
ID	0.999	0.201	2.715	1.830–4.030	<0.001 *
IDA	1.467	0.368	4.338	2.108–8.927	<0.001 *
Model 2					
ID	0.984	0.201	2.674	1.803–3.966	<0.001 *
IDA	1.361	0.369	3.901	1.893–8.042	<0.001 *
Model 3					
ID	0.769	0.232	2.157	1.369–3.399	0.001 *
IDA	1.434	0.437	4.196	1.780–9.887	0.001 *

[a] SE, standard error of mean; OR, odds ratio; 95% CI, 95% confidence interval; [b] Model 1: Not adjusted; Model 2: Adjusted for gestational week, birthweight, sex, body weight percentile, body length percentile, age; Model 3: Adjusted for gestational week, birthweight, sex, body weight percentile, body length percentile, age of infants, as well as mothers' BMI, gestational weight gain, education level, and hemoglobin level before delivery; * $p < 0.05$.

4. Discussion

The period of infancy constitutes a critical window of growth and brain development, and thus, micronutrient deficiencies during this period may have adverse effects on neurocognitive functions. Iron deficiency is the most prevalent nutritional deficiency among infants in developing countries. Women of childbearing age are at risk of iron deficiency because of poor iron content in the diet, increased demand for iron during pregnancy, and iron loss during menstruation and childbirth. In addition, breastfed infants are vulnerable to developing ID because of rapid growth, depletion of their iron endowment, and low iron content in breast milk and in some complementary foods. In our study, among the 509 mother–infant dyads who submitted complete data, 3.7% and 2.7% of the infants aged below six months had ID and IDA, respectively. However, in infants aged above six months, the prevalence of ID and IDA rapidly increased to 20.4% and 6.6%, respectively. Analysis of the maternal hematologic data revealed that anemia was not detected in the mothers during the routine prenatal examination. The basic characteristics of all infants (Normal, ID, IDA) were similar except for the chronological age and feeding type.

The prevalence of ID and IDA varies greatly among countries worldwide. In India, the prevalence of ID in infants aged 3, 4, and 5 months was 5.4%, 21.4%, and 36.4%, respectively, whereas that of IDA was 4.6%, 16.7%, and 11.4%, respectively [19]. In Turkey, Germany, and Brazil, the prevalence of ID in infants aged four months were 19.8%, 6%, and 5.7%, the prevalence of IDA in those infants were 9.5%, 0%, and 3.4%, respectively [20–22]. The prevalence of ID and IDA in infants before six months of age in our study was concordant with that observed in Germany and Brazil. In Spain, the prevalence of ID and IDA was 9.6% and 4.3%, respectively, in 12-month-old infants [23]. The prevalence of ID was 14.0%, and that of IDA was 9.4% in infants aged 9–12 months in Estonia [24]. In Saudi Arabia, out of the 274 infants aged 6–24 months studied, 126 (51%) were diagnosed as having IDA [25]. Among 619 Korean infants aged 8–15 months old, ID and IDA were diagnosed in 174 (28.1%) and 87 infants (14.0%), respectively [26]. The prevalence of ID and IDA in two cohorts of infants aged nine months old in China was 2.8% and 20.7% and 12.0% and 31.2%, respectively [27]. The prevalence of ID and IDA in infants above six months of age in our study was concordant with that observed in China and Korea.

Breast milk is considered the best food for infants, because it is highly nutritious for infant growth and contains maternal antibodies that provide defense against pathogens. A recent study indicated that human breast milk has very little iron (0.5 mg/L at one month and 0.29 mg/L at 3–5 months) [28]. Our data revealed that the average iron content of breast milk from the mothers of the infants was 0.21 ± 0.06 mg/L. Although iron in human breast milk has higher bioavailability, it may not be sufficient for infants. Therefore, infants' body iron stores meet most requirements for breast-fed infants during the first six months of life. A study concluded that a normal, healthy, full-term infant has sufficient amounts of iron until approximately 4–6 months of age [29]. Our results revealed that the prevalence of ID and IDA in infants aged 1–6 months was 3.7% and 2.7%, respectively, and these infants were all in aged 4–6 month and breastfed. Hence, breastfeeding for more than four months can slightly increase the risk of ID and IDA with lower iron stores.

Studies have indicated that the risk factors for the development of ID included small-for-gestational-age, infants below 10th percentile weight for gestation, infants of diabetic mothers, very-low-birth weight preterm neonates (VLBW, <1500 g at birth) and infants with lower iron stores [30,31]. Therefore, although the iron status of our subjects seems to be more related to iron intake, studies have shown the smoking, obesity, and childbirth by caesarean section also affected the iron status of infants [32]. These factors were not considered in the present study. In the absence of inflammation, serum ferritin measurement is the most specific test to determine total iron content stored in the body. Our data revealed that infants in ID and IDA groups with lower serum ferritin levels reflected depleted iron stores. Another indicator of iron deficiency was TS. In cases of iron deficiency, serum iron is reduced, and TIBC is increased, resulting in a substantial reduction in TS. A threshold of 16% is generally used to screen for iron deficiency. Our data revealed that subjects with ID and IDA had a TS below the threshold and TS in IDA group was lower than that in ID group.

Another possible reason causing iron depletion in infants below six months of age could be maternal iron deficiency during pregnancy, which results in offspring with inadequate iron storage in the body. Some studies have found little or no correlation between maternal and neonatal iron status, whereas, others have suggested that the fetus was vulnerable to maternal ID [33,34]. Mothers of IDA infants had lower Hb level, although there were no statistical differences. We further analyzed the correction between infants Hb level and mothers Hb level, and the results were not correlated. Although the mother's iron nutrition status during pregnancy may affect the child's iron nutrition status, our results revealed that feeding still mainly affects the infant's iron nutrition status. In addition, the timing of umbilical cord clamping affects iron stores in the newborn. A study indicated that delay in cord clamping increases the red blood cell volume and iron stores in infants [35]. Hence, cord clamping could be a feasible solution to improve the iron status of infants.

The WHO recommends exclusive breastfeeding of infants for the first six months of life. Thereafter, infants should receive complementary foods with continued breastfeeding up to two years of age or above. Taiwan's health policy also follows this recommendation. In this study, among 328 infants below six months of age, only 17 were introduced to complementary food. Most of these foods were cereals or fruit juices that had low iron content. Thus, in addition to prenatal storage, formula milk contributed more iron to the infants below six months of age. Although human milk has a high bioavailability of iron, the iron content was so low that exclusive breastfeeding increased the risk of ID and IDA. We determined that the total iron intake was positively correlated with Hb level in infants below six months of age, thereby indicating that although prenatal storage was crucial to maintain iron status, additional dietary iron intake can improve the Hb levels and prevent ID and IDA, especially in infants aged 4–6 months. Evidence from randomized control trials suggests that the rate of IDA in breastfed infants could be positively altered by the introduction of solids at four months of age [36]. The American Academy of Pediatrics recommends that exclusively breastfed, full-term infants receive 1 mg/kg of iron supplements per day from the age of four months [37]. Taiwan's maternal and child policy particularly emphasizes the benefits of breastfeeding. The exclusive breastfeeding rate for infants at six months in Taiwan increased from 20.1% in 2004 to 50.2% in 2011 [38]. Therefore, introducing complementary food early or providing iron supplementation is imperative for infants aged 4–6 months who are exclusively breastfed.

Although infants aged 7–12 months were provided complementary foods, the iron intake from complementary foods was not different among the normal, ID, and IDA groups. Notably, milk was the major source of iron. Upon further analysis of data, we observed that up to 70% of infants with ID and 90% of infants with IDA were still breastfed. This result indicated that infants who are still breastfed for more than six months do not obtain adequate iron from breast milk. This suggests that mothers who still breastfeed after six months could provide high-quality iron-rich foods to reduce the prevalence of ID and IDA.

When we reported the iron status of infants to their mothers, most of the mothers presented their infants had good growth and not aware of the insufficient iron intake and that it increased the risk of ID or IDA. Conversely, infants who used commercial formulas instead of breast milk had better iron status because most commercial formulas are iron-fortified. Future health policies should educate mothers to prepare high-quality iron-rich foods or provide iron supplementation for breastfed infants.

The maximum iron requirement for infants aged 4–12 months is approximately 1 mg/kg or 10 mg/day. The average full-term infant requires 8 mg of iron daily from approximately six months of age [39]. Our data demonstrated that the median iron intake of infants aged 1–6 months was 3.49 mg/day, and the median iron intake of infants aged 7–12 months was 6.47 mg/day, which could reach the normal iron nutritional status. Infants with IDA had normal growth and no obvious symptoms except for pallor were observed, and no infants were suspected of having anemia by caregivers. Therefore, the presentation of iron deficiency is subtle and can be detected accurately only by medical personnel.

Although our results determined that breastfeeding was associated with an increased the prevalence of ID and/or IDA, the advantages of breast milk are recognized and unquestionable. Thus, more attention should be paid to the problem of iron deficiency in infants, and strategies should be proposed, including improving maternal iron status, introducing high-quality complementary food early, and even providing iron supplement to breastfed infants. The Pediatrics Association of Taiwan revised the guidelines for breastfed infants in 2016. The content includes the following: (1) Encourage full-term infants to start breastfeeding as soon as possible after birth, (2) Continue to breastfeed until one year of age. After one year of age, the mother may continue to breastfeed the infants, (3) Breastfed infants should be started on complementary foods at 4–6 months of age. If no complementary foods are added after four months, oral iron supplementation should be started at 1 mg/kg/day. Iron deficiency affects the development of cognition, nerves, and behavior, some of which are long-term and irreversible [40]. In this study, all infants with ID and IDA improved iron status and anemia after medical iron supplementation and regular checkups by pediatricians.

The strength of the present work is that it is the first to look at the association between breastfeeding and ID and IDA during infancy in Taiwan. The results can be used as a reference for nutrition policymakers. However, the study had some limitations. First, this was a cross-sectional study that was unable to clarify the effects of longitudinal nutritional status on the development of ID and IDA. Second, the sample size was relatively small, and all participants lived in northern Taiwan, which might limit the generalizability of the results. Therefore, additional large-sample, multicenter studies are required. Third, we only prioritized examining several clinical iron markers that are more likely related to iron status. Fourth, the lack of information regarding the initiation of complementary feeding, that could significantly impact iron status in infants. Nevertheless, further studies are warranted, including those for following up infants with iron deficiency in the first year to analyze whether it affects their cognition function and growth, as well as whether early introduction of high-quality iron-rich complementary foods can improve the iron status of infants.

5. Conclusions

Our data revealed that exclusive breastfeeding increases the prevalence of ID and IDA in infants aged 4–6 months, and prolonged breastfeed above six months can significantly increase the prevalence of ID and IDA. Although iron in breast milk has good bioavailability, its low iron content results in insufficient iron intake in infants and increases the risk of anemia. Hence, health policies should encourage the early introduction of iron-rich complementary foods and educate mothers to prepare high-quality complementary foods to reduce the risk of anemia, especially in infants above six months. In addition, if no complementary foods are added after four months, oral iron supplementation should be started in breastfeeding infants.

Author Contributions: Conceptualization, S.-C.L. and C.-M.C.; methodology: All; data curation: S.-C.M., Y.-L.C., L.-Y.T., Y.-T.K., I.-M.C. and Y.-C.C.; validation: S.-C.M., C.-K.S. and M.-L.C.; drafting of the manuscript: S.-C.L.; critical revision of the manuscript: C.-M.C. and S.-C.M.; final approval of the version to be published: S.-C.L. All authors have read and agreed to the published version of the manuscript.

Funding: This study was supported by the Ministry of Health and Welfare (DOH101-HP-4204 and DOH102-HP-4203).

Acknowledgments: We thank the participants and the medical staff for their participation. This manuscript was edited by Wallace Academic Editing.

Conflicts of Interest: The authors have no conflicts of interest to declare.

References

1. Lessen, R.; Kavanagh, K. Position of the Academy of Nutrition and Dietetics: Promoting and Supporting Breastfeeding. *J. Acad. Nutr. Diet.* **2015**, *115*, 444–449. [CrossRef] [PubMed]
2. Fewtrell, M.; Wilson, D.C.; Booth, I.; Lucas, A. Six months of exclusive breast feeding: How good is the evidence? *BMJ* **2011**, *342*, c5955. [CrossRef] [PubMed]
3. Monajemzadeh, S.; Zarkesh, M. Iron deficiency anemia in infants aged 12-15 months in Ahwaz, Iran. *Indian J. Pathol. Microbiol.* **2009**, *52*, 182–184. [CrossRef]
4. Özdemir, N. Iron deficiency anemia from diagnosis to treatment in children. *Turk Pediatri Ars.* **2015**, *50*, 11–19. [CrossRef]
5. Qasem, W.A.; Friel, J.K. An Overview of Iron in Term Breast-Fed Infants. *Clin. Med. Insights Pediatr.* **2015**, *9*, 79–84. [CrossRef]
6. McLean, E.; Cogswell, M.; Egli, I.; Wojdyla, D.; de Benoist, B. Worldwide prevalence of anaemia, WHO Vitamin and Mineral Nutrition Information System, 1993–2005. *Public Health Nutr.* **2009**, *12*, 444–454. [CrossRef]
7. Steinbicker, A.U.; Muckenthaler, M.U. Out of Balance—Systemic Iron Homeostasis in Iron-Related Disorders. *Nutrients* **2013**, *5*, 3034–3061. [CrossRef]
8. Lozoff, B.; Smith, J.B.; Clark, K.M.; Perales, C.G.; Rivera, F.; Castillo, M. Home intervention improves cognitive and social-emotional scores in iron-deficient anemic infants. *Pediatrics* **2010**, *126*, e884–e894. [CrossRef]
9. Allen, L.H. Anemia and iron deficiency: Effects on pregnancy outcome. *Am. J. Clin. Nutr.* **2000**, *71*, 1280S–1284S. [CrossRef] [PubMed]
10. Grant, C.C.; Wall, C.R.; Brewster, D.; Nicholson, R.; Whitehall, J.; Super, L.; Pitcher, L. Policy statement on iron deficiency in pre-school-aged children. *J. Paediatr. Child Health* **2007**, *43*, 513–521. [CrossRef] [PubMed]
11. Cao, C.; O'brien, K.O. Pregnancy and iron homeostasis: An update. *Nutr. Rev.* **2013**, *71*, 35–51. [CrossRef] [PubMed]
12. Ejezie, F.; Nwagha, U.; Ikekpeazu, E.; Ozoemena, O.; Onwusi, E. Assessment of iron content of breast milk in preterm and term mothers in enugu urban. *Ann. Med. Health Sci. Res.* **2011**, *1*, 85–90. [PubMed]
13. Friel, J.; Qasem, W.; Cai, C. Iron and the Breastfed Infant. *Antioxidants* **2018**, *7*, 54. [CrossRef] [PubMed]
14. Erick, M. Breast milk is conditionally perfect. *Med. Hypotheses* **2018**, *111*, 82–89. [CrossRef]
15. Wang, F.; Liu, H.; Wan, Y.; Li, J.; Chen, Y.; Zheng, J.; Huang, T.; Li, D. Prolonged Exclusive Breastfeeding Duration Is Positively Associated with Risk of Anemia in Infants Aged 12 Months. *J. Nutr.* **2016**, *146*, 1707–1713. [CrossRef]
16. Tsai, S.-F.; Chen, S.-J.; Yen, H.-J.; Hung, G.-Y.; Tsao, P.-C.; Jeng, M.-J.; Lee, Y.-S.; Soong, W.-J.; Tang, R.-B. Iron Deficiency Anemia in Predominantly Breastfed Young Children. *Pediatr. Neonatol.* **2014**, *55*, 466–469. [CrossRef]
17. Lyu, L.C.; Lee, F.J.; Chen, H.Y.; Fang, L.J.; Chiang, H.J. Test-weighing and nutrient intakes of breast milk feeding for Taiwanese infants from 1 to 12 months of age. *Nutr. Sci. J.* **2011**, *3*, 87–98.
18. Cheng, X.Z.; Jin, C.; Zhang, K.C. Determination of trace elements in waste beer yeasts by ICP-MS with microwave digestion. *Guang Pu Xue Yu Guang Pu Fen Xi = Guang Pu* **2008**, *28*, 2421–2424.
19. Krishnaswamy, S.; Bhattarai, D.; Bharti, B.; Bhatia, P.; Das, R.; Bansal, D. Iron deficiency and iron deficiency anemia in 3–5 months-old, Breastfed Healthy Infants. *Indian J. Pediatr.* **2017**, *84*, 505–508. [CrossRef]
20. Arvas, A.; Elgormus, Y.; Gur, E.; Alikasifoglu, M.; Celebi, A. Iron status in breast-fed full-term infants. *Turk. J. Pediatr.* **2000**, *42*, 22–26.
21. Dube, K.; Schwartz, J.; Mueller, M.J.; Kalhoff, H.; Kersting, M. Iron intake and iron status in breastfed infants during the first year of life. *Clin. Nutr.* **2010**, *29*, 773–778. [CrossRef] [PubMed]
22. Marques, R.F.; Taddei, J.A.; Lopez, F.A.; Braga, J.A. Breastfeeding exclusively and iron deficiency anemia during the first 6 months of age. *Rev. Assoc. Médica Bras.* **2014**, *60*, 18–22. [CrossRef] [PubMed]
23. Trave, T.D.; Vélaz, L.D. Prevalence of iron deficiency in healthy 12-month-old infants. *An. Esp. Pediatr.* **2002**, *57*, 209–214.
24. Vendt, N.; Grünberg, H.; Leedo, S.; Tillmann, V.; Talvik, T. Prevalence and causes of iron deficiency anemias in infants aged 9 to 12 months in Estonia. *Medicina* **2007**, *43*, 947. [CrossRef]

25. Al Hawsawi, Z.M.; Al-Rehali, S.A.; Mahros, A.M.; Al-Sisi, A.M.; Al-Harbi, K.D.; Yousef, A.M. High prevalence of iron deficiency anemia in infants attending a well-baby clinic in northwestern Saudi Arabia. *Saudi Med. J.* **2015**, *36*, 1067–1070. [CrossRef]
26. Hong, J.; Chang, J.Y.; Shin, S.; Oh, S. Breastfeeding and Red Meat Intake Are Associated with Iron Status in Healthy Korean Weaning-age Infants. *J. Korean Med Sci.* **2017**, *32*, 974–984. [CrossRef]
27. Clark, K.M.; Li, M.; Zhu, B.; Liang, F.; Shao, J.; Zhang, Y.; Ji, C.; Zhao, Z.; Kaciroti, N.; Lozoff, B. Breastfeeding, mixed, or formula feeding at 9 months of age and the prevalence of iron deficiency and iron deficiency anemia in two cohorts of infants in China. *J. Pediatr.* **2017**, *181*, 56–61. [CrossRef]
28. Cai, C.; Harding, S.; Friel, J. Breast milk iron concentrations may be lower than previously reported: Implications for exclusively breastfed infants. *Matern. Pediatr. Nutr.* **2015**, *2*, 2.
29. Domellof, M.; Braegger, C.; Campoy, C.; Colomb, V.; Decsi, T.; Fewtrell, M.; Hojsak, I.; Mihatsch, W.; Molgaard, C.; Shamir, R.; et al. Iron requirements of infants and toddlers. *J. Pediatr. Gastroenterol. Nutr.* **2014**, *58*, 119–129. [CrossRef]
30. Mukhopadhyay, K.; Yadav, R.K.; Kishore, S.S.; Garewal, G.; Jain, V.; Narang, A. Iron status at birth and at 4 weeks in term small-for-gestation infants in comparison with appropriate-for-gestation infants. *J. Matern.-Fetal Neonatal Med.* **2011**, *24*, 886–890. [CrossRef]
31. Rao, R.; Georgieff, M.K. Iron therapy for preterm infants. *Clin. Perinatol.* **2009**, *36*, 27–42. [CrossRef] [PubMed]
32. McCarthy, E.K.; Kenny, L.C.; Hourihane, J.O.B.; Irvine, A.D.; Murray, D.M.; Kiely, M.E. Impact of maternal, antenatal and birth-associated factors on iron stores at birth: Data from a prospective maternal–infant birth cohort. *Eur. J. Clin. Nutr.* **2017**, *71*, 782. [CrossRef] [PubMed]
33. Ervasti, M.; Sankilampi, U.; Heinonen, S.; Punnonen, K. Early signs of maternal iron deficiency do not influence the iron status of the newborn, but are associated with higher infant birthweight. *Acta Obs. Gynecol. Scand.* **2009**, *88*, 83–90. [CrossRef] [PubMed]
34. Sweet, D.G.; Savage, G.; Tubman, T.R.; Lappin, T.R.; Halliday, H.L. Study of maternal influences on fetal iron status at term using cord blood transferrin receptors. *Arch. Dis. Child. Fetal Neonatal. Ed.* **2001**, *84*, F40–F43. [CrossRef]
35. Chaparro, C.M.; Neufeld, L.M.; Tena Alavez, G.; Eguia-Liz Cedillo, R.; Dewey, K.G. Effect of timing of umbilical cord clamping on iron status in Mexican infants: A randomised controlled trial. *Lancet* **2006**, *367*, 1997–2004. [CrossRef]
36. Qasem, W.; Fenton, T.; Friel, J. Age of introduction of first complementary feeding for infants: A systematic review. *BMC Pediatr.* **2015**, *15*, 107. [CrossRef]
37. Baker, R.D.; Greer, F.R. Diagnosis and prevention of iron deficiency and iron-deficiency anemia in infants and young children (0–3 years of age). *Pediatrics* **2010**, *126*, 1040–1050. [CrossRef]
38. Chiou, S.-T.; Chen, L.-C.; Yeh, H.; Wu, S.-R.; Chien, L.-Y. Early Skin-to-Skin Contact, Rooming-in, and Breastfeeding: A Comparison of the 2004 and 2011 National Surveys in Taiwan. *Birth* **2014**, *41*, 33–38. [CrossRef]
39. Schulman, I. Iron Requirements in Infancy. *JAMA J. Am. Med. Assoc.* **1961**, *175*, 118–123. [CrossRef]
40. Carter, R.C.; Jacobson, J.L.; Burden, M.J.; Armony-Sivan, R.; Dodge, N.C.; Angelilli, M.L.; Lozoff, B.; Jacobson, S.W. Iron deficiency anemia and cognitive function in infancy. *Pediatrics* **2010**, *126*, e427–e434. [CrossRef]

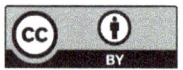

© 2020 by the authors. Licensee MDPI, Basel, Switzerland. This article is an open access article distributed under the terms and conditions of the Creative Commons Attribution (CC BY) license (http://creativecommons.org/licenses/by/4.0/).

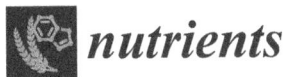

Article

The Effectiveness of Different Doses of Iron Supplementation and the Prenatal Determinants of Maternal Iron Status in Pregnant Spanish Women: ECLIPSES Study

Lucía Iglesias Vázquez [1], Victoria Arija [1,2,*], Núria Aranda [1], Estefanía Aparicio [1], Núria Serrat [3], Francesc Fargas [4], Francisca Ruiz [4], Meritxell Pallejà [2], Pilar Coronel [5], Mercedes Gimeno [5] and Josep Basora [2,6]

1. Department of Preventive Medicine and Public Health, Faculty of Medicine and Health Sciences, Universitat Rovira i Virgili, 43201 Reus, Spain; lucia.iglesias@urv.cat (L.I.V.); nuria.aranda@urv.cat (N.A.); estefania.aparicio@urv.cat (E.A.)
2. Tarragona–Reus Research Support Unit, Jordi Gol University Institute for Primary Care Research, 43202 Tarragona, Spain; meritxell.palleja@urv.cat (M.P.); josep.basora@urv.cat (J.B.)
3. Clinical Laboratory, University Hospital Joan XXIII, Institut Català de la Salut, Generalitat de Catalunya, 43005 Tarragona, Spain; nserrat.tarte.ics@gencat.cat
4. Sexual and Reproductive Health Service of Reus–Tarragona, Institut Català de la Salut, Generalitat de Catalunya, 43202 Tarragona, Spain; ffargas.tarte.ics@gencat.cat (F.F.); paqui.r.d@hotmail.com (F.R.)
5. Meiji Pharma Spain S.A. (formerly Tedec-Meiji Farma S.A.) Alcalá de Henares, 28802 Madrid, Spain; p.coronel@tedecmeiji.com (P.C.); m.gimeno@tedecmeiji.com (M.G.)
6. CIBERobn (Center for Biomedical Research in Physiopathology of Obesity and Nutrition), Instituto de Salud Carlos III, 28029 Madrid, Spain
* Correspondence: victoria.arija@urv.cat; Tel.: +97-7759334

Received: 16 September 2019; Accepted: 7 October 2019; Published: 10 October 2019

Abstract: Iron deficiency (ID), anemia, iron deficiency anemia (IDA) and excess iron (hemoconcentration) harm maternal–fetal health. We evaluated the effectiveness of different doses of iron supplementation adjusted for the initial levels of hemoglobin (Hb) on maternal iron status and described some associated prenatal determinants. The ECLIPSES study included 791 women, randomized into two groups: Stratum 1 (Hb = 110–130g/L, received 40 or 80mg iron daily) and Stratum 2 (Hb > 130g/L, received 20 or 40mg iron daily). Clinical, biochemical, and genetic information was collected during pregnancy, as were lifestyle and sociodemographic characteristics. In Stratum 1, using 80 mg/d instead of 40 mg/d protected against ID on week 36. Only women with ID on week 12 benefited from the protection against anemia and IDA by increasing Hb levels. In Stratum 2, using 20 mg/d instead of 40 mg/d reduced the risk of hemoconcentration in women with initial serum ferritin (SF) ≥ 15 µg/L, while 40 mg/d improved SF levels on week 36 in women with ID in early pregnancy. Mutations in the *HFE* gene increased the risk of hemoconcentration. Iron supplementation should be adjusted to early pregnancy levels of Hb and iron stores. Mutations of the *HFE* gene should be evaluated in women with high Hb levels in early pregnancy.

Keywords: iron supplementation; pregnancy; randomized controlled trial; serum ferritin; hemoglobin; iron status; iron stores; *HFE* gene

1. Introduction

Iron requirements increase during pregnancy. Since dietary sources cannot always prevent iron deficit, iron supplements are usually prescribed to women who plan to become pregnant.

However, there is no consensus on the ideal iron dosage during pregnancy. Anemia is the most common and widespread nutritional disorder globally and a significant public health problem [1,2]. Anemia is attributed to iron deficiency (ID) in half of the cases in the general population [1,3] and in up to 90% of cases of pregnant women [4]. Studies show that an inadequate iron status during pregnancy can lead to adverse mother–child outcomes. In the mother, iron deficiency, anemia, and iron deficiency anemia (IDA) have been associated with preeclampsia, preterm delivery, and even miscarriage, and in the child with fetal growth restriction, low birth weight and impaired cognitive development [5–10]. Furthermore, some studies have underscored the importance of timing of ID and IDA, since some long–term consequences, especially regarding the development and functioning of the child's brain, are irreversible, even after correcting iron levels [11,12]. As a result, it is essential to maintain good nutritional care even before getting pregnant, as well as throughout the whole gestation, to ensure an optimal health status for mother and baby.

In addition to participating as enzymatic cofactor in a wide range of metabolic reactions, iron is indispensable for the synthesis of hemoglobin (Hb), the synthesis and methylation of DNA, and oxygen transport [13,14]. The increase in blood volume and the formation of new tissue during pregnancy are the main mechanisms underlying the increased iron requirements [15–17]. Crucially, iron has a key role in neuronal proliferation, myelination, and the synthesis of several neurotransmitters during the development of the fetal brain [11,18]. Despite concerns about the state of prenatal iron, which caused the launch of public health policies to address iron deficiency [19], it is estimated that in Europe, around 25% of pregnant women become anemic during pregnancy [2,3,19]. The prevalence of ID is greater than the prevalence of IDA, and it often develops during the later months of pregnancy, even in women with sufficient iron stores at the start of the pregnancy [20]. In addition, while diet and supplementation are the main sources of iron, the maternal iron status is influenced by many other biological, lifestyle, and even social factors. According to published research, genetic alterations, ethnicity, obstetric history, toxic habits (i.e., smoking or alcohol), and socioeconomic status (SES) could have a defining role [21–25].

On the other hand, unnecessary or excessive iron supplementation might generate high levels of Hb, also known as the risk of hemoconcentration, in the second and third trimesters of pregnancy. This condition, which affects between 8.7% and 42% of pregnancies in industrialized countries [26,27], increases oxidative stress and blood viscosity, causing placental infarction and hindering the perfusion of oxygen and nutrients to the fetus [28–31]. Although hemoconcentration can be as harmful as iron deficiency for maternal health and children's health, in clinical practice, iron supplementation is usually not adjusted to fit iron status.

The primary aim of this study was to evaluate the effectiveness of iron supplements during pregnancy in different doses adjusted to the Hb levels of the first trimester. As secondary outcomes, we described the percentage of ID, anemia, IDA, and risk of hemoconcentration in a large sample of pregnant Spanish women and the prenatal factors associated with maternal iron status at the end of pregnancy.

2. Materials and Methods

2.1. Study Design

The ECLIPSES study [32] was a community randomized controlled trial (RCT) conducted in the province of Tarragona (Catalonia, Spain) between 2013 and 2017. The 791 participants were contacted in their primary care centers during the first routine visit with midwives and were included in the trial according to the following inclusion criteria: over 18 years of age, gestation time ≤12 weeks, no lab indication of anemia (Hb ≥ 110 g/L on week 12), ability to understand the official State languages (Spanish or Catalan), and the ability to understand the characteristics of the study. Women with multiple pregnancy, adverse obstetric history, those who had taken >10 mg iron daily during the three months prior to week 12 of gestation, and those who reported a previous severe illness (immunosuppression) or chronic disease that could affect their nutritional status (cancer, diabetes, malabsorption, or liver disease) were excluded. A signed informed consent was obtained from all participants.

The participants were allocated into two strata according their initial Hb levels on week 12 of pregnancy, as follows:

(1) Stratum 1: women with initial Hb levels between 110 and 130 g/L were prescribed 40 or 80 mg/d of iron supplementation.

(2) Stratum 2: women with initial Hb levels > 130 g/L were prescribed 40 or 20 mg/d iron supplementation. Although in clinical practice, only plasma Hb and serum ferritin (SF) levels are measured, we suspected that women with initial Hb > 130 g/L could have some alteration in the *HFE* gene which would predispose them to iron overload.

In addition to the recruitment visit before the 12th week of gestation, the study consisted of three visits throughout the pregnancy: at the 12th, 24th, and 36th weeks of gestation. Separately, the women attended routine pregnancy visits with their midwives and obstetricians.

During the first visit (12th week), the midwives delivered the supplements to the participants according to the intervention group to which they had been assigned. The prescription of each dose of supplements within the groups was randomized and triple blinded. The laboratories Tedec–Meiji made the same box for all different doses of supplements, so that the laboratory technicians, the clinical staff and the researchers did not know the dose of iron received by each woman until the study ended. Women were advised to take one pill per day until the next visit, at which time they had to return any left-over pills to evaluate adherence. An independent investigator compared the number of pills left over with the compliance reported by the participants. Good compliance was considered for women who reported having forgotten to take the supplement less than twice per week at every visit of the study. When they reported forgetting two or more times per week in any of the visits, compliance was considered low.

If women developed anemia in the middle of pregnancy (24th week), they received the usual treatment for anemia.

The sample size was calculated according to previous data from our research group [9,33], taking into account the risk of IDA and hemoconcentration during the third trimester of pregnancy as principal variables [32]. The study was designed in agreement with the Declaration of Helsinki/Tokyo. All procedures involving human subjects were approved by Clinical Research Ethics Committee of the Jordi Gol University Institute for Primary Care Research (*Institut d' Investigació en Atenció Primària; IDIAP*), the Pere Virgili Health Research Institute (*Institut d'Investigació Sanitària Pere Virgili; IISPV*), and the Spanish Agency for Medicines and Medical Devices (*Agencia Española del Medicamento y Productos Sanitarios; AEMPS*). Signed, informed consent was obtained from all women participating in the study. This clinical trial was registered at www.clinicaltrialsregister.eu as EudraCT number 2012-005480-28 and at www.clinicaltrials.gov with identification number NCT03196882.

2.2. Data Collection

2.2.1. Baseline Data (on Week 12 of Gestation)

Midwives and researchers of the study (dietitians) compiled clinical and obstetrical data from participants during the first visit. They obtained the following information during the personal interview and from specific questionnaires: date of birth, weight, height, blood pressure, parity (yes/no), number of previous children, planned pregnancy (yes/no), previous use of contraceptives (yes/no), and type of contraceptives. Medical and surgical history and obstetric data were also recorded.

Maternal age was classified as <25 years, 25–34 years, and ≥35 years. Each maternal pre–pregnancy body mass index (BMI, Kg/cm^2) was categorized as underweight (BMI < 18.5), normal weight (BMI 18.5–24.9), overweight (BMI 25–29.9), or obese (BMI ≥ 30).

The dietary assessment was obtained using a short food frequency questionnaire (FFQ) validated in our population [34] and filled by participants at each visit of the study. From this information, we were able to calculate the percentage of adherence to the Mediterranean diet [35], considered a high–quality dietary pattern. In addition, women were asked about their use of multivitamin supplements, including >10mg iron, which constituted an exclusion criteria for this study.

Lifestyle habits before conception were also recorded, including alcohol intake and smoking. To assess smoking, we used the Fagerström test [36] and women were classified as smokers and non-smokers at the first visit of the study. The International Physical Activity Questionnaire (IPAQ) [37] was used to record the physical activity (PA) of participants. They reported the time spent doing exercise of different intensity (vigorous, moderate or a walk lasting at least 10 minutes) during the previous week; the information was recorded as "days per week" in which physical activity of each intensity was performed, and the "hours" and "minutes" dedicated in each of those days. Women also reported amount of time spent sitting during a typical day. We used these data to calculate the metabolic equivalents of task.

Sociodemographic data of participants and their partners were also recorded. The educational level was classified into four groups: unfinished primary school (<12 years old), primary school (up to 12 years old), secondary school (up to 18 years old) and higher education, which included university and vocational studies. Regarding occupational status, women were classified as students, employed or unemployed. Women in employment were asked about their profession, which was classified following the Catalan Classification of Occupations (CCO-2011) [38]. All this information was used to calculate the family's socioeconomic status (SES).

Regarding ethnicity, five categories were used: Caucasian, Latin American, Asian, Arab, and Black.

Blood samples were taken on week 12 of gestation to perform blood and genetics tests. Hematological parameters (Hb, mean corpuscular volume (MCV), and hematocrit) and some specific biochemical markers (serum ferritin (SF) and C–reactive protein (CRP)) were measured, and genetic mutations of the *HFE* gene (C282Y, H63D, and S65C) were checked for. The samples were stored in the BioBank for future use.

2.2.2. Data Recorded during Scheduled Study Visits

Diet and physical activity were also evaluated at 24th and 36th weeks of gestation. In addition, blood was collected during both visits to analyze routine blood parameters, including Hb levels. On week 36, SF levels were also measured.

Any adverse effect from the supplementation was recorded and included in the statistical analyses.

2.2.3. Definition of Iron Status

Anemia was defined as Hb < 110 g/L at 12th and 36th weeks and Hb < 105 g/L at 24th week of gestation. ID was defined as SF < 15 µg/L and IDA as anemia and one of the following criteria: SF < 15 µg/L or MCV < 70 fL. SF levels ≥ 15 µg/L was considered as non–deficient or normal iron stores.

2.3. Statistical Analysis

All statistical analyses were performed for the population by intention to treat (ITT) and per-protocol. The population by ITT considered all the participants that were initially included in the study; the per-protocol population, however, consisted only of those participants who complied with the protocol of the study. In the latter, therefore, we excluded women who developed anemia on visit 2, at 24 weeks of gestation.

All analyses were performed separating the sample by stratum; i.e., according to the Hb levels in the first visit of the study. Student's *t*-test and ANOVA were used to describe continuous variables (mean and SD), and the chi-squared test for categorical variables (percentages). Natural logarithm (Ln) transformation was applied to normalize the distribution of SF, increasing the validity of analyses, and using the median and interquartile ranges (IQR).

Multivariate regression models (multiple linear regressions and logistic regressions) were used to assess the effect of different doses of iron supplementation, along with other prenatal predictors, on maternal iron status on week 36 of pregnancy. The models were adjusted for the following variables: maternal age, parity, socioeconomic status, use of hormonal contraception prior to getting pregnant, planned pregnancy, smoking habit, alcohol intake, pre–pregnancy maternal BMI, gestational weight gain, Hb on week 12 of gestation, SF on week 12 of gestation, CRP on week 12 of gestation, *HFE* gene genotypes, maternal ethnic origin, physical activity as weekly mean of metabolic equivalent of task (METs), and adherence to Mediterranean diet.

Furthermore, adjusted multivariate regression models were performed for each stratum, separating women with and without ID in the first trimester in order to explore whether iron supplementation acted differently according to iron reserves at the beginning of pregnancy. They were adjusted for the same variables previously mentioned, except for SF on week 12 of gestation. To avoid information overload, the tables only show the statistically significant regression models.

SPSS (version 25.0 for Windows; SPSS Inc., Chicago, IL, USA) was used for statistical analyses. Statistical significance was set at $p < 0.05$.

3. Results

Of the total of 791 pregnant women included in the study at week 12 of pregnancy (529 from Stratum 1 and 262 from Stratum 2), the data shown in this article are based on the population by ITT, which consisted of of 534 women with data on week 36 (354 from Stratum 1 and 180 from Stratum 2). Attrition was due to: voluntary abandonment (22.75%); miscarriage (1.64%); emergence of exclusion criteria during pregnancy (5.82%), including serious or chronic illness that could affect the nutritional development (e.g., cancer, diabetes, and malabsorption); and participants lost to follow up (2.28%). Attrition was proportional in both Strata, as shown in the Flowchart (Figure 1). In the supplementary materials, we also show the analyses for the per-protocol population, which excluded anemic women at 24th week of gestation (11.7% in Stratum 1 and 2.7% in Stratum 2).

Table 1 shows the biological, lifestyle, and sociodemographic characteristics of participants at baseline. Compared with Stratum 1, women from Stratum 2 had a statistically significant higher baseline weight (64.83 and 67.17 kg, respectively, $p = 0.017$) and pre–pregnancy BMI (24.66 and 25.82, respectively, $p = 0.001$), and had gained significantly less weight during gestation (11.11 and 9.69 kg, respectively, $p = 0.030$). These differences did not translate into a significant effect on maternal iron status in the multivariate analyses. Table 1 also shows a trend ($p = 0.075$) toward a higher percentage of women with previous pregnancies in Stratum 1 (62.3%) than in Stratum 2 (55.7%). No significant differences in baseline characteristics were detected between women who dropped out of the study and women who reached the end of the intervention (Table S1).

We excluded the S65C mutation in the *HFE* gene from the multivariate analyses because of its low prevalence in our sample. For the same reason, subjects who were homozygous and heterozygous for H63D, together with the combined heterozygote H63D/C282Y, were grouped as "carrier of the H63D mutation." We compared, therefore, three categories of mutation of the *HFE* gene in the multivariate analyses: wild type (WT/WT), heterozygous for C282Y/WT, and carrier of the H63D mutation. A similar situation occurred with maternal ethnic origin: we excluded Asian and Black subjects from subsequent analyses due to the low representation in the studied population, and only three final categories were considered: Caucasian, Arab, and Latin American.

Since diet is expected to influence iron status, adherence to the Mediterranean diet was compared among the different study groups (Figure 2), but no significant differences were found.

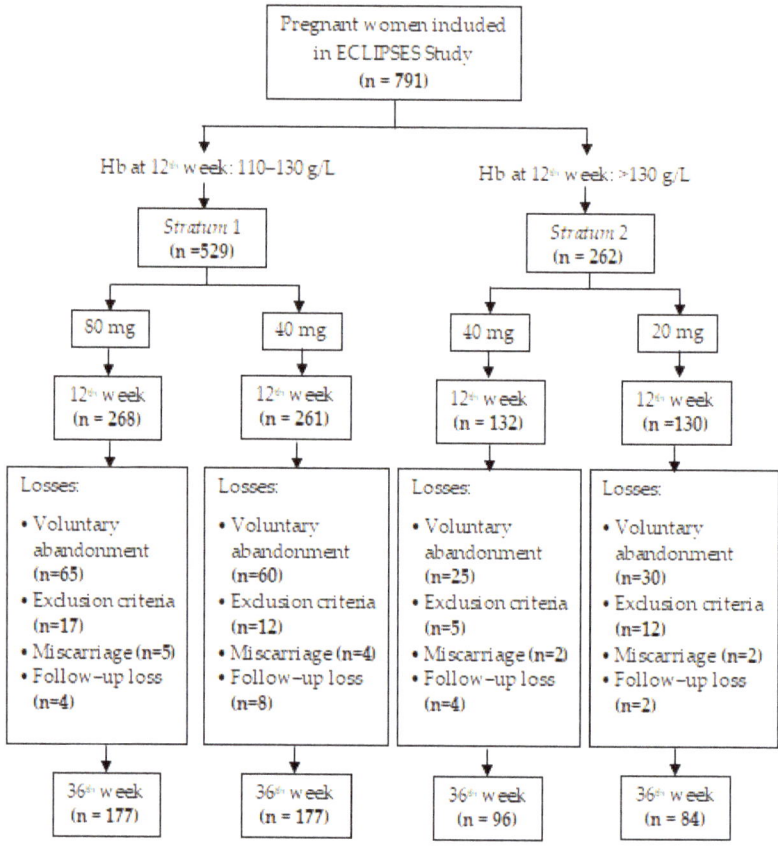

Figure 1. Flowchart of the study.

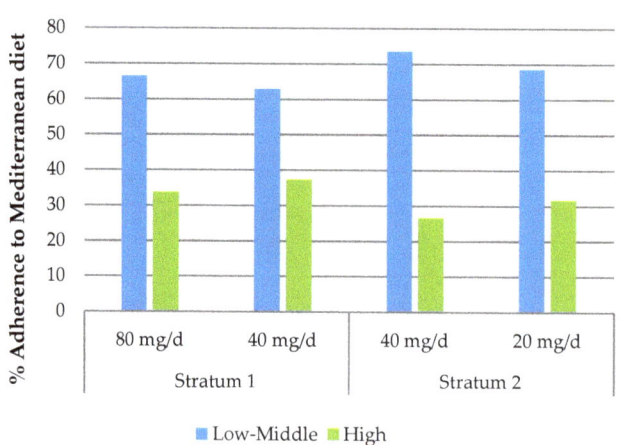

Figure 2. Adherence to the Mediterranean diet in the different groups of iron supplementation.

Table 1. Baseline characteristics of the study population.

	Stratum 1 (n = 529)		Stratum 2 (n = 262)		p
	Mean	SD	Mean	SD	
Age, years	30.40	5.07	30.21	5.28	0.613
Weight, Kg	64.83	11.31	67.17	13.60	0.017
Pre–pregnancy BMI, Kg/m^2	24.66	4.13	25.82	5.08	0.001
Gestational weight gain, Kg	11.11	8.17	9.69	9.47	0.030
	% (n)		% (n)		
Smoking	16.6 (88)		20.2 (53)		0.214
Parity	62.3 (329)		55.7 (146)		0.075
Planned pregnancy	79.8 (422)		80.5 (211)		0.801
Use of hormonal contraception	18.3 (97)		18.1 (47)		0.929
Pre–pregnancy BMI					
Underweight	1.3 (7)		2.3 (6)		0.314
Normal weight	60.9 (322)		51.5 (135)		0.012
Overweight	25.7 (136)		27.9 (73)		0.518
Obesity	12.1 (64)		18.3 (48)		0.018
HFE gene mutation	31.7 (130)		32.53 (68)		0.834
HFE genotype					
WT/WT	67.3 (280)		66.2 (141)		0.779
C282Y/WT	3.8 (16)		2.8 (6)		0.506
Carrier of H63D mutation	27.4 (114)		29.1 (62)		0.652
Carrier of S65C mutation	1.4 (6)		1.9 (4)		0.679
Family socioeconomic status					
Low	16.4 (87)		15.6 (41)		0.774
Middle	66.7 (353)		67.6 (177)		0.816
High	16.8 (89)		16.8 (44)		0.991
Maternal ethnic origin					
Caucasian	82.8 (405)		82.9 (203)		0.991
Asian	0.2 (1)		0.8 (2)		0.221
Arab	7.8 (38)		8.2 (20)		0.853
Black	1.8 (9)		0.4 (1)		0.114
Latin American	7.4 (36)		7.7 (19)		0.849
Adherence to Mediterranean diet					
Low–Middle	64.7 (342)		71.0 (186)		0.075
High	35.3 (187)		29.0 (76)		0.075

BMI: body mass index; WT: wild type. Sample size HFE genotype = 629; sample size maternal ethnic origin = 734.

We also performed a bivariate analysis comparing the percentage of women with and without risk of hemoconcentration on week 36 of gestation based on their initial Hb levels and HFE genotypes. As shown in Figure 3, we found that the H63D mutation in the HFE gene was significantly more prevalent among women from Stratum 2 (initial Hb levels > 130 g/L) who developed iron overload, compared with women who completed the pregnancy without risk of hemoconcentration (41.4% and 19.8%, respectively, $p = 0.045$). Similar results were obtained regarding the S65C mutation, which was observed in 6.9% of women who showed risk of hemoconcentration at the end of gestation, compared to 0.8% of women with normal Hb levels in the last trimester ($p = 0.031$). On the other hand, women with wild type (WT) genotype, i.e., without mutations in the HFE gene, were significantly more prevalent in the group from Stratum 2 who finished the pregnancy without risk of excess iron, than among women with Hb levels above 130 g/L on week 36 of gestation (74.6% and 51.7%, respectively, $p = 0.015$).

In Table 2 we describe and compare the blood tests results of women on weeks 12 and 36 of gestation among the intervention groups; a significant difference ($p = 0.042$) was observed in SF levels at week 36 between 80 and 40 mg/d iron in Stratum 1 (median: 17.19, IQR: 11.53, and median: 14.70, IQR: 9.37, respectively) in the non–adjusted bivariate analyses. Table 2 also shows that the prevalence of ID on week 36 was significantly higher ($p = 0.012$) in the group receiving 40 mg iron per day (51%)

than in women receiving 80 mg daily (38.2%). No other significant differences were observed between groups regarding prevalence of various iron states, although the risk of hemoconcentration in the third trimester of pregnancy showed a tendency to be higher among women who received 40 mg daily of iron (24%) than those receiving 20 mg of iron per day (13.1%). The same results were obtained in the per–protocol population (Table S2).

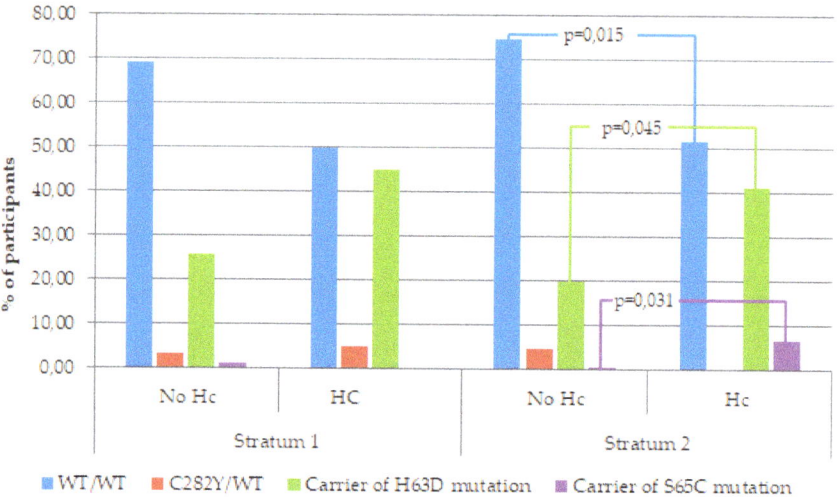

Figure 3. Percentage of women with and without risk of hemoconcentration (Hc) on week 36 of pregnancy, according to their initial hemoglobin (Hb) levels and *HFE* genotypes.

Multivariate analyses were performed to explore the effectiveness of iron dosages evaluated in Stratum 1 (80 mg/d and 40 mg/d) and Stratum 2 (40 mg/d and 20 mg/d), as well as the impact of several possible prenatal determinant factors. The results of the adjusted multivariate analyses for Stratum 1, summarized in Table 3, show that taking an iron supplement of 40 mg/d instead of 80 mg/d significantly reduced SF levels ($p = 0.026$) and doubled the risk of ID ($p = 0.022$) at the end of pregnancy. In contrast, the intervention with different doses of iron did not significantly change Hb levels ($p = 0.718$), the risk of anemia ($p = 0.166$), or IDA ($p = 0.299$). SF levels in early pregnancy were positively associated with Hb levels (β: 1.70; SE: 0.66; $p = 0.010$) and SF levels (β: 0.60, SE: 0.04, $p < 0.001$) in the third trimester. Additionally, maternal age 35 years and above increased SF in week 36 of pregnancy (β: 0.21; SE: 0.07; $p = 0.002$). Increasing early pregnancy levels of SF showed a protective effect against ID (OR: 0.29; 95%CI: 0.19–0.45; $p < 0.001$), anemia (OR: 0.54; 95%CI: 0.32–0.90; $p = 0.018$), and IDA (OR: 0.32; 95%CI: 0.17–0.59; $p < 0.001$). No differences were observed between the iron dosages evaluated in Stratum 1 in relation to the risk of hemoconcentration at week 36 of gestation after adjusting for possible confounders ($p = 0.481$). The adjusted multiple linear regression model for the risk of hemoconcentration was not statistically significant ($p = 0.071$). Moreover, in Stratum 1, when the regression models were performed separating women with and without ID on week 12 (Table 4), we observed that only in women with ID, the dose of 80 mg/d instead of 40 mg/d increased Hb levels in the third trimester (β: 8.81; SE: 2.40; $p = 0.001$), protecting women against anemia and IDA (OR: 0.03; 95%CI: 0.01–0.60; $p = 0.021$, for both cases).

Table 2. Blood tests results of participants on week 36 of gestation according to supplementation dose.

	Stratum 1			Stratum 2		
	80 g/d	40 g/d	p	40 g/d	20 g/d	p
		12th week				
Hemoglobin (g/L)	123.26 (5.32)	123.44 (4.77)	0.689	135.68 (4.59)	136.61 (4.44)	0.098
Serum ferritin (µg/L)	38.95 (26.10)	38.20 (25.05)	0.740	38.50 (28.98)	40.75 (30.00)	0.965
Mean corpuscular volume (fL)	87.08 (6.36)	87.30 (6.63)	0.696	88.53 (3.43)	88.54 (3.74)	0.980
C-reactive protein (mg/L)	0.73 (0.62)	0.74 (0.72)	0.815	0.72 (0.54)	0.70 (0.53)	0.779
Iron deficiency (%)	14.2 (38)	14.2 (37)	0.999	14.4 (19)	12.3 (16)	0.620
		36th week				
Hemoglobin (g/L)	117.63 (7.55)	117.21 (8.35)	0.622	123.07 (10.19)	121.04 (8.85)	0.157
Serum ferritin (µg/L)	17.19 (11.53)	14.70 (9.38)	0.042	11.10 (8.10)	11.00 (6.80)	0.798
Mean corpuscular volume (fL)	89.31 (6.87)	88.19 (12.06)	0.261	90.23 (4.19)	89.61 (4.11)	0.299
C-reactive protein (mg/L)	0.76 (0.74)	0.71 (0.64)	0.470	0.70 (0.69)	0.75 (0.56)	0.593
Iron deficiency (%)	38.2 (71)	51 (98)	0.012	66 (68)	69.7 (62)	0.590
Iron deficiency anemia (%)	8.5 (15)	9.6 (17)	0.711	7.3 (7)	11.9 (10)	0.291
Anemia (%)	11.9 (21)	13 (23)	0.747	8.3 (8)	11.9 (10)	0.426
Hemoconcentration (%)	6.8 (12)	7.9 (14)	0.684	24 (23)	13.1 (11)	0.063

Continuous variables expressed as means (SD), except for serum ferritin, which is expressed as median (interquartile range). Categorical variables expressed in percentages (n).

Table 3. The effects of the intervention with iron supplementation (40 or 80 mg/day) throughout pregnancy on hemoglobin and serum ferritin levels and on the risk of iron deficiency (ID), anemia, iron deficiency anemia (IDA), and hemoconcentration on the third trimester in women from Stratum 1.

Hemoglobin levels				
Independent variables	β	SE	p	Model
[a] Intervention (0:80 mg/d, 1:40 mg/d)	−0.42	0.85	0.622	$R^2 = -0.002$ $p = 0.622$
[b] Intervention (0:80 mg/d, 1:40 mg/d)	0.33	0.92	0.718	$R^2 = 0.031$ $p = 0.050$
Hemoglobin on week 12 of pregnancy	0.25	0.10	0.015	
Serum ferritin on week 12 of pregnancy	1.70	0.66	0.010	
Serum ferritin levels				
Independent variables	β	SE	p	Model
[a] Intervention (0:80 mg/d, 1:40 mg/d)	−0.10	0.06	0.085	$R^2 = 0.004$ $p = 0.085$
[c] Intervention (0:80 mg/d, 1:40 mg/d)	−0.12	0.05	0.026	$R^2 = 0.436$ $p < 0.001$
Serum ferritin on week 12 of pregnancy	0.60	0.04	<0.001	
Maternal age (0:25–34 years, 1:<25 years)	0.05	0.08	0.559	
Maternal age (0:25–34 years, 1:≥35 years)	0.21	0.07	0.002	
Iron deficiency (0:no, 1:yes)				
Independent variables	OR	95% CI	p	Model
[a] Intervention (0:80 mg/d, 1:40 mg/d)	1.69	1.12–2.54	0.012	R^2 Nagelkerke = 0.022 $p = 0.012$
[c] Intervention (0:80 mg/d, 1:40 mg/d)	1.82	1.09–3.03	0.022	R^2 Nagelkerke = 0.241 $p < 0.001$
Serum ferritin on week 12 of pregnancy	0.29	0.19–0.45	<0.001	
Anemia (0:no, 1:yes)				
Independent variables	OR	95% CI	p	Model
[a] Intervention (0:80 mg/d, 1:40 mg/d)	1.11	0.59–2.09	0.747	R^2 Nagelkerke = 0.001 $p = 0.747$
[b] Intervention (0:80 mg/d, 1:40 mg/d)	1.70	0.80–3.61	0.166	R^2 Nagelkerke = 0.146 $p = 0.027$
Planned pregnancy (0:no, 1:yes)	3.57	1.00–12.80	0.050	
Serum ferritin on week 12 of pregnancy	0.54	0.32–0.90	0.018	

Table 3. Cont.

Iron–deficiency anemia (0:no, 1:yes)				
Independent variables	OR	95% CI	p	Model
[a] Intervention (0:80 mg/d, 1:40 mg/d)	1.15	0.55–2.38	0.711	R^2 Nagelkerke = 0.001 $p = 0.711$
[b] Intervention (0:80 mg/d, 1:40 mg/d) Serum ferritin on week 12 of pregnancy	1.58 0.32	0.67–3.71 0.17–0.59	0.299 <0.001	R^2 Nagelkerke = 0.19 $p = 0.004$
Hemoconcentration (0:no, 1:yes)				
Independent variables	OR	95% CI	p	Model
[a] Intervention (0:80 mg/d, 1:40 mg/d)	1.18	0.53–2.63	0.684	R^2 Nagelkerke = 0.001 $p = 0.684$
[b] Intervention (0:80 mg/d, 1:40 mg/d) Genotype HFE (0:WT/WT, 1: carrier of H63D) Genotype HFE (0:WT/WT, 1: C282Y/WT) Parity (0:no, 1:yes)	1.44 3.28 1.93 0.26	0.52–3.97 0.09–6.68 0.21–18.02 0.09–0.76	0.481 0.026 0.566 0.014	R^2 Nagelkerke = 0.166 $p = 0.071$

a Crude model. b Adjusted for: iron supplementation dosage, maternal age, use of hormonal contraception, pre–pregnancy maternal body mass index, gestational weight gain, HFE genotypes, maternal ethnic origin, hemoglobin on week 12, serum ferritin on week 12, c–reactive protein on week 12, socioeconomic status, weekly mean METS on week 12, smoking habit, alcohol intake, planned pregnancy, parity, mean caloric intake during pregnancy, and adherence to a Mediterranean diet. c Adjusted for: model b, except for hemoglobin on week 12.

Table 4. The effect of the intervention with iron supplementation in Stratum 1 (0:80 mg/d, 1:40 mg/d) throughout pregnancy on maternal iron status on the third trimester, according to their initial iron stores.

SF < 15 µg/L				
Hemoglobin levels	β	SE	p	Model
Crude model	−7.06	2.43	0.006	$R^2 = 0.129$ $p = 0.006$
[a] Adjusted model	−8.81	2.40	0.001	$R^2 = 0.32$ $p = 0.003$
Iron deficiency (0:no, 1:yes)	OR	95% CI	p	Model
Crude model	3.10	0.93–10.39	0.066	R^2 Nagelkerke = 0.091 $p = 0.060$
[b] Adjusted model	4.51	0.78–26.08	0.092	R^2 Nagelkerke = 0.429 $p = 0.013$
Anemia (0:no, 1:yes)	OR	95% CI	p	Model
Crude model	5.50	1.05–28.75	0.043	R^2 Nagelkerke = 0.145 $p = 0.025$
[a] Adjusted model	29.14	1.67–508.56	0.021	R^2 Nagelkerke = 0.596 $p = 0.020$
Iron–deficiency anemia (0:no, 1:yes)	OR	95% CI	p	Model
Crude model	5.50	1.05–28.75	0.043	R^2 Nagelkerke = 0.145 $p = 0.025$
[a] Adjusted model	29.14	1.67–508.56	0.021	R^2 Nagelkerke = 0.596 $p = 0.020$
SF≥15 µg/L				
Hemoglobin levels	β	SE	p	Model
Crude model	0.75	0.88	0.395	$R^2 = -0.001$ $p = 0.395$
[a] Adjusted model	0.42	0.96	0.664	$R^2 = 0.035$ $p = 0.031$

a Adjusted for: iron supplementation dosage, maternal age, use of hormonal contraception, pre–pregnancy maternal body mass index, gestational weight gain, HFE gene genotypes, maternal ethnic origin, hemoglobin on week 12, c–reactive protein on week 12, socioeconomic status, weekly mean of METS on week 12, smoking habit, alcohol intake, planned pregnancy, parity, mean caloric intake during pregnancy, and adherence to Mediterranean diet. b Adjusted for: model a, except for hemoglobin on week 12.

Similarly, Table 5 shows the results of multivariate analyses performed after selecting women from Stratum 2. Adjusting for possible confounding factors, we found that a daily iron supplementation of 20 mg as opposed to 40 mg during pregnancy reduced the risk of hemoconcentration by 69% ($p = 0.035$) without increasing the risk of any iron deficit states studied at the end of pregnancy. Similarly to Stratum 1, higher SF levels on week 12 of gestation were positively correlated with SF levels (β: 0.42; SD: 0.06; $p < 0.001$) in the last months. Increasing SF levels in early pregnancy protected, therefore, against ID (OR: 0.36; 95%CI: 0.19–0.68; $p = 0.002$), anemia and IDA (OR: 0.26; 95%CI: 0.08–0.66; $p = 0.023$, for both cases). Furthermore, the analyses showed the effect of maternal age on iron status on week 36, with women under 25 years presenting reduced SF levels (β: −0.28; SE: 0.11; $p = 0.013$), and women 35 years and older at lower risk of ID (OR: 0.37; 95%CI: 0.16–0.91; $p = 0.029$) than women between 25 and 34 years of age. It was also found that the middle–high SES, compared with low SES, protected against anemia and IDA (OR: 0.06; 95%CI: 0.01–0.40; $p = 0.003$, for both cases) in women who started pregnancy with Hb levels above 130 g/L. Regarding iron overload, in addition to the aforementioned effect of the low iron dose, higher Hb levels early in pregnancy and being a carrier of the H63D mutation significantly increased Hb levels on week 36 (β: 0.72; SE: 0.16, and β: 3.93; SE: 1.74, respectively) and the risk of hemoconcentration (OR: 1.20; 95%CI: 1.08–1.33, and OR: 3.09; 95%CI: 1.10–8.71, respectively). When the multivariate analyses were applied to the sample of women from Stratum 2, categorized according their initial iron stores, we found that compared to 20 mg, 40 mg of iron per day increased SF on week 36 (β: 0.39; SE: 0.15; $p = 0.014$) only in women with iron deficiency, while 20 mg/d reduced the risk of hemoconcentration (OR: 0.25; 95%CI: 0.07–0.85; $p = 0.027$) in women with initial iron stores within the normal range (Table 6).

Table 5. The effects of the intervention with iron supplementation (40 or 20 mg/day) throughout pregnancy on hemoglobin and serum ferritin levels and on the risk of ID, anemia, IDA, and hemoconcentration on the third trimester in women from Stratum 2.

Hemoglobin levels				
Independent variables	β	SE	p	Model
[a] Intervention (0:40 mg/d, 1:20 mg/d)	−1.91	1.44	0.188	$R^2 = 0.004$ $p = 0.188$
[b] Intervention (0:40 mg/d, 1:20 mg/d) Genotype HFE (0:WT/WT, 1: carrier of H63D) Genotype HFE (0:WT/WT, 1: C282Y/WT) Hemoglobin on week 12 of pregnancy	−2.50 3.93 1.34 0.72	1.47 1.74 3.70 0.16	0.092 0.025 0.718 <0.001	$R^2 = 0.116$ $p = 0.003$
Serum ferritin levels				
Independent variables	β	SE	p	Model
[a] Intervention (0:40 mg/d, 1:20 mg/d)	0.02	0.07	0.734	$R^2 = -0.003$ $p = 0.734$
[c] Intervention (0:40 mg/d, 1:20 mg/d) Maternal age (0:25–34 years, 1:<25 years) Maternal age (0:25–34 years, 1:≥35 years) Serum ferritin on week 12 of pregnancy	0.01 −0.28 0.12 0.42	0.08 0.11 0.10 0.06	0.954 0.013 0.221 <0.001	$R^2 = 0.218$ $p < 0.001$
Low iron stores (0:no, 1:yes)				
Independent variables	OR	95% CI	p	Model
[a] Intervention (0:40 mg/d, 1:20 mg/d)	1.18	0.64–2.17	0.590	R^2 Nagelkerke = 0.002 $p = 0.590$
[c] Intervention (0:40 mg/d, 1:20 mg/d) Maternal age (0:25–34 years, 1:<25 years) Maternal age (0:25–34 years, 1:≥35 years) Serum ferritin on week 12 of pregnancy	1.45 3.07 0.37 0.36	0.69–3.02 0.78–12.12 0.16–0.91 0.19–0.68	0.326 0.109 0.029 0.002	R^2 Nagelkerke = 0.229 $p = 0.003$

Table 5. Cont.

Anemia (0:no, 1:yes)				
Independent variables	OR	95% CI	p	Model
[a] Intervention (0:40 mg/d, 1:20 mg/d)	1.48	0.56–3.96	0.428	R^2 Nagelkerke = 0.007 $p = 0.426$
[b] Intervention (0:40 mg/d, 1:20 mg/d) SES (0:low; 1:middle + high) Serum ferritin on week 12 of pregnancy	2.01 0.06 0.26	0.44–9.09 0.01–0.40 0.08–0.66	0.364 0.003 0.023	R^2 Nagelkerke = 0.468 $p = 0.002$
Iron–deficiency anemia (0:no, 1:yes)				
Independent variables	OR	95% CI	p	Model
[a] Intervention (0:40 mg/d, 1:20 mg/d)	1.78	0.62–4.74	0.295	R^2 Nagelkerke = 0.013 $p = 0.291$
[b] Intervention (0:40 mg/d, 1:20 mg/d) SES (0:low; 1:middle + high) Serum ferritin on week 12 of pregnancy	2.01 0.06 0.26	0.44–9.09 0.01–0.40 0.08–0.66	0.364 0.003 0.023	R^2 Nagelkerke = 0.468 $p = 0.002$
Hemoconcentration (0:no, 1:yes)				
Independent variables	OR	95% CI	p	Model
[a] Intervention (0:40 mg/d, 1:20 mg/d)	0.48	0.22–1.05	0.067	R^2 Nagelkerke = 0.031 $p = 0.060$
[b] Intervention (0:40 mg/d, 1:20 mg/d) Hemoglobin on week 12 of pregnancy Genotype HFE (0:WT/WT, 1: carrier of H63D) Genotype HFE (0:WT/WT, 1: C282Y/WT)	0.31 1.20 3.09 0.00	0.11–0.92 1.08–1.33 1.10–8.71 .	0.035 0.001 0.033 0.999	R^2 Nagelkerke = 0.282 $p = 0.004$

a Crude model. b Adjusted for: iron supplementation dosage, maternal age, use of hormonal contraception, pre–pregnancy maternal body mass index, gestational weight gain, HFE gene genotypes, maternal ethnic origin, hemoglobin on week 12, serum ferritin on week 12, c–reactive protein on week 12, socioeconomic status, weekly mean of METS on week 12, smoking habit, alcohol intake, planned pregnancy, parity, mean caloric intake during pregnancy, and adherence to a Mediterranean diet. c Adjusted for: model b, except for hemoglobin on week 12.

Table 6. The effect of the intervention with iron supplementation on Stratum 2 (0:40 mg/d, 1:20 mg/d) throughout pregnancy regarding maternal iron status in the third trimester, according to initial iron stores.

SF<15 µg/L				
Serum ferritin levels	β	SE	p	Model
Crude model	−0.24	0.14	0.083	$R^2 = 0.061$ $p = 0.083$
[b] Adjusted model	−0.39	0.15	0.014	$R^2 = 0.344$ $p = 0.021$
Iron deficiency (0:no, 1:yes)	OR	95% CI	p	Model
Crude model	6.11	0.60–62.23	0.126	R^2 Nagelkerke = 0.163 $p = 0.085$
[b] Adjusted model	42.09	0.00–50.00	0.614	R^2 Nagelkerke = 0.924 $p = 0.001$
SF≥15 µg/L				
Hemoglobin levels	β	SE	p	Model
Crude model	−1.75	1.54	0.260	$R^2 = 0.002$ $p = 0.260$
[a] Adjusted model	−2.00	1.56	0.200	$R^2 = 0.184$ $p < 0.001$

Table 6. Cont.

Serum ferritin levels	β	SE	p	Model
Crude model	0.06	0.08	0.455	$R^2 = -0.002$ $p = 0.455$
[b] Adjusted model	0.08	0.09	0.368	$R^2 = 0.077$ $p = 0.008$
Anemia (0:no, 1:yes)	OR	95% CI	p	Model
Crude model	1.34	0.43–4.20	0.611	R^2 Nagelkerke = 0.004 $p = 0.611$
[a] Adjusted model	1.02	0.20–5.10	0.984	R^2 Nagelkerke = 0.383 $p = 0.007$
Iron–deficiency anemia (0:no, 1:yes)	OR	95% CI	p	Model
Crude model	1.63	0.50–5.39	0.421	R^2 Nagelkerke = 0.010 $p = 0.417$
[a] Adjusted model	1.02	0.20–5.10	0.984	R^2 Nagelkerke = 0.383 $p = 0.007$
Hemoconcentration (0:no, 1:yes)	OR	95% CI	p	Model
Crude model	0.46	0.20–1.06	0.068	R^2 Nagelkerke = 0.035 $p = 0.061$
[a] Adjusted model	0.25	0.07–0.85	0.027	R^2 Nagelkerke = 0.261 $p = 0.001$

a Adjusted for: iron supplementation dosage, maternal age, use of hormonal contraception, pre–pregnancy maternal body mass index, gestational weight gain, *HFE* gene genotypes, maternal ethnic origin, hemoglobin on week 12, C–reactive protein on week 12, socioeconomic status, weekly mean of METS on week 12, smoking habit, alcohol intake, planned pregnancy, parity, mean caloric intake during pregnancy, and adherence to a Mediterranean diet. b Adjusted for: model a, except for hemoglobin on week 12.

In the multivariate analyses of Stratum 2, the results for the per–protocol and for the ITT populations were the same (Table S4); for Stratum 1, the regression models for Hb levels, anemia and IDA lost statistical significance when women who were anemic at mid–pregnancy were removed from the sample. However, the results about the effects on SF levels and ID were the same as for the ITT population (Table S3).

4. Discussion

Despite the wealth of research on prenatal iron supplementation, there is a lack of consensus on the optimal iron dosage in relation to the characteristics of each woman. Consequently, we were determined to investigate the effectiveness of different doses of iron supplementation on preventing iron deficiency and excess iron in the last trimester of gestation. To our knowledge, few publications address the interplay of early maternal iron status and the effect of prenatal iron supplementation [39].

Firstly, we observed that the prevalence of ID found in both strata of our study population (38.2%–69.70%) was in the range of the European estimates for pregnant women published in the most recent reports [2,3]; regarding the prevalence of anemia (8.3%–13%) and IDA (7.3%–11.9%), our results were considerably lower than the estimates of the same reports (24.5% and 35%, respectively). In relation to the risk of hemoconcentration, we observed that its prevalence (~13%) was similar to previous reports from Spain by Arija et al. [27] and within the wide range reported in European countries (8.7% to 42%) [26]. We should underscore that most research focuses on iron deficiency, and only few studies have described the prevalence of excess iron; consequently, the estimates on iron overload are less updated and not as established. As expected, we observed a significantly higher prevalence of risk of hemoconcentration in Stratum 2 (13.1% for 20 mg/d and 24% for 40 mg/d) than in Stratum 1 (6.8% for 80 mg/d and 7.9% for 40 mg/d) at the end of pregnancy. This difference supports our hypothesis that women with normal–high initial Hb levels were at greater risk of iron overload, possibly due to the persistent effect that genetic alterations in the *HFE* gene exert on iron levels [40,41]. Our results also show a higher prevalence of *HFE* gene mutations in women from Stratum 2 at risk of hemoconcentration on week 36, as opposed to the higher prevalence of the wild type genotype in women who finished the pregnancy without that risk (see Figure 2). This highlights the influence of the genetic alteration in the *HFE* gene on the risk of iron overload in women with initial Hb levels > 130 g/L. Moreover, within Stratum 2, we found that the percentage of women at risk of hemoconcentration on week 36 in the group of 20 mg of iron per day was fifty percent less than in the group receiving 40 mg daily (13.1% and 24%, respectively, $p = 0.063$), confirming our hypothesis that low iron doses are the best option in this case.

To clarify the effectiveness of different doses of prenatal iron supplementation on maternal iron status, the multivariate analyses were adjusted for several associated variables, including obstetric, biological, and socioeconomic conditions, as well as *HFE* gene genotype and iron–related blood parameters. In this regard, in women from Stratum 1 who began the gestation with Hb levels between 110 and 130 g/L, we observed that a daily dosage of 80 mg iron, as opposed to 40 mg, improved SF levels (b: 0.12, $p = 0.026$) and protected against ID (OR: 0.55, $p = 0.022$) at the end of pregnancy. Furthermore, when we explored the effect of iron supplementation in women within Stratum 1 according their initial iron reserves, we found that the higher dose of iron (80 mg/d) reduced the risk of anemia and IDA (OR: 0.03 and $p = 0.021$, for both cases) during the last months of gestation in women with iron–deficiency (SF < 15 µg/L, 14.2%) at the start of the pregnancy. In contrast, no significant effect was observed in women with SF ≥ 15 µg/L on week 12. These results respond to the physiological regulation of intestinal iron absorption in accordance with iron reserves, by which the body strongly regulates iron absorption when stores are sufficient [42,43]. On the contrary, and in agreement with Milman et al. [44], we did not find additional effects of high doses of iron in women with correct iron reserves at the beginning of the study. We can conclude that the usual prescribed dose of 40 mg daily would be effective in women with optimal initial iron reserves, but not in women with iron deficiency in early pregnancy.

On the other hand, in Stratum 2 (initial Hb levels >130 g/L), women who received a daily dosage of 20 mg iron, compared with the group that received 40 mg, reduced the risk of hemoconcentration in the third trimester (OR: 0.31, $p = 0.035$), without increasing the risk of iron deficit. In this case, we should underscore that the risk of iron overload trebles in carriers of the H63D mutation of the *HFE* gene (OR: 3.09, $p = 0.033$). Accordingly, we would advise to prescribe low doses of iron to women with normal–high Hb (>130 g/L) levels in early pregnancy. Interestingly, the baseline prevalence of ID was higher than expected in this group (13.4%); similarly to *Stratum* 1, the different doses produced different results regarding iron status, which varied in accordance with the initial iron stores. The protective effect of 20 mg iron per day against the risk of hemoconcentration (OR: 0.25, $p = 0.027$) was only observed in women with sufficient iron reserves in early pregnancy (SF ≥ 15 µg/L).

Based on these findings, we emphasize that iron supplementation during pregnancy should be adapted to the initial iron status of each woman, assessed not only by Hb levels but also by SF levels, to prevent both iron deficiency and iron overload at the end of gestation. These conclusions are in agreement with the valuable contributions of Milman et al. [45,46], Casanueva et al. [47], and Peña-Rosas and Viteri [26], who advocate adapting prenatal iron supplementation in view that both iron deficit and hemoconcentration have been associated with negative effects on maternal–child health [5–10,28–30].

Generally, in clinical practice only Hb levels are measured to monitor maternal iron status during pregnancy. However, while detecting anemia, Hb levels fail to diagnose ID. Our results show that the effects of iron supplementation vary as a function of initial iron reserves, indicating the importance of detecting ID at the beginning of the gestation. We advocate for the routine measurement of SF levels during antenatal checks. We also underscore that mutations in the *HFE* gene should be studied in women with normal–high Hb levels at the beginning of pregnancy to avoid excessive iron supply.

Indeed, in relation to this, it is known that there is a racial difference in the prevalence of alterations in the HFE gene, being greater in the populations of northern Europe than in the Mediterranean countries [24]. This adds even more weight to the premise that it is necessary to evaluate the individual characteristics of women to prescribe the most efficient prenatal iron supplementation in each case.

In this study, the multivariate analyses have also revealed some prenatal determinants of maternal iron status at the end of pregnancy. For instance, high SF levels on week 12 were associated with the increase of Hb and SF levels on week 36 in both strata, reducing the risk of all iron deficiency states: 71% and 64% lower risk of ID, 68% and 74% lower risk of IDA, and 46% and 74% lower risk of anemia for Stratum 1 and Stratum 2, respectively (see Tables 3 and 4). The results show that SF levels on week 36 increased with maternal age, and in Stratum 2, maternal age was also linked to the risk of ID in the third trimester of gestation, although to our knowledge, the underlying mechanism of this association is not yet elucidated. We found a protective role of middle–high SES against anemia and IDA (OR: 0.06, $p = 0.003$, for both cases), specifically in women from Stratum 2. This finding coincides with previous reports that conclude that low–income status is a risk factor for iron deficiency, presenting as ID, anemia and IDA, especially in developing countries [23,48,49]. This observation stresses that a low SES might be associated with less healthy lifestyles and under-attendance to antenatal care [50,51]. Also in agreement with other studies [40,52,53], we found that the H63D mutation in the HFE gene increased Hb levels (b: 3.93, $p = 0.025$) and trebled the risk of hemoconcentration (OR: 3.09, $p = 0.033$) on week 36. It is well established that mutations in the HFE gene are highly prevalent in Caucasian populations and that they are linked to iron overload [3,54]. It has been suggested that HFE gene mutations increase intestinal iron absorption [41,55]. In our study, therefore, the results suggest that the presence of some mutation in the HFE gene would increase iron absorption in women with initial Hb levels >130mg/L. Unexpectedly, maternal iron status was not significantly associated with diet in the multivariate analyses in any strata. Similarly, comparative analyses, including adherence to the Mediterranean diet failed to show significant differences between different supplementation groups. This result suggests that the diet was very similar among all the women in the study. Finally, the trend for a higher percentage of parity in Stratum 1 (62.3%) than in Stratum 2 (55.7%) suggests that previous births could weaken the iron status of women at the beginning of pregnancy. Interestingly, in the multivariate analyses parity seemed to reduce by 74% the risk of hemoconcentration in women of Stratum 1, but the results in the regression model were not statistically significant ($p = 0.071$).

Understanding that the prenatal iron supplementation has a different effect on maternal iron status at the end of pregnancy according to initial levels of Hb and SF could contribute to improving public health policies and to adapting clinical practices to the population groups at risk. Taking into consideration other associated prenatal determinants of maternal iron status can also improve antenatal care. In view of the evidence presented in this study, we emphasize firstly, the importance of full iron reserves before pregnancy, in preparation for the high cost of iron during gestation; and secondly, we recommend that clinicians adapt iron supplementation to the initial levels of Hb and iron reserves (see Figure 4). To assess the presence of genetic mutations in the HFE gene in women with normal–high Hb levels and full iron reserves at the beginning of pregnancy can help to reduce the risk of hemoconcentration in this group.

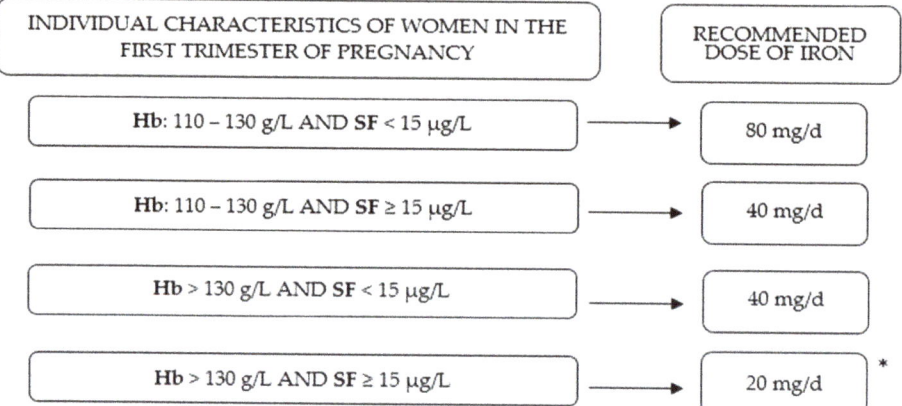

* In this group, it is recommended the determination of mutations in the HFE gene

Figure 4. Adaptation of prenatal iron supplementation according the individual characteristics of women in the first trimester of pregnancy.

Strengths and Limitations

The main strengths of the current community RCT are the large sample size ($n = 791$) and the extensive data collection regarding sociodemographic conditions, clinical information, obstetric data, and lifestyle, including diet and physical activity. In addition, testing for *HFE* gene mutations has added valuable information on the effect of genetic variability on iron metabolism and on the possible impact of personalized iron supplementation. Methodologically, we were able to evaluate the progression of iron status by monitoring blood parameters at different stages of pregnancy. However, some limitations must be taken into account when interpreting the findings of this study. Firstly, the notable dropout rate, although this is not uncommon in community interventions such as ours, which require several visits. No woman dropped out due to gastrointestinal side effects, since we used ferrimanitol ovalbumin instead of ferrous sulfate in our study. Another limitation was the lack of SF measurements in the 24th week of pregnancy, which would have strengthened the results. Since women gave birth in hospitals, data on maternal iron status at delivery were not available for inclusion.

5. Conclusions

In conclusion, we advise routine monitoring of Hb and SF during antenatal check–ups. These tools can be used in clinical practice to prescribe the optimal dose of iron supplements, with the ultimate aim of achieving the best pregnancy outcomes. In addition, the study of mutations in the *HFE* gene in women with normal–high Hb levels at the beginning of pregnancy could reduce the risk of hemoconcentration. Further studies are needed to assess the effect of mutations in the *HFE* gene on the maternal iron status and its interplay with prenatal iron supplementation to determine if there is a real need to use supplements in these cases. Future studies should also assess whether, in addition to the benefits for pregnant women, the supplementation with different doses of iron have benefits for their children.

Supplementary Materials: The following are available online at http://www.mdpi.com/2072-6643/11/10/2418/s1, Table S1: Baseline characteristics of the population lost trhought the study; Table S2: Biochemical characteristics of participants at 36th week of gestation according to dose of supplementation (by protocol); Table S3: Effect of the intervention with iron supplementation (40 or 80 mg/day) through pregnancy on hemoglobin and serum ferritin levels and on the risk of ID, anemia, IDA and hemoconcentration at third trimester in women from Stratum 1 (by protocol); Table S4: Effect of the intervention with iron supplementation (40 or 20 mg/day) through pregnancy on hemoglobin and serum ferritin levels and on the risk of ID, anemia, IDA and hemoconcentration at third trimester in women from Stratum 2 (by protocol).

Author Contributions: Conceptualization: V.A. and N.A.; data curation: L.I.V., N.A., E.A., and M.P.; formal analysis: L.I.V.; funding: V.A., N.A., E.A., N.S., and F.F.; investigation: L.I.V., V.A., N.A., E.A., N.S., F.F., F.R., and J.B.; project administration: V.A. and J.B.; resources: V.A., P.C., M.G., and J.B.; supervision: V.A.; data visualization: L.I.V.; writing (original draft): L.I.V.; writing (review and editing): L.I.V. and V.A.

Funding: This research was funded by the Health Research Fund of the Ministry of Health and Consumer Affairs (Madrid, Spain) (Instituto de Salud Carlos III, Fondo de Investigación Sanitaria, Ministerio de Sanidad y Consumo) with the grant number PI12/02777.

Acknowledgments: We thank to Meiji Pharma Spain S.A. –formerly Tedec-Meiji Farma S.A– (Pilar Coronel and Mercedes Gimeno) for logistic assistance and for providing free iron supplements. Research Group in Nutrition and Mental Health (NUTRISAM), Universitat Rovira i Virgili (Victoria Arija, Josepa Canals, Estefanía Aparicio, Núria Aranda, Cristina Bedmar, Carmen Hernández, Lucía Iglesias, Cristina Jardí and Núria Voltas). Sexual and Reproductive Health Care Services (ASSIR) of Tarragona, Spain (Francesc Fargas, Francisca Ruiz, Gemma March, Susana Abajo) and team of midwives recruiting for the study (Irene Aguilar, Sònia Aguiles, Rosa Alzúria, Judit Bertrán, Carmen Burgos, Elisabet Bru, Montserrat Carreras, Beatriz Fernández, Carme Fonollosa, María Leiva, Demetria Patricio, Teresa Pinto, María Ramírez, Eusebia Romano and Inés Sombreo). Jordi Gol University Institute for Primary Care Research (IDIAP) (Josep Basora and Meritxell Pallejà from the Research Unit in Tarragona; and Rosa Morros, Helena Pere and Anna García Sangenis from the Central Unit in Barcelona). Laboratory of the Institut Català de la Salut (Núria Serrat).

Conflicts of Interest: The authors declare no conflict of interest. The sponsors had no role in the design, execution, interpretation, or writing of the study.

References

1. De Benoist, B.; McLean, E.; Egli, I.; Cogswell, M. *Worldwide Prevalence of Anaemia 1993–2005: WHO Global Database on Anaemia*; WHO: Geneva, Switzerland, 2008.
2. World Health Organization. *The Global Prevalence of Anaemia in 2011*; WHO: Geneva, Switzerland, 2015.
3. Milman, N.; Taylor, C.L.; Merkel, J.; Brannon, P.M. Iron status in pregnant women and women of reproductive age in Europe. *Am. J. Clin. Nutr.* **2017**, *106*, 1655S–1662S. [CrossRef] [PubMed]
4. The Global Library of Women's Medicine. Available online: https://www.glowm.com/Critical_current_issue/page/25 (accessed on 22 May 2019).
5. Radlowski, E.C.; Johnson, R.W. Perinatal iron deficiency and neurocognitive development. *Front. Hum. Neurosci.* **2013**, *7*, 585. [CrossRef] [PubMed]
6. Hernández-Martínez, C.; Canals, J.; Aranda, N.; Ribot, B.; Escribano, J.; Arija, V. Effects of iron deficiency on neonatal behavior at different stages of pregnancy. *Early Hum. Dev.* **2011**, *87*, 165–169. [CrossRef] [PubMed]
7. Rahmati, S.; Azami, M.; Badfar, G.; Parizad, N.; Sayehmiri, K. The relationship between maternal anemia during pregnancy with preterm birth: A systematic review and meta-analysis. *J. Matern. Fetal Neonatal Med.* **2018**, 1–11. [CrossRef] [PubMed]
8. Figueiredo, A.C.M.G.; Gomes-Filho, I.S.; Silva, R.B.; Pereira, P.P.S.; Mata, F.A.F.D.; Lyrio, A.O.; Souza, E.S.; Cruz, S.S.; Pereira, M.G. Maternal anemia and low birth weight: A systematic review and meta–analysis. *Nutrients* **2018**, *10*, 601. [CrossRef] [PubMed]
9. Ribot, B.; Aranda, N.; Viteri, F.E.; Hernández-Martínez, C.; Canals, J.; Arija, V. Depleted iron stores without anaemia early in pregnancy carries increased risk of lower birthweight even when supplemented daily with moderate iron. *Hum. Reprod.* **2012**, *27*, 1260–1266. [CrossRef] [PubMed]
10. Vallée, L. Fer et neurodéveloppement. *Arch. Pediatr.* **2017**, *24*, 5S18–5S22. [CrossRef]
11. Todorich, B.; Pasquini, J.M.; Garcia, C.I.; Paez, P.M.; Connor, J.R. Oligodendrocytes and myelination: The role of iron. *Glia* **2009**, *57*, 467–478. [CrossRef] [PubMed]
12. Beard, J. Iron Deficiency alters brain development and functioning. *J. Nutr.* **2003**, *133*, 1468S–1472S. [CrossRef] [PubMed]
13. Abbaspour, N.; Hurrell, R.; Kelishadi, R. Review on iron and its importance for human health. *J. Res. Med. Sci.* **2014**, *19*, 164–174. [PubMed]
14. Gupta, C.P. Role of Iron (Fe) in Body. *IOSR J. Appl. Chem.* **2014**, *7*, 38–46. [CrossRef]
15. Marangoni, F.; Cetin, I.; Verduci, E.; Canzone, G.; Giovannini, M.; Scollo, P.; Corsello, G.; Poli, A. Maternal diet and nutrient requirements in pregnancy and breastfeeding. An Italian Consensus Document. *Nutrients* **2016**, *8*, 629. [CrossRef] [PubMed]

16. Bothwell, T. Iron requirements in pregnancy and strategies to meet them. *Am. J. Clin. Nutr.* **2000**, *72*, 257S–264S. [CrossRef] [PubMed]
17. Kominiarek, M.A.; Rajan, P. Nutrition recommendations in pregnancy and lactation. *Med. Clin. N. Am.* **2016**, *100*, 1199–1215. [CrossRef] [PubMed]
18. Piñero, D.J.; Connor, J.R. Iron in the brain: An important contributor in normal and diseased states. *Neuroscientist* **2000**, *6*, 435–453. [CrossRef]
19. Stevens, G.A.; Finucane, M.M.; De-Regil, L.M.; Paciorek, C.J.; Flaxman, S.R.; Branca, F.; Peña-Rosas, J.P.; Bhutta, Z.A.; Ezzati, M. Global, regional, and national trends in haemoglobin concentration and prevalence of total and severe anaemia in children and pregnant and non-pregnant women for 1995–2011: A systematic analysis of population–Representative data. *Lancet Glob. Heal.* **2013**, *1*, 16–25. [CrossRef]
20. Allen, L.H. Anemia and iron deficiency: Effects on pregnancy outcome. *Am. J. Clin. Nutr.* **2000**, *71*, 1280S–1284S. [CrossRef]
21. Ghio, A.J.; Hilborn, E.D.; Stonehuerner, J.G.; Dailey, L.A.; Carter, J.D.; Richards, J.H.; Crissman, K.M.; Foronjy, R.F.; Uyeminami, D.L.; Pinkerton, K.E. Particulate matter in cigarette smoke alters iron homeostasis to produce a biological effect. *Am. J. Respir. Crit. Care Med.* **2008**, *178*, 1130–1138. [CrossRef]
22. Miller, E.M. The reproductive ecology of iron in women. *Am. J. Phys. Anthropol.* **2016**, *159*, S172–S195. [CrossRef]
23. Balarajan, Y.; Ramakrishnan, U.; Özaltin, E.; Shankar, A.H.; Subramanian, S.V. Anaemia in low-income and middle-income countries. *Lancet* **2011**, *378*, 2123–2135. [CrossRef]
24. Beutler, E.; Felitti, V.; Gelbart, T.; Waalen, J. Haematological effects of the C282Y HFE mutation in homozygous and heterozygous states among subjects of northern and southern European ancestry. *Br. J. Haematol.* **2003**, *120*, 887–893. [CrossRef]
25. Gordeuk, V.R.; Brannon, P.M. Ethnic and genetic factors of iron status in women of reproductive age. *Am. J. Clin. Nutr.* **2017**, *106*, S1594–S1599. [CrossRef] [PubMed]
26. Peña-Rosas, J.P.; Viteri, F.E. Effects and safety of preventive oral iron or iron+folic acid supplementation for women during pregnancy. *Cochrane Database Syst. Rev.* **2009**, CD004736. [CrossRef]
27. Arija, V.; Ribot, B.; Aranda, N. Prevalence of iron deficiency states and risk of haemoconcentration during pregnancy according to initial iron stores and iron supplementation. *Public Health Nutr.* **2013**, *16*, 1371–1378. [CrossRef] [PubMed]
28. Rayman, M.P.; Barlis, J.; Evans, R.W.; Redman, C.W.G.; King, L.J. Abnormal iron parameters in the pregnancy syndrome preeclampsia. *Am. J. Obstet. Gynecol.* **2002**, *187*, 412–418. [CrossRef] [PubMed]
29. Gaillard, R.; Eilers, P.H.C.; Yassine, S.; Hofman, A.; Steegers, E.A.P.; Jaddoe, V.W.V. Risk factors and consequences of maternal anaemia and elevated haemoglobin levels during pregnancy: A population-based prospective cohort study. *Paediatr. Perinat. Epidemiol.* **2014**, *28*, 213–226. [CrossRef]
30. Aranda, N.; Hernández-Martínez, C.; Arija, V.; Ribot, B.; Canals, J. Haemoconcentration risk at the end of pregnancy: Effects on neonatal behaviour. *Public Health Nutr.* **2017**, *20*, 1405–1413. [CrossRef] [PubMed]
31. Aranda, N.; Ribot, B.; Viteri, F.E.; Cavallé, P.; Arija, V. Predictors of haemoconcentration at delivery: Association with low birth weight. *Eur. J. Nutr.* **2013**, *52*, 1631–1639. [CrossRef] [PubMed]
32. Arija, V.; Fargas, F.; March, G.; Abajo, S.; Basora, J.; Canals, J.; Ribot, B.; Aparicio, E.; Serrat, N.; Hernández-Martínez, C.; et al. Adapting iron dose supplementation in pregnancy for greater effectiveness on mother and child health: Protocol of the ECLIPSES randomized clinical trial. *BMC Pregnancy Childbirth* **2014**, *14*, 33. [CrossRef]
33. Aranda, N.; Ribot, B.; Garcia, E.; Viteri, F.E.; Arija, V. Pre-pregnancy iron reserves, iron supplementation during pregnancy, and birth weight. *Early Hum. Dev.* **2011**, *87*, 791–797. [CrossRef]
34. Trinidad Rodríguez, I.; Fernández Ballart, J.; Cucó Pastor, G.; Biarnés Jordà, E.; Arija Val, V. Validation of a short questionnaire on frequency of dietary intake: Reproducibility and validity. *Nutr. Hosp.* **2008**, *23*, 242–252.
35. Trichopoulou, A.; Costacou, T.; Bamia, C.; Trichopoulos, D. Adherence to a Mediterranean diet and survival in a Greek population. *N. Engl. J. Med.* **2003**, *348*, 2599–2608. [CrossRef] [PubMed]
36. Fagerström, K.O. Measuring degree of physical dependence to tobacco smoking with reference to individualization of treatment. *Addict. Behav.* **1978**, *3*, 235–241. [CrossRef]

37. Craig, C.L.; Marshall, A.L.; Sjöström, M.; Bauman, A.E.; Booth, M.L.; Ainsworth, B.E.; Pratt, M.; Ekelund, U.; Yngve, A.; Sallis, J.F.; et al. International physical activity questionnaire: 12-country reliability and validity. *Med. Sci. Sports Exerc.* **2003**, *35*, 1381–1395. [CrossRef] [PubMed]
38. Classificació catalana d'ocupacions 2011 (CCO–2011). Adaptació de la CNO–2011. Available online: https://www.idescat.cat/serveis/biblioteca/docs/cat/cco2011.pdf (accessed on 22 May 2019).
39. Brannon, P.M.; Taylor, C.L. Iron supplementation during pregnancy and infancy: Uncertainties and implications for research and policy. *Nutrients* **2017**, *9*, 1327. [CrossRef] [PubMed]
40. Aranda, N.; Viteri, F.E.; Montserrat, C.; Arija, V. Effects of C282Y, H63D, and S65C HFE gene mutations, diet, and life-style factors on iron status in a general Mediterranean population from Tarragona, Spain. *Ann. Hematol.* **2010**, *89*, 767–773. [CrossRef] [PubMed]
41. Philpott, C.C. Molecular aspects of iron absorption: Insights into the role of HFE in hemochromatosis. *Hepatology.* **2002**, *35*, 993–1001. [CrossRef]
42. Fisher, A.L.; Nemeth, E. Iron homeostasis during pregnancy. *Am. J. Clin. Nutr.* **2017**, *106*, S1567–S1574. [CrossRef]
43. Anderson, G.J.; Frazer, D.M. Current understanding of iron homeostasis. *Am. J. Clin. Nutr.* **2017**, *106*, S1559–S1566. [CrossRef]
44. Milman, N.; Bergholt, T.; Eriksen, L.; Byg, K.E.; Graudal, N.; Pedersen, P.; Hertz, J. Iron prophylaxis during pregnancy—How much iron is needed? A randomized dose-response study of 20–80 mg ferrous iron daily in pregnant women. *Acta Obstet. Gynecol. Scand.* **2005**, *84*, 238–247. [CrossRef]
45. Milman, N.; Byg, K.E.; Bergholt, T.; Eriksen, L.; Hvas, A.M. Body iron and individual iron prophylaxis in pregnancy—Should the iron dose be adjusted according to serum ferritin? *Ann. Hematol.* **2006**, *85*, 567–573. [CrossRef] [PubMed]
46. Milman, N. Oral iron prophylaxis in pregnancy: Not too little and not too much! *J. Pregnancy* **2012**, *2012*, 514345. [CrossRef]
47. Casanueva, E.; Viteri, F.E.; Mares-Galindo, M.; Meza-Camacho, C.; Loría, A.; Schnaas, L.; Valdés-Ramos, R. Weekly iron as a safe alternative to daily supplementation for nonanemic pregnant women. *Arch. Med. Res.* **2006**, *37*, 674–682. [CrossRef] [PubMed]
48. ACC/SCN. *Fourth Report on the World Nutrition Situation: Nutrition Throughout the Life Cycle*; ACC/SCN in collaboration with IFPRI: Geneva, Switzerland, 2000.
49. Alwan, N.A.; Hamamy, H. Maternal iron status in pregnancy and long-term health outcomes in the offspring. *J. Pediatr. Genet.* **2015**, *4*, 111–123. [PubMed]
50. Lindquist, A.; Kurinczuk, J.; Redshaw, M.; Knight, M. Experiences, utilisation and outcomes of maternity care in England among women from different socio-economic groups: Findings from the 2010 National Maternity Survey. *BJOG Int. J. Obstet. Gynecol.* **2015**, *122*, 1610–1617. [CrossRef] [PubMed]
51. Larson, C.P. Poverty during pregnancy: Its effects on child health outcomes. *Paediatr. Child. Health* **2007**, *12*, 673. [CrossRef] [PubMed]
52. Benyamin, B.; Esko, T.; Ried, J.S.; Radhakrishnan, A.; Vermeulen, S.H.; Traglia, M.; Gögele, M.; Anderson, D.; Broer, L.; Podmore, C.; et al. Novel loci affecting iron homeostasis and their effects in individuals at risk for hemochromatosis. *Nat. Commun.* **2014**, *5*, 4926. [CrossRef] [PubMed]
53. Adams, P.C.; Reboussin, D.M.; Barton, J.C.; McLaren, C.E.; Eckfeldt, J.H.; McLaren, G.D.; Dawkins, F.W.; Acton, R.T.; Harris, E.L.; Gordeuk, V.R.; et al. Hemochromatosis and iron-overload screening in a racially diverse population. *N. Engl. J. Med.* **2005**, *352*, 1769–1778. [CrossRef] [PubMed]
54. Hollerer, I.; Bachmann, A.; Muckenthaler, M.U. Pathophysiological consequences and benefits of HFE mutations: 20 years of research. *Haematologica* **2017**, *102*, 809–817. [CrossRef] [PubMed]
55. Nemeth, E.; Ganz, T. Regulation of iron metabolism by hepcidin. *Annu. Rev. Nutr.* **2006**, *26*, 323–342. [CrossRef]

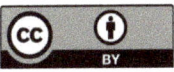

© 2019 by the authors. Licensee MDPI, Basel, Switzerland. This article is an open access article distributed under the terms and conditions of the Creative Commons Attribution (CC BY) license (http://creativecommons.org/licenses/by/4.0/).

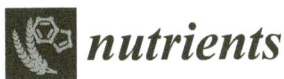

Article

Fermented Goat Milk Consumption Enhances Brain Molecular Functions during Iron Deficiency Anemia Recovery

Jorge Moreno-Fernández [1,2], Inmaculada López-Aliaga [1,2], María García-Burgos [1,2], María J.M. Alférez [1,2,*] and Javier Díaz-Castro [1,2]

1. Department of Physiology, Faculty of Pharmacy, Campus Universitario de Cartuja, E-18071 Granada, Spain; jorgemf@ugr.es (J.M.-F.); milopez@ugr.es (I.L.-A.); mariagb@ugr.es (M.G.-B.); javierdc@ugr.es (J.D.-C.)
2. Institute of Nutrition and Food Technology "José Mataix Verdú", University of Granada, E-18071 Granada, Spain
* Correspondence: malferez@ugr.es; Tel.: +34-958-243883

Received: 30 July 2019; Accepted: 18 September 2019; Published: 7 October 2019

Abstract: Iron deficiency anemia (IDA) is one of the most prevalent nutritional deficiencies worldwide. Iron plays critical roles in nervous system development and cognition. Despite the known detrimental consequences of IDA on cognition, available studies do not provide molecular mechanisms elucidating the role of iron in brain functions during iron deficiency and recovery with dairy components. In this study, 100 male Wistar rats were placed on a pre-experimental period of 40 days and randomly divided in two groups: a control group receiving a normal-Fe diet, (45 mg/kg), and an Fe-deficient group receiving a low-Fe diet (5 mg/kg). At day 40, 10 rats per group were sacrificed to anemia control, and 80 rats were divided into eight experimental groups fed with fermented goat or cow milk-based diets, with normal Fe content or Fe overload (450 mg/kg) for 30 days. IDA decreased most of the parameters related to brain molecular functions, namely dopamine, irisin, MAO-A, oxytocin, β-endorphin, and α-MSH, while it increased synaptophysin. These alterations result in an impairment of brain molecular functions. In general, during anemia recovery, fermented goat milk diet consumption increased dopamine, oxytocin, serotonin, synaptophysin, and α-MSH, and decreased MAO-A and MAO-B, suggesting a potential neuroprotective effect in brain functions, which could enhance brain molecular functions.

Keywords: iron deficiency anemia; fermented goat milk; brain molecular functions; neuroprotective effect

1. Introduction

Despite the global progress achieved in nutrition and science development, iron deficiency (ID) remains the most prevalent nutritional deficiency worldwide, affecting between 4–6 billion people. ID is also the main cause of anemia. Two billion people, more than 25% of the world's population, has manifestations of iron deficiency anemia (IDA) [1]. Among its many physiological functions, iron plays key roles in nervous system development and function, via biochemical processes involved in brain structure and functions. There are several studies on the effects of ID on brain development and functions [2,3], and on the link between iron status and cognitive function [4,5]. In this sense, iron is involved in the adequate myelination of the white matter, hippocampus development, and neurotransmitter homeostasis, with neurophysiological and behavioral outcomes showing relations to iron status at several life stages [6]. Behavioral performance and brain functions, as measured by electroencephalography, are sensitive to iron status [5].

Moreover, several studies showed that anemia may be associated with impairment in cerebral blood flow and oxygen metabolism, impaired cognitive function, confusion, loss of concentration, impaired memory, and low mental alertness [7]. Acute anemia results in the slowing of data-processing ability and memory impairment in humans [8]. In addition, cognitive ability is improved by erythropoietin [9].

Recent studies found several evidences that iron supplementation improved attention and concentration [5,10], as well as cognitive function [4]. These improvements in psychological symptoms appear to be mediated by an enhancement of oxygen transport to the brain [11].

In the scientific literature, raised awareness about the effects of nutrition on brain molecular functions exists, although few studies have examined the cognitive effects of fermented milks on cognitive function, and none of them linked to iron status. Currently, dairy products are increasingly consumed to prevent cognitive impairment and dementia [12]. Recent evidence suggests that the inclusion of dairy products in a balanced diet might have several positive effects on cognitive health in advanced age [13].

On the other hand, we have reported previously that fermented goat milk consumption is beneficial in IDA due to the improvement in the key proteins of intestinal iron metabolism, enhancing the digestive and metabolic utilization of iron, increasing iron deposits in target organs, and favoring the recovery of hematological parameters [14]. However, despite the known detrimental consequences of IDA on cognition, research linking iron status to brain functions has largely been ignored, and available studies are mainly focused on psychological tests evaluating cognitive function, concentration, memory, and alertness without providing molecular mechanisms elucidating the role of iron in brain functions during ID and recovery with dairy components. Hence, taking into account all these considerations, we set out to investigate the impact of fermented goat or cow milk-based diets (with normal or overload iron content) consumption during IDA recovery on the brain molecular functions in animal models.

2. Materials and Methods

2.1. Fermentation and Dehydration of the Milks

Fermented milks were prepared following the previously described method [15].

2.2. Animals

One hundred male *Wistar* albino breed rats (3 weeks of age and weighing about 34.56 ± 6.35 g) were included in this study. Experimental procedures were carried out in agreement with the guidelines about animal welfare and experimentation (Declaration of Helsinki; Directive 2010/63/EU).

Individual, ventilated, and thermos-regulated cages were used to randomly allocate the rats.

The room temperature (22.5 °C), humidity (60%), and a 12-h light-dark cycle were automatically controlled. Animal weight was taken as a variable factor, and numbers randomly assigned were generated (Microsoft Excel, 2016 (Microsoft, Redmond, WA, USA). Subsequently, the mean of the 100 weights were compared by a one-way ANOVA. The groups were formed to obtain a probability level of $p = 0.09$. The animals of each group had initial weights of 34.28 ± 5.12 g, 34.39 ± 5.01 g, 36.27 ± 4.58 g, 35.23 ± 6.12 g, 36.13 ± 6.37 g, 35.29 ± 6.01 g, 36.13 ± 5.13 g, 37.92 ± 6.21 g, 33.88 ± 6.11 g and 35.53 ± 5.76 g ($p > 0.05$), respectively. Diet intake was controlled, pair feeding all the animals, and bidistilled water was available ad libitum.

2.3. Experimental Design

Figure 1 features the experimental design of the study. During the pre-experimental period (PEP), ($n = 100$) rats were divided into two groups: the control group receiving the AIN 93G diet with a normal Fe diet ($n = 50$, 44.8 mg/kg by analysis) [16], and the anemic group receiving the same diet, but with a low Fe content ($n = 50$, 6.1 mg/kg by analysis), induced experimentally during 40 days by a method developed previously by our research group [17]. On day 40 of the study, 2 aliquots of blood were collected from the caudal vein of each rat. One of them had Ethylenediaminetetraacetic acid (EDTA) to measure all the hematological parameters, and the other one was centrifuged (1500× g,

4 °C, 15 min) without anticoagulant to separate the serum and subsequent analysis of serum iron, total iron-binding capacity (TIBC), ferritin, and hepcidin.

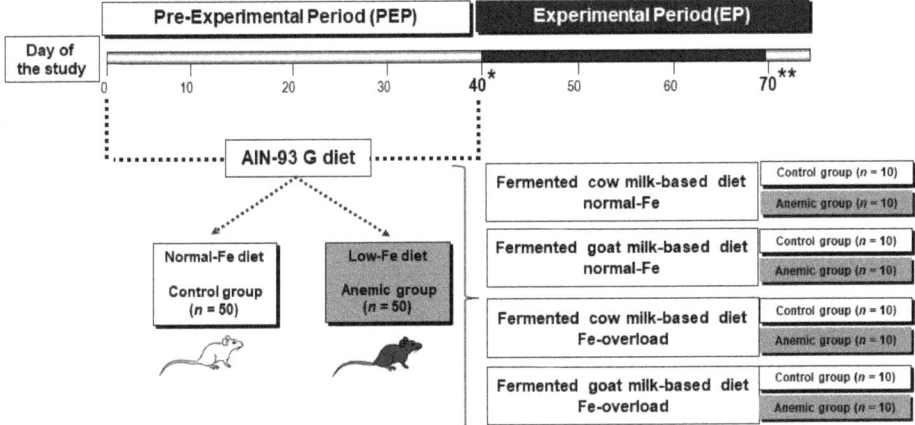

Figure 1. The study experimental design. * 10 control and 10 anemic rats were totally bled out by cannulation of the abdominal aorta. ** 80 animals were totally bled out by cannulation of the abdominal aorta. AIN-93 G diet, Standard diet from the American Institute of Nutrition (for the growth phase).

When the induction of the anemia period finalized (day 40 of the study), 10 rats per group were sacrificed, and the remaining 80 animals subsequently started the experimental period (EP) in which the control ($n = 40$) and anemic groups ($n = 40$) were further fed for 30 days with a fermented cow milk or fermented goat milk-based diet, with normal Fe content (45 mg·kg^{-1}) or Fe overloaded content (450 mg·kg^{-1}) to induce chronic Fe overload [18] prepared with fermented cow or goat milk, as previously reported [14].

At the end of the PEP and the end of EP, 20 and 80 animals respectively were anesthetized intraperitoneally with sodium pentobarbital (Sigma-Aldrich Co., St. Louis, MO, USA) and totally bled out. Blood aliquots with EDTA were analyzed to measure the hematological parameters, and the rest of the blood was centrifuged (1500× g, 4 °C, 15 min) without anticoagulant to separate the red blood cells from the serum and to determine the parameters related to iron status. The brain was removed immediately, weighed, and was split into two portions (which included parts of both hemispheres) and placed on cold saline buffer. Brain samples were homogenized in phosphate-buffered saline (PBS), pH 7.4 by the homogenizer. Protease inhibitor cocktail (Sigma-Aldrich Co., St. Louis, MO, USA) was used. The homogenate was centrifuged at 2000× g for 15 min at 4 °C. Thereafter, supernatants were divided into aliquots, and were stored at −80 °C for further analysis of parameters related to brain molecular functions. The remaining part was frozen in liquid nitrogen and immediately stored at −80 °C. This aliquot was used for precipitation with acetonitrile to proceed the neuropeptide assessment with Milliplex MAP assay.

2.4. Hematological Test

The hematological parameters were measured using an automated hematology analyzer Sysmex K-1000D (Sysmex, Tokyo, Japan).

2.5. Iron Assessments

Serum iron, total iron-binding capacity (TIBC), and transferrin saturation were determined using Sigma Diagnostics Iron and TIBC reagents (Sigma, St Louis, MO, USA). Concentrations of serum ferritin (µg·L^{-1}) and serum hepcidin (Hepcidin-25 ng·mL^{-1}) were determined using a rat ELISA Kit

(Biovendor GmbH, Heidelberg, Germany) for TIBC and another commercial kit for serum ferritin (DRG Instruments GmbH, Marburg, Germany).

2.6. Dopamine

Dopamine levels in brain homogenate were measured using a commercial enzyme immunoassay kit (MyBioSource, San Diego, CA, USA). Once the tissues were homogenized, the resulting suspension was subjected to ultrasonication. After that, the homogenates were centrifugated for 15 min at $1500\times g$. Measurements in duplicate were used to determine intra-assay variability.

2.7. Serotonin

The level of serotonin in brain homogenate was determined using a commercially available enzyme immunoassay ELISA Kit (MyBioSource, San Diego, CA, USA). One hundred microliters of the homogenate were added to duplicate wells in the ELISA plate, which was then processed according to the directions of the manufacturer.

2.8. MAO-A and MAO-B

To determine monoamine oxidase A and B (MAO-A and MAO-B) brain homogenate levels, a commercial rat ELISA kit was performed (Wuhan Fine Biological Technology Co., Ltd., Wuhan, China). After brain homogenization, the resulting suspension was sonicated with an ultrasonic cell disrupter to break the cell membranes. After that, the homogenates were centrifugated for 5 min at $5000\times g$. Then, the concentration of MAO-A and MAO-B was determined by measuring the absorbance at 450 nm (Bio-tek, Winooski, VT, USA).

2.9. Irisin

Irisin levels in brain homogenate were measured using a commercial kit (Wuhan Fine Biological Technology Co., Ltd., Wuhan, China). To further break the cells, the homogenate suspension was sonicated with an ultrasonic cell disrupter. The homogenates were then centrifuged for 5 min at $5000\times g$, and absorbance from each sample was measured in duplicate using a spectrophotometric microplate reader at a wavelength of 450 nm (Bio-tek, Winooski, VT, USA).

2.10. Synaptophysin

Synaptophysin in brain homogenate was measured using a commercial ELISA kit (USCN Life Science, Euromedex, Souffelweyersheim, France). After addition of the substrate solution, the intensity of color developed is reverse proportional to the concentration of synaptophysin in the sample. Plates were read spectrophotometrically (Bio-tek, Winooski, VT, USA) at 450 nm.

2.11. Neuropeptides Assessment

α-Melanocyte-stimulating hormone (α-MSH), β-endorphin, neurotensin, oxytocin, and substance P on acetonitrile-precipitated brain homogenate extracts were determined, using the RMNPMAG-83K Milliplex MAP Rat Neuropeptide Magnetic Bead Panel (Millipore Corporation, City, TX, USA). The plate was read on a LABScan 100 analyzer (Luminex Corporation, Austin, TX, USA) with xPONENT software (Luminex Corporation, Austin, TX, USA) for data acquisition. Neuropeptides on acetonitrile-precipitated brain homogenate extracts were determined by comparing the mean of duplicate samples with the standard curve for each assay.

2.12. Statistical Analysis

These analyses were carried out using the SPSS computer program (version 24.0, 2016, SPSS Inc., Chicago, IL, USA). To test differences between groups (normal Fe versus low Fe) during the PEP, Student's *t* test was used. Individual means were tested by pairwise comparison with Tukey's multiple comparison test when main effects and their interactions were significant. Two-way ANOVA was performed to determine the effects of type of diet, anemia, and iron content in the diet. $p < 0.05$ was set as significant.

3. Results

Iron deprivation during the pre-experimental period markedly decreased all the hematological parameters in the anemic group compared to the controls ($p < 0.001$); meanwhile, red cell distribution width, platelets count, total iron-binding capacity, and hepcidin were higher ($p < 0.001$), and the white blood cell count remained unchanged (Table 1).

Table 1. Hematological parameters from control and anemic rats (pre-experimental period).

	Normal-Fe Control Group ($n = 50$)	Low-Fe Anemic Group ($n = 50$)
Hemoglobin concentration (g·L^{-1})	130.62 ± 2.77	60.46 ± 2.77 *
Red blood cells (10^{12}·L^{-1})	7.11 ± 0.22	3.19 ± 0.30 *
Hematocrit (%)	41.13 ± 1.03	13.12 ± 1.33 *
Mean corpuscular volume (fL)	54.92 ± 0.52	37.21 ± 0.37 *
Mean corpuscular hemoglobin (pg)	20.01 ± 0.15	14.22 ± 0.53 *
Mean corpuscular hemoglobin concentration (g·dL^{-1})	36.12 ± 0.37	30.56 ± 0.73 *
Red cell distribution width (%)	16.33 ± 0.45	19.67 ± 0.35 *
Platelets (10^9·L^{-1})	731 ± 70.11	2123 ± 112 *
White blood cells (10^9·L^{-1})	8.32 ± 0.41	8.45 ± 0.59
Lymphocytes (10^6·mL^{-1})	7.76 ± 0.51	5.62 ± 0.77 *
Fe (µg·L^{-1})	1342 ± 97.31	607 ± 55.22 *
Total iron-binding capacity (µg·L^{-1})	2623 ± 179	18002 ± 539 *
Transferrin saturation (%)	49.22 ± 5.86	4.01 ± 0.45 *
Ferritin (µg·L^{-1})	79.54 ± 2.23	49.12 ± 1.58 *
Hepcidin (ng·mL^{-1})	13.25 ± 0.32	15.42 ± 0.68 *

Data are shown as the mean values ± Standard error of the mean. * Significantly different from the control group ($p < 0.001$, Student's t test).

With both fermented milk-based diets, the hematological parameters showed a recovery after supplying the normal-Fe or Fe-overload fermented milk-based diets (EP). Serum hepcidin decreased in control and anemic animals fed fermented goat milk (normal iron content or Fe overload) in comparison with fermented cow milk ($p < 0.001$). Serum iron increased in the Fe-overload groups in all experimental conditions ($p < 0.01$). Fe overload also increased hemoglobin ($p < 0.001$), hematocrit ($p < 0.01$), total iron-binding capacity ($p < 0.01$), transferrin saturation ($p < 0.01$), and serum ferritin ($p < 0.01$) (Table 2).

IDA decreased most of the parameters related to brain molecular functions, namely dopamine ($p < 0.05$), MAO-A, oxytocin, irisin, α-MSH, and β-endorphin ($p < 0.001$), while it increased synaptophysin ($p < 0.001$) (Table 3).

With regard to the brain molecular function parameters studied after IDA recovery (EP), Table 4 shows that 30 days after supplying the fermented milk-based diets, fermented goat milk consumption increased dopamine in both groups of animals with normal Fe with respect to fermented cow milk ($p < 0.01$), while it decreased this parameter in the Fe-overload control animals ($p < 0.01$). Fermented goat milk decreased MAO-A in both groups of animals: those in the Fe-overload group ($p < 0.001$) and in the control group fed normal Fe ($p < 0.05$). It also decreased the MAO-B in both groups of animals fed fermented goat milk with normal Fe ($p < 0.001$) levels. Synaptophysin increased in all the groups fed fermented goat milk either, with normal Fe or Fe overload ($p < 0.001$ for the control groups, and ($p < 0.01$ for the anemic groups, except for anemic animals fed fermented goat milk with normal Fe, in which we observed a reduction ($p < 0.01$). α-MSH increased in all the groups fed fermented goat milk ($p < 0.001$ for normal Fe and $p < 0.01$ for Fe overload).

Table 2. Hematological parameters from control and anemic rats fed for 30 days with fermented cow or goat milk-based diets with normal Fe content or Fe overload ($n = 10$ animals per group).

	Fe Content	Fermented Cow Milk Diet		Fermented Goat Milk Diet		Two-Way ANOVA		
		Control Group	Anemic Group	Control Group	Anemic Group	Diet	Anemia	Fe Content
Hemoglobin concentration (g·L^{-1})	Normal	127.73 ± 2.35	128.42 ± 2.43	131.91 ± 2.44	130.01 ± 2.39	NS[1]	NS	<0.001
	Overload	141.97 ± 2.53 [C]	140.18 ± 2.87 [C]	141.43 ± 2.77 [C]	145.62 ± 2.92 [BC]	<0.05	NS	
Red blood cells (10^{12}·L^{-1})	Normal	7.21 ± 0.18	7.16 ± 0.20	7.35 ± 0.22	7.32 ± 0.19	NS	NS	<0.05
	Overload	7.01 ± 0.19	7.19 ± 0.19	8.12 ± 0.28 [AC]	7.21 ± 0.22	<0.01	NS	
Hematocrit (%)	Normal	40.22 ± 1.12	39.22 ± 1.01	41.87 ± 1.41 [A]	43.05 ± 1.11 [B]	<0.01	NS	<0.01
	Overload	39.87 ± 1.25	45.11 ± 2.34 [C]	44.75 ± 1.51 [AC]	44.91 ± 1.41 [C]	<0.05	NS	
Mean corpuscular volume (fL)	Normal	57.28 ± 0.54	55.28 ± 0.53	57.41 ± 0.57	55.22 ± 0.54	NS	NS	NS
	Overload	56.90 ± 0.60	53.39 ± 0.54	56.62 ± 0.54	56.33 ± 0.51 [B]	<0.05	NS	
Platelets (10^9·L^{-1})	Normal	935.62 ± 72.11	961.53 ± 67.33	929.21 ± 78.11	937.32 ± 68.53	NS	NS	NS
	Overload	939.22 ± 71.24	963.29 ± 70.21	936.12 ± 79.76	942.12 ± 70.25	NS	NS	
Serum Fe (µg·L^{-1})	Normal	1323 ± 81.88	1347 ± 85.33	1362 ± 88.22	1332 ± 91.13	NS	NS	<0.01
	Overload	1576 ± 98.56 [C]	1592 ± 96.25 [C]	1552 ± 97.89 [C]	1569 ± 95.76 [C]	NS	NS	
Total iron-binding capacity (µg·L^{-1})	Normal	2782 ± 153	2788 ± 142	2791 ± 143	2786 ± 152	NS	NS	<0.01
	Overload	3151 ± 167 [C]	3234 ± 171 [C]	3241 ± 166 [C]	3188 ± 169 [C]	NS	NS	
Transferrin saturation (%)	Normal	46.22 ± 0.91	45.50 ± 0.87	46.79 ± 0.78	46.89 ± 0.91	NS	NS	<0.01
	Overload	47.85 ± 1.21 [C]	47.62 ± 1.12 [C]	48.96 ± 1.11 [C]	48.79 ± 1.07 [C]	NS	NS	
Serum ferritin (µg·L^{-1})	Normal	83.11 ± 1.56	83.77 ± 1.29	84.31 ± 1.65	82.24 ± 1.82	NS	NS	<0.01
	Overload	86.95 ± 1.88 [C]	85.98 ± 1.76 [C]	86.96 ± 1.83 [C]	87.03 ± 1.79 [C]	NS	NS	
Serum hepcidin (ng·mL^{-1})	Normal	16.21 ± 0.61	16.37 ± 0.53	14.11 ± 0.58 [A]	14.33 ± 0.61 [B]	<0.01	NS	NS
	Overload	16.42 ± 0.58	16.39 ± 0.51	15.07 ± 0.58 [A]	14.22 ± 0.57 [B]	<0.01	NS	

Data are shown as the mean values ± SEM. [1] NS, not significant. [A] Mean values from control group fed with fermented cow milk diet were significantly different ($p < 0.05$, Tukey's test). [B] Mean values from the anemic group fed with fermented cow milk diet were significantly different ($p < 0.05$, Tukey's test). [C] Mean values from the corresponding group fed with normal Fe content were significantly different ($p < 0.05$, Tukey's test).

Table 3. Brain molecular function parameters in brain homogenate (pg mL^{-1}) from control and anemic rats (pre-experimental period).

	Normal-Fe Control Group ($n = 10$)	Low-Fe Anemic Group ($n = 10$)
Dopamine	1970.00 ± 180.21	1560.01 ± 90.05 *
Serotonin	9179.0 ± 174.9	9409.0 ± 1813.5
MAO-A	7856.3 ± 225.2	6622.3 ± 212.7 **
MAO-B	267.96 ± 25.85	219.85 ± 10.81
Neurotensin	513.40 ± 48.18	442.61 ± 37.63
Oxytocin	249.71 ± 21.22	181.85 ± 17.86 **
Irisin	21.17 ± 1.19	16.74 ± 0.90 **
Synaptophysin	771.79 ± 36.97	1121.37 ± 28.62 **
α-MSH	616.34 ± 20.52	200.58 ± 44.29 **
β-Endorphin	2431.5 ± 126.0	1308.3 ± 186.6 **

Data are shown as the mean values ± SEM. Significantly different from the control group (* $p < 0.05$, ** $p < 0.001$, Student's t test). MAO, Monoamine oxidase; α-MSH, α-Melanocyte-stimulating hormone.

Anemia decreased the dopamine in animals fed fermented goat or cow milk with Fe overload ($p < 0.05$ and $p < 0.001$ respectively), MAO-A and MAO-B in the animals fed fermented cow milk ($p < 0.001$ for normal Fe and $p < 0.05$ for Fe overload), and goat milk with Fe overload ($p < 0.001$ MAO-A and $p < 0.05$ MAO-B). Anemia increased neurotensin in the normal-Fe groups fed fermented cow milk ($p < 0.001$). Oxytocin increased in the anemic animals fed fermented cow milk with normal Fe ($p < 0.01$), and decreased in animals fed both types of fermented milk with Fe overload ($p < 0.001$). Serotonin increased in anemic animals fed both milk-based diets with normal Fe ($p < 0.001$) in comparison with control animals. Synaptophysin increased in the anemic animals fed fermented cow milk ($p < 0.01$), and decreased in the anemic animals fed fermented goat milk ($p < 0.001$) in both normal and Fe overload. Anemia decreased α-MSH levels in all the groups fed both milk-based diets either with normal Fe or Fe overload ($p < 0.001$). Anemia decreased β-endorphin levels in the animals fed both fermented milks with normal Fe ($p < 0.001$) (Table 4).

Fe overload increased dopamine levels in both groups of animals fed fermented cow milk diet ($p < 0.01$), and increased MAO-A levels in the control groups fed both milk-based diets ($p < 0.001$), while it decreased this parameter in the anemic group fed fermented goat milk ($p < 0.001$). Fe overload also increased MAO-B levels in all the groups fed both types of fermented milk ($p < 0.01$), except for the anemic groups fed fermented cow milk. Fe overload increased neurotensin in the control group fed fermented cow milk ($p < 0.01$), and decreased this parameter in the anemic group fed the same diet ($p < 0.01$). For the mice in the Fe-overload groups, oxytocin increased in control animals fed both fermented milk diets ($p < 0.01$) and decreased in anemic animals fed both fermented milk diets ($p < 0.001$). Fe overload caused a marked reduction in serotonine levels in control and anemic rats fed both milk-based diets ($p < 0.001$). Synaptophysin decreased in the control groups and anemic rats fed fermented cow milk ($p < 0.001$), and increased in the animals fed fermented goat milk ($p < 0.001$). Fe overload increased α-MSH levels in the groups fed fermented cow milk ($p < 0.001$), and decreased this hormone in the groups fed fermented goat milk ($p < 0.01$). β-Endorphin decreased in the control animals fed fermented cow or goat milk with Fe overload ($p < 0.001$) (Table 4).

Table 4. Brain molecular function parameters in brain homogenate (pg mL^{-1}) from control and anemic rats fed for 30 days with fermented cow or goat milk-based diets with normal Fe content or Fe overload (n = 10 animals per group).

	Fe Content	Fermented Cow Milk Diet		Fermented Goat Milk Diet		Two-Way ANOVA		
		Control Group	Anemic Group	Control Group	Anemic Group	Diet	Anemia	Fe Content
Dopamine	Normal	1210.00 ± 40.01	980.14 ± 30.07	1710.10 ± 16.07 [A]	1320.11 ± 11.23 [B]	<0.01	NS	<0.05
	Overload	3130.02 ± 22.14 [D]	1440.21 ± 30.12 [CD]	1400.02 ± 60.04 [A]	1260 ± 40.33 [C]	<0.01	<0.01	
Serotonin	Normal	33651.9 ± 3334.5	61341.9 ± 5820.1 [C]	39278.9 ± 4571.7	82050.5 ± 2995.1 [BC]	<0.05	<0.001	<0.001
	Overload	26346.4 ± 2943.3 [D]	29564.3 ± 2806.3 [D]	20981.4 ± 852.7 [D]	23688.0 ± 962.7 [D]	NS	NS	
MAO-A	Normal	8220.1 ± 261.5	7279.3 ± 298.6 [C]	7390.3 ± 211.9 [A]	6716.7 ± 483.3 [B]	<0.05	<0.05	<0.01
	Overload	13935.1 ± 282.3 [D]	7152.6 ± 498.0 [C]	8403.7 ± 353.4 [AD]	4001.8 ± 168.3 [BCD]	<0.001	<0.001	
MAO-B	Normal	260.96 ± 10.81	237.89 ± 11.57 [C]	215.13 ± 10.10 [A]	208.93 ± 10.07 [B]	<0.001	<0.05	<0.01
	Overload	327.70 ± 9.56 [D]	259.96 ± 6.68 [C]	305.24 ± 9.01 [D]	267.52 ± 7.90 [CD]	NS	<0.01	
Neurotensin	Normal	317.98 ± 11.94	405.37 ± 18.23 [C]	336.36 ± 21.37	373.21 ± 10.15	NS	<0.05	<0.05
	Overload	360.77 ± 12.67 [D]	345.61 ± 12.80 [D]	355.79 ± 10.39	341.56 ± 9.98	NS	NS	
Oxytocin	Normal	145.57 ± 9.27	173.42 ± 33.90 [C]	182.41 ± 7.27 [A]	177.74 ± 1.87	<0.05	<0.05	<0.001
	Overload	217.27 ± 3.58 [D]	86.95 ± 0.13 [CD]	225.52 ± 3.94 [D]	89.85 ± 1.57 [CD]	NS	<0.01	
Irisin	Normal	16.75 ± 0.70	15.96 ± 0.35	19.18 ± 1.26	17.24 ± 1.03	NS	NS	NS
	Overload	19.32 ± 0.60	16.66 ± 0.85	17.58 ± 0.79	15.64 ± 0.70	NS	NS	
Synaptophysin	Normal	836.97 ± 31.40	907.33 ± 27.57 [C]	1091.02 ± 26.92 [A]	730.09 ± 20.44 [BC]	<0.001	<0.01	<0.001
	Overload	552.01 ± 40.56 [D]	789.02 ± 49.59 [CD]	1290.56 ± 51.89 [AD]	883.40 ± 24.74 [BCD]	<0.001	<0.001	
α-MSH	Normal	310.87 ± 14.95	86.28 ± 1.38 [C]	1162.05 ± 9.07 [A]	494.28 ± 22.64 [BC]	<0.001	<0.001	<0.001
	Overload	669.74 ± 33.48 [D]	251.69 ± 18.04 [CD]	726.85 ± 21.86 [AD]	312.54 ± 9.40 [BCD]	<0.01	<0.001	
β-Endorphin	Normal	2426.5 ± 79.4	744.3 ± 39.9 [C]	2551.9 ± 131.7	671.3 ± 36.4 [C]	NS	<0.01	<0.05
	Overload	741.6 ± 41.3 [D]	688.6 ± 40.9	1344.2 ± 71.5 [AD]	640.1 ± 34.0 [C]	<0.05	NS	

Data are shown as the mean values ± SEM. NS, not significant. [A] Mean values from control group fed a fermented cow milk diet were significantly different (p < 0.05, Tukey's test). [B] Mean values from anemic group fed a fermented cow milk diet were significantly different (p < 0.05, Tukey's test). [C] Mean values of anemic animals were significantly different (p < 0.05, Tukey's test). [D] Mean values from the corresponding group fed with normal Fe content were significantly different (p < 0.05, Student's t test). MAO, Monoamine oxidase; α-MSH, α-Melanocyte-stimulating hormone.

4. Discussion

A better characterization of the events in the pathophysiology of IDA and the influence on nervous system molecular functions and homeostasis during the recovery of this deficiency would led to new nutritional strategies improving brain molecular functions and the other deleterious effects of the pathology. The animal model used in the current study simulates physiological deficiencies to iron and anemia recovery, and therefore argues that the response to brain functions can be modulated by dietary components.

The results of the current study reveal a clear impairment in some brain molecular functions due to IDA, because most of the parameters studied were impaired. ID manifests as alterations in cognitive function, behavior, and mood [19]. Iron is a cofactor of many metabolic processes as well as the synthesis of aminergic neurotransmitters; it plays a major function in brain development, and has a key role in myelinogenesis and synaptogenesis. Several mechanisms regarding the influence of iron deficiency on brain functions have been reported: the decrease in oxygen-carrying capacity of the blood could result in hypoperfusion of the brain, which could lead to an imbalance in oxidative/antioxidant status and inflammatory responses, causing neurodegenerative processes [20]. Furthermore, anemia induces renal changes, leading to lower erythropoietin levels as well as increasing the risk of neural degeneration, as this hormone has neuroprotective effects in situations of hypoxia [21]. Thus, IDA induces pathological changes in brain tissue and vessels, leading to reduced oxygen transportation as well as impaired synaptic functioning [22].

Dopamine levels have been heavily examined in patients suffering from IDA, and it is well established that this neurotransmitter is implicated in learning, memory, and attention, as well as several hormonal pathways, stress responses, addiction, and emotional behavior [23]. IDA leads to diminished central dopaminergic transmission and receptor trafficking, with the D2 receptor particularly affected [24]. Other evidence of biochemical abnormalities during IDA include decreased concentrations of thyroid hormones, as we have previously reported [25], increasing the levels of circulating catecholamines. This involves beta adrenergic receptors and affects the availability of glucose, impairing synaptic plasticity and changes in dendritic structure that lead to a loss of neurons [26], indicating that IDA can alter neurotransmitter metabolism.

Surprisingly, milk-based diets have really different effects on dopamine and serotonin, which are both monoamines that have iron-dependent synthesis pathways. In general, there is consensus in the scientific literature reporting a negative effect of ID on dopamine functions and synthesis [27], which coincides with our results during the anemia induction. However, conflicting results exist on the effects of ID on serotonin levels in rats. ID decreases serotonin due to a down-regulation of several biosynthesis pathways in young rats [28]. On the contrary, an increase in serotonin levels during ID has been reported in adults, reflecting a down-regulation of serotonin metabolism [29]. Serotonin transporters are reduced in the striatum of ID mice [30]. Additionally, gestational ID reduces serotonin uptake by synaptic vesicles in offspring, which is a process that can be normalized after four weeks of iron replenishment [31]. However, in other studies, ID had no effect on serotonin levels or metabolism in newborns or adults [32], and serotonin levels in the prefrontal cortex of the ID rats did not differ from controls [33]. These reported results in serotonin homeostasis appear conflicting, and hint at underlying additional mechanisms of the iron–monoamine relationship [2]. Therefore, although ID did not changed serotonin levels, the differences during iron repletion could be attributed to the different behavior of serotonin mentioned above, and the enhancement of the digestive and metabolic utilization of iron in fermented goat milk [14]. Moreover, a limitation of the study is the lack of a regional analysis of the brain molecules studied, which could help to specify the effect of fermented dairy products on brain functions, and could explain these results.

It has been reported that irisin promotes the differentiation of human embryonic stem cell-derived neural cells into neurons, as well as increased mature neuronal and astrocyte markers together with the improved expression of neurotrophic factors in the brain [34]. Therefore, the decrease of irisin levels in this study due to IDA reveals impairment in the molecular mechanisms driving neuron homeostasis. Moreover, the decrease recorded in MAO-A can be explained because iron is a key factor for MAO activity, and monoamine neurotransmitter synthesis requires the iron-dependent enzymes tyrosine and tryptophan hydroxylase, which is a finding that has been correlated with later behavioral consequences in juvenile monkeys, influencing brain function [35]. IDA also decreased oxytocin, which is a hypothalamic neuropeptide involved in regulating social behavior, and has a key role in physiological conditions and brain diseases. It has been reported that CO exerts an inhibitory tone on oxytocin secretion [36], and it is well known that CO output is increased during IDA. Additionally, IDA also decreased α-MSH which has been proven as an anti-inflammatory and neuroprotective hormone in animal studies [37] and β-endorphin, which has an important role in the development of the non-synaptic or paracrine communication between neurons [38], revealing the impairment of brain molecular functions.

On the other hand, synaptophysin increased during IDA. This interesting result can be explained because synaptobrevin II is a vesicular protein receptor that is essential for neurotransmitter release; therefore, its correct trafficking to synaptic vesicles is critical to render them fusion-competent. Synaptophysin binds to synaptobrevin II in the synaptic vesicles and facilitates its retrieval during endocytosis. Under physiological conditions, the expression of synaptophysin in a 1:2 ratio with synaptobrevin II is sufficient to fully rescue normal synaptobrevin II trafficking. The balance between synaptophysin and synaptobrevin II is critical for the exocytotic release of neurotransmitters [39]. Since as previously mentioned, anemia is associated with an impairment in cerebral blood flow and oxygen metabolism, as well as low neurotransmitter release [7], the overexpression of synaptophysin could be a compensatory mechanism to cope with the low neurotransmitter release from the synaptic vesicles during this condition.

In general, an improvement of nervous system molecular functions has been observed after anemia recovery with fermented goat milk (including dopamine, oxytocin, serotonin, α-MSH, and synaptophysin), which can be explained by several factors, including the better recovery of IDA with this dairy product.

Previous studies of our research group showed an increased expression of some key iron metabolism proteins such as duodenal cytochrome b, divalent metal transporter 1, and ferroportin 1 in rats fed fermented goat milk compared to fermented cow milk. These proteins enable overcoming the effects of IDA, increasing iron bioavailability in target organs and efficient iron repletion after IDA [14], and have significant implications in the brain molecular mechanisms related to cognitive functions.

On the other hand, synaptophysin is considered a reliable biomarker for synaptic density and synaptogenesis [40]. Synaptophysin is also correlated with a loss or increase in synaptic densities in studies of aging and neurodegenerative disorders [41]. In the current study, the production of synaptophysin was significantly increased in the rats consuming fermented goat milk, because as previously reported [42], the production of neurotrophic factors, as well as the survival of neuronal synapses and the retention of cognitive function is increased when the inflammation is suppressed.

In this sense, we have previously reported that in control and anemic rats, interleukin (IL)-1β, IL-2, IL-12p70, IP-10 and tumour necrosis factor (TNF)-α (pro-inflammatory cytokines) decrease after fermented goat milk consumption, and levels of IL-4, IL-13 and IL-10 (pro-inflammatory cytokines) [43] increase. These results are due to the better nutritional characteristics of fermented goat milk, in comparison with fermented cow milk, playing a potential role of this dairy product as a high nutritional value food with anti-inflammatory properties. It has also been reported that TNF-α produced by microglia exacerbates the neurodegenerative diseases [44]. In the brain, microglia mainly regulate immunological phenomena; as a result, it seems that fermented goat milk may regulate also the microglial inflammatory response, leading to a suppression of the inflammatory signaling and neuronal degeneration. Chronic inflammation in the brain exacerbates the pathological condition and cognitive functions decline in many neurodegenerative processes, which is due to neurotrophic factors that are suppressed by inflammation and are toxic to neurons [45,46].

Increased awareness of the role of oxidative stress in the pathogenesis of neurodegenerative processes has highlighted the issue of whether oxidative damage is a fundamental step in the pathogenesis or instead results from disease-associated pathology. Recently, it has been reported that oxidative damage results in amyloid deposition in the brain, resulting in neuronal cell death and neurodegenerative diseases [47,48]. In this sense, we have previously reported [49,50] that fermented goat milk increased some antioxidant enzymes in brain tissue as well as total antioxidant status and melatonin, even in the case of Fe overload. These increases limit the oxidative damage to the brain biomolecules (lipids, protein DNA, prostaglandins) and protect the nervous tissue of the oxidative-induced cell death that induces neurodegenerative processes.

In the current study, iron overload increased dopamine levels in the brain with a fermented cow milk based-diet, and it has been previously reported that iron accumulation relates to dopamine, comprising a toxic couple that is reliant on interacting with other biomolecules, and causes selective neurodegeneration in some areas of the brain [51]. MAO-A levels were increased in control animals consuming both types of fermented milk with iron overload; an enzyme catalyzes the oxidative deamination of monoamine neurotransmitters, increasing the production of reactive oxygen species and oxidative stress, which is potentially a risk factor for neuronal loss and neurodegenerative disorders [52]. Iron excess also reduced β-endorphin in the control animals, which has several activities such as analgesic, immunostimulatory, stress busting, and anti-inflammatory, as well as having a key role in the adequate neurological responses [53]. These deleterious effects of iron overload are in accordance with previous reports revealing that iron supplementation results in brain accumulation and subsequent toxicity, increasing oxidative damage up to a level that natural defenses fail, and at which neuronal apoptotic rates are exacerbated [54].

We have previously reported that except for alanine, in which the differences were not statistically significant, all other amino acids were higher in fermented goat milk than in fermented cow milk, including glycine threonine and tyrosine [15], and it has been reported that orally administered β-lactopeptide of glycine-threonine-tryptophan-tyrosine inhibits the activity of monoamine oxidase in the brain [55]. It has also been reported that the MAO inhibitor reduces reactive oxygen species and suppresses some neurodegenerative diseases [56]. In addition, the inhibitory activity of MAO reduces the activation of nuclear factor kappa B (NF-κB) and suppresses NF-κB-regulated pro-inflammatory responses [57], which supports the results obtained with the animals fed fermented goat milk. In the current study, an increase in α-MSH was also recorded in all groups fed fermented goat milk. α-MSH is a hormone that functions as a neurotransmitter and neuromodulator; it is involved in significant neuronal circuitry, and is also a mediator of immunity and inflammation. At the molecular level, these effects of α-MSH are mediated via the inhibition of the activation of transcription factors such as NF-κB [58], reducing once more the pro-inflammatory responses in the nervous system and suppressing some pathways that lead to neurodegenerative environments.

5. Conclusions

In conclusion, by using an animal model of severe iron deficiency, the current study has showed a relation between iron status and brain molecular parameters related to key functions during anemia instauration and recovery. The alterations recorded in the biomarker-related brain functions studied may result in impairments in behavioral and cognitive functions during severe iron deficiency anemia. In addition, the results of the current study reveal that in general, during anemia recovery, a fermented goat milk-based diet, normal iron, or iron overload inhibits MAO activities, and increases serotonin, synaptophysin, and α-MSH levels. It also has been implicated in the suppression of inflammatory responses, an improvement in iron metabolism, and a reduction of evoked oxidative stress, as observed in previous studies. Taken together, all these results suggest a potential neuroprotective effect of fermented goat milk, which could enhance brain molecular functions, although further studies are needed to confirm these findings.

Author Contributions: I.L.-A. and J.D.-C. designed the study. J.M.-F., J.D.-C., M.J.M.A. and M.G.-B. performed the experiments, analyzed the data, and wrote the manuscript. All the authors approved the final version of the manuscript and agree to be accountable for all aspects of the work in ensuring that questions related to the accuracy or integrity of any part of the work are appropriately investigated and resolved. All persons designated as authors qualify for authorship, and all those who qualify for authorship are listed.

Funding: This study was supported by the Excellence Research Project (P11-AGR-7648) from the Regional Government of Andalusia.

Acknowledgments: J.M.-F. and M.G.-B. were supported by a fellowship from the Ministry of Education, Culture and Sport (Spain), and are grateful to the Excellence Ph.D. Program "Nutrición y Ciencias de los Alimentos" from the University of Granada. The authors also thank S.S. for her efficient support in the revision with the English language.

Conflicts of Interest: The authors declare no conflict of interest.

References

1. Kyu, H.H.; Pinho, C.; Wagner, J.A.; Brown, J.C.; Bertozzi-Villa, A.; Charlson, F.J.; Coffeng, L.E.; Dandona, L.; Erskine, H.E.; Ferrari, A.J.; et al. Global and National Burden of Diseases and Injuries Among Children and Adolescents Between 1990 and 2013: Findings From the Global Burden of Disease 2013 Study. *JAMA Pediatrics* **2016**, *170*, 267–287. [CrossRef]
2. Beard, J.L.; Connor, J.R. Iron status and neural functioning. *Ann. Rev. Nutr.* **2003**, *23*, 41–58. [CrossRef] [PubMed]
3. Cusick, S.E.; Georgieff, M.K.; Rao, R. Approaches for Reducing the Risk of Early-Life Iron Deficiency-Induced Brain Dysfunction in Children. *Nutrients* **2018**, *10*, 227. [CrossRef] [PubMed]
4. Murray-Kolb, L.E.; Wenger, M.J.; Scott, S.P.; Rhoten, S.E.; Lung'aho, M.G.; Haas, J.D. Consumption of Iron-Biofortified Beans Positively Affects Cognitive Performance in 18- to 27-Year-Old Rwandan Female College Students in an 18-Week Randomized Controlled Efficacy Trial. *J. Nutr.* **2017**, *147*, 2109–2117. [CrossRef] [PubMed]
5. Wenger, M.J.; DellaValle, D.M. Effect of iron deficiency on simultaneous measures of behavior, brain activity, and energy expenditure in the performance of a cognitive task. *Nutr. Neurosci.* **2019**, *22*, 196–206. [CrossRef] [PubMed]
6. Murray-Kolb, L.E. Iron and brain functions. *Curr. Opin. Clin. Nutr. Metab. Care* **2013**, *16*, 703–707. [CrossRef] [PubMed]
7. Pickett, J.L.; Theberge, D.C.; Brown, W.S.; Schweitzer, S.U.; Nissenson, A.R. Normalizing hematocrit in dialysis patients improves brain function. *Am. J. Kidney Dis. Off. J. Natl. Kidney Found.* **1999**, *33*, 1122–1130. [CrossRef]
8. Nissenson, A.R. Epoetin and cognitive function. *Am. J. Kidney Dis. Off. J. Natl. Kidney Found.* **1992**, *20*, 21–24. [PubMed]
9. Moreno, F.; Sanz-Guajardo, D.; Lopez-Gomez, J.M.; Jofre, R.; Valderrabano, F. Increasing the Hematocrit Has a Beneficial Effect on Quality of Life and Is Safe in Selected Hemodialysis Patients. *J. Am. Soc. Nephrol.* **2000**, *11*, 335.
10. Falkingham, M.; Abdelhamid, A.; Curtis, P.; Fairweather-Tait, S.; Dye, L.; Hooper, L. The effects of oral iron supplementation on cognition in older children and adults: A systematic review and meta-analysis. *Nutr. J.* **2010**, *9*, 4. [CrossRef]
11. Bahrami, A.; Khorasanchi, Z. Anemia is associated with cognitive impairment in adolescent girls: A cross-sectional survey. *Appl. Neuropsychol. Child* **2019**, 1–7. [CrossRef] [PubMed]
12. Camfield, D.A.; Owen, L.; Scholey, A.B.; Pipingas, A.; Stough, C. Dairy constituents and neurocognitive health in ageing. *Br. J. Nutr.* **2011**, *106*, 159–174. [CrossRef] [PubMed]
13. Crichton, G.E.; Murphy, K.J.; Bryan, J. Dairy intake and cognitive health in middle-aged South Australians. *Asia Pac. J. Clin. Nutr.* **2010**, *19*, 161–171. [PubMed]
14. Moreno-Fernandez, J.; Diaz-Castro, J.; Pulido-Moran, M.; Alferez, M.J.; Boesch, C.; Sanchez-Alcover, A.; Lopez-Aliaga, I. Fermented Goat's Milk Consumption Improves Duodenal Expression of Iron Homeostasis Genes during Anemia Recovery. *J. Agric. food Chem.* **2016**, *64*, 2560–2568. [CrossRef] [PubMed]

15. Moreno-Fernandez, J.; Diaz-Castro, J.; Alferez, M.J.; Hijano, S.; Nestares, T.; Lopez-Aliaga, I. Production and chemical composition of two dehydrated fermented dairy products based on cow or goat milk. *J. Dairy Res.* **2016**, *83*, 81–88. [CrossRef] [PubMed]
16. Reeves, P.G.; Nielsen, F.H.; Fahey, G.C., Jr. AIN-93 purified diets for laboratory rodents: Final report of the American Institute of Nutrition ad hoc writing committee on the reformulation of the AIN-76A rodent diet. *J. Nutr.* **1993**, *123*, 1939–1951. [CrossRef]
17. Pallares, I.; Lisbona, F.; Aliaga, I.L.; Barrionuevo, M.; Alferez, M.J.; Campos, M.S. Effect of iron deficiency on the digestive utilization of iron, phosphorus, calcium and magnesium in rats. *Br. J. Nutr.* **1993**, *70*, 609–620. [CrossRef] [PubMed]
18. Raja, K.B.; Simpson, R.J.; Peters, T.J. Intestinal iron absorption studies in mouse models of iron-overload. *Br. J. Haematol.* **1994**, *86*, 156–162. [CrossRef] [PubMed]
19. Lozoff, B.; Beard, J.; Connor, J.; Barbara, F.; Georgieff, M.; Schallert, T. Long-lasting neural and behavioral effects of iron deficiency in infancy. *Nutr. Rev.* **2006**, *64*, S34–S43. [CrossRef]
20. Zlokovic, B.V. Neurovascular pathways to neurodegeneration in Alzheimer's disease and other disorders. *Nat. Rev. Neurosci.* **2011**, *12*, 723. [CrossRef]
21. Hasselblatt, M.; Ehrenreich, H.; Siren, A.L. The brain erythropoietin system and its potential for therapeutic exploitation in brain disease. *J. Neurosurg. Anesthesiol.* **2006**, *18*, 132–138. [CrossRef] [PubMed]
22. Munoz, P.; Humeres, A. Iron deficiency on neuronal function. *Biometals Int. J. Role Met. Ions Biol. Biochem. Med.* **2012**, *25*, 825–835. [CrossRef] [PubMed]
23. Nieoullon, A. Dopamine and the regulation of cognition and attention. *Prog. Neurobiol.* **2002**, *67*, 53–83. [CrossRef]
24. Unger, E.L.; Wiesinger, J.A.; Hao, L.; Beard, J.L. Dopamine D2 receptor expression is altered by changes in cellular iron levels in PC12 cells and rat brain tissue. *J. Nutr.* **2008**, *138*, 2487–2494. [CrossRef] [PubMed]
25. Moreno-Fernandez, J.; Diaz-Castro, J. Iron Deficiency and Neuroendocrine Regulators of Basal Metabolism, Body Composition and Energy Expenditure in Rats. *Nutrients* **2019**, *11*, 631. [CrossRef] [PubMed]
26. McEwen, B.S.; Sapolsky, R.M. Stress and cognitive function. *Curr. Opin. Neurobiol.* **1995**, *5*, 205–216. [CrossRef]
27. Youdim, M.B.; Ben-Shachar, D.; Yehuda, S. Putative biological mechanisms of the effect of iron deficiency on brain biochemistry and behavior. *Am. J. Clin. Nutr.* **1989**, *50*, 607–617. [CrossRef] [PubMed]
28. Shukla, A.; Agarwal, K.N.; Chansuria, J.P.; Taneja, V. Effect of latent iron deficiency on 5-hydroxytryptamine metabolism in rat brain. *J. Neurochem.* **1989**, *52*, 730–735. [CrossRef]
29. Finch, C.A.; Miller, L.R.; Inamdar, A.R.; Person, R.; Seiler, K.; Mackler, B. Iron deficiency in the rat. Physiological and biochemical studies of muscle dysfunction. *J. Clin. Investig.* **1976**, *58*, 447–453. [CrossRef]
30. Morse, A.C.; Beard, J.L.; Azar, M.R.; Jones, B.C. Sex and Genetics are Important Cofactors in Assessing the Impact of Iron Deficiency on the Developing Mouse Brain. *Nutr. Neurosci.* **1999**, *2*, 323–335. [CrossRef]
31. Kaladhar, M.; Rao, B.S. Effect of maternal iron deficiency in rat on serotonin uptake in vitro by brain synaptic vesicles in the offspring. *J. Neurochem.* **1983**, *40*, 1768–1770. [CrossRef] [PubMed]
32. Youdim, M.B.; Ben-Shachar, D. Minimal brain damage induced by early iron deficiency: Modified dopaminergic neurotransmission. *Isr. J. Med. Sci.* **1987**, *23*, 19–25. [PubMed]
33. Li, Y.; Kim, J.; Buckett, P.D.; Böhlke, M.; Maher, T.J.; Wessling-Resnick, M. Severe postnatal iron deficiency alters emotional behavior and dopamine levels in the prefrontal cortex of young male rats. *J. Nutr.* **2011**, *141*, 2133–2138. [CrossRef] [PubMed]
34. Wrann, C.D. FNDC5/irisin—Their role in the nervous system and as a mediator for beneficial effects of exercise on the brain. *Brain Plast.* **2015**, *1*, 55–61. [CrossRef] [PubMed]
35. Golub, M.S.; Hogrefe, C.E. Fetal iron deficiency and genotype influence emotionality in infant rhesus monkeys. *J. Nutr.* **2015**, *145*, 647–653. [CrossRef] [PubMed]
36. Kostoglou-Athanassiou, I.; Forsling, M.L.; Navarra, P.; Grossman, A.B. Oxytocin release is inhibited by the generation of carbon monoxide from the rat hypothalamus-further evidence for carbon monoxide as a neuromodulator. *Brain Res. Mol. Brain Res.* **1996**, *42*, 301–306. [CrossRef]
37. Singh, M.; Mukhopadhyay, K. Alpha-melanocyte stimulating hormone: An emerging anti-inflammatory antimicrobial peptide. *BioMed Res. Int.* **2014**, *2014*, 874610. [CrossRef]
38. Veening, J.G.; Barendregt, H.P. The effects of beta-endorphin: State change modification. *Fluids Barriers CNS* **2015**, *12*, 3. [CrossRef]

39. Gordon, S.L.; Harper, C.B.; Smillie, K.J.; Cousin, M.A. A Fine Balance of Synaptophysin Levels Underlies Efficient Retrieval of Synaptobrevin II to Synaptic Vesicles. *PLoS ONE* **2016**, *11*, e0149457. [CrossRef]
40. Alladi, P.A.; Wadhwa, S.; Singh, N. Effect of prenatal auditory enrichment on developmental expression of synaptophysin and syntaxin 1 in chick brainstem auditory nuclei. *Neuroscience* **2002**, *114*, 577–590. [CrossRef]
41. Joca, S.R.; Guimaraes, F.S.; Del-Bel, E. Inhibition of nitric oxide synthase increases synaptophysin mRNA expression in the hippocampal formation of rats. *Neurosci. Lett.* **2007**, *421*, 72–76. [CrossRef] [PubMed]
42. Ano, Y.; Ozawa, M.; Kutsukake, T.; Sugiyama, S.; Uchida, K.; Yoshida, A.; Nakayama, H. Preventive effects of a fermented dairy product against Alzheimer's disease and identification of a novel oleamide with enhanced microglial phagocytosis and anti-inflammatory activity. *PLoS ONE* **2015**, *10*, e0118512. [CrossRef] [PubMed]
43. Lopez-Aliaga, I.; Garcia-Pedro, J.D.; Moreno-Fernandez, J.; Alferez, M.J.M.; Lopez-Frias, M.; Diaz-Castro, J. Fermented goat milk consumption improves iron status and evokes inflammatory signalling during anemia recovery. *Food Funct.* **2018**, *9*, 3195–3201. [CrossRef] [PubMed]
44. Lourenco, M.V.; Ledo, J.H. Targeting Alzheimer's pathology through PPARgamma signaling: Modulation of microglial function. *J. Neurosci. Off. J. Soc. Neurosci.* **2013**, *33*, 5083–5084. [CrossRef] [PubMed]
45. Xia, M.Q.; Qin, S.X.; Wu, L.J.; Mackay, C.R.; Hyman, B.T. Immunohistochemical study of the beta-chemokine receptors CCR3 and CCR5 and their ligands in normal and Alzheimer's disease brains. *Am. J. Pathol.* **1998**, *153*, 31–37. [CrossRef]
46. Mrak, R.E.; Griffin, W.S. Potential inflammatory biomarkers in Alzheimer's disease. *J. Alzheimer's Dis. JAD* **2005**, *8*, 369–375. [CrossRef]
47. Cheignon, C.; Tomas, M.; Bonnefont-Rousselot, D.; Faller, P.; Hureau, C.; Collin, F. Oxidative stress and the amyloid beta peptide in Alzheimer's disease. *Redox Biol.* **2018**, *14*, 450–464. [CrossRef]
48. Chi, H.; Chang, H.-Y.; Sang, T.-K. Neuronal cell death mechanisms in major neurodegenerative diseases. *Int. J. Mol. Sci.* **2018**, *19*, 3082. [CrossRef]
49. Moreno-Fernandez, J.; Diaz-Castro, J.; Alferez, M.J.; Nestares, T.; Ochoa, J.J.; Sanchez-Alcover, A.; Lopez-Aliaga, I. Fermented goat milk consumption improves melatonin levels and influences positively the antioxidant status during nutritional ferropenic anemia recovery. *Food Funct.* **2016**, *7*, 834–842. [CrossRef]
50. Moreno-Fernandez, J.; Diaz-Castro, J.; Alferez, M.J.; Boesch, C.; Nestares, T.; Lopez-Aliaga, I. Fermented goat milk improves antioxidant status and protects from oxidative damage to biomolecules during anemia recovery. *J. Sci. Food Agric.* **2017**, *97*, 1433–1442. [CrossRef]
51. Hare, D.J.; Double, K.L. Iron and dopamine: A toxic couple. *Brain J. Neurol.* **2016**, *139*, 1026–1035. [CrossRef] [PubMed]
52. Naoi, M.; Riederer, P.; Maruyama, W. Modulation of monoamine oxidase (MAO) expression in neuropsychiatric disorders: Genetic and environmental factors involved in type A MAO expression. *J. Neural Transm.* **2016**, *123*, 91–106. [CrossRef] [PubMed]
53. Shrihari, T.G. BETA—Endorphins—A Novel Natural Holistic Healer. *J. Microb. Biochem. Technol.* **2018**, *10*, 25–26.
54. Miwa, C.P.; de Lima, M.N.; Scalco, F.; Vedana, G.; Mattos, R.; Fernandez, L.L.; Hilbig, A.; Schroder, N.; Vianna, M.R. Neonatal iron treatment increases apoptotic markers in hippocampal and cortical areas of adult rats. *Neurotox. Res.* **2011**, *19*, 527–535. [CrossRef]
55. Ano, Y.; Ayabe, T.; Kutsukake, T.; Ohya, R.; Takaichi, Y.; Uchida, S.; Yamada, K.; Uchida, K.; Takashima, A.; Nakayama, H. Novel lactopeptides in fermented dairy products improve memory function and cognitive decline. *Neurobiol. Aging* **2018**, *72*, 23–31. [CrossRef]
56. Nagatsu, T.; Sawada, M. Molecular mechanism of the relation of monoamine oxidase B and its inhibitors to Parkinson's disease: Possible implications of glial cells. *J. Neural Transm. Suppl.* **2006**, *71*, 53–65.
57. Son, B.; Jun, S.Y.; Seo, H.; Youn, H.; Yang, H.J.; Kim, W.; Kim, H.K.; Kang, C.; Youn, B. Inhibitory effect of traditional oriental medicine-derived monoamine oxidase B inhibitor on radioresistance of non-small cell lung cancer. *Sci. Rep.* **2016**, *6*, 21986. [CrossRef]
58. Luger, T.A.; Scholzen, T.E.; Brzoska, T.; Bohm, M. New insights into the functions of alpha-MSH and related peptides in the immune system. *Ann. N. Y. Acad. Sci.* **2003**, *994*, 133–140. [CrossRef]

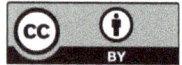

© 2019 by the authors. Licensee MDPI, Basel, Switzerland. This article is an open access article distributed under the terms and conditions of the Creative Commons Attribution (CC BY) license (http://creativecommons.org/licenses/by/4.0/).

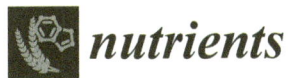

Review

Iron Homeostasis Disruption and Oxidative Stress in Preterm Newborns

Genny Raffaeli [1,†], Francesca Manzoni [1,2,†], Valeria Cortesi [1,2], Giacomo Cavallaro [1], Fabio Mosca [1,2] and Stefano Ghirardello [1,*]

1. Fondazione IRCCS Ca' Granda Ospedale Maggiore Policlinico, NICU, 20122 Milano, Italy; genny.raffaeli@unimi.it (G.R.); francescamanzoni.unimi@gmail.com (F.M.); valeria.cortesi92@gmail.com (V.C.); giacomo.cavallaro@policlinico.mi.it (G.C.); fabio.mosca@unimi.it (F.M.)
2. Department of Clinical Sciences and Community Health, Università degli Studi di Milano, 20122 Milano, Italy
* Correspondence: stefano.ghirardello@mangiagalli.it; Tel.: +39-2-5503-2234; Fax: +39-2-5503-221
† Co-first authorship.

Received: 30 April 2020; Accepted: 25 May 2020; Published: 27 May 2020

Abstract: Iron is an essential micronutrient for early development, being involved in several cellular processes and playing a significant role in neurodevelopment. Prematurity may impact on iron homeostasis in different ways. On the one hand, more than half of preterm infants develop iron deficiency (ID)/ID anemia (IDA), due to the shorter duration of pregnancy, early postnatal growth, insufficient erythropoiesis, and phlebotomy losses. On the other hand, the sickest patients are exposed to erythrocytes transfusions, increasing the risk of iron overload under conditions of impaired antioxidant capacity. Prevention of iron shortage through placental transfusion, blood-sparing practices for laboratory assessments, and iron supplementation is the first frontier in the management of anemia in preterm infants. The American Academy of Pediatrics recommends the administration of 2 mg/kg/day of oral elemental iron to human milk-fed preterm infants from one month of age to prevent ID. To date, there is no consensus on the type of iron preparations, dosages, or starting time of administration to meet optimal cost-efficacy and safety measures. We will identify the main determinants of iron homeostasis in premature infants, elaborate on iron-mediated redox unbalance, and highlight areas for further research to tailor the management of iron metabolism.

Keywords: iron; redox unbalance; prematurity; transfusion; anemia; blood-sparing

1. Iron Homeostasis and Prematurity

Iron is an essential micronutrient that plays a pivotal role in early development, being involved in hemoglobin synthesis, oxygen delivery, electron transfer, energy metabolism, and cell differentiation [1]. Nowadays, there is consistent evidence about the relationship between in utero iron supply and subsequent cognitive and neurobehavioral outcomes [2,3]. Iron homeostasis is a balance between iron absorption, storage, and recycle by erythroid precursors. The total body iron is distributed into three compartments [4]. The majority of total body iron (at least two-thirds) is within erythrocytes, in the form of hemoglobin (Hb). A small part (about 15%) is "storage iron", mostly kept within ferritin or hemosiderin in liver and spleen, ready to be mobilized [5–7]; the remainder (10%) is non-heme-non-storage tissue-circulating iron. The latter is bound to serum transferrin, an iron chelator that keeps iron in a soluble, inert, reduced state, preventing toxic oxidative reactions [7]. Hepcidin is a peptide hormone acting as a negative feedback regulator of iron metabolism, by modulating the expression of ferroportin, which is an iron-exporter transmembrane protein of enterocytes and macrophages. Hepcidin synthesis in the hepatocytes is determined by circulating and stored iron, inflammation, and erythropoietin. In the event of high iron levels or inflammation, hepatic hepcidin release is increased and ferroportin expression is downregulated. Conversely, anemia, hypoxia, and low iron levels are associated with reduced hepcidin expression, leading to the increased activity of ferroportin and the mobilization of iron reserves [4,6]. Iron deficiency (ID) is a relevant public health problem and is the most common single-element deficiency worldwide, affecting around 2 billion people globally [1,8]. Both pre-existing anemia and increased iron requirements during pregnancy make pregnant women particularly vulnerable to develop iron deficiency anemia (IDA) [2]. It is estimated that maternal IDA affects approximately 30–50% of pregnant women in developing countries and less than 1% in developed countries where iron supplementation is part of routine care [9]. There are no conclusive results about the relationship between maternal and neonatal iron status. Past studies showed that early maternal sideropenic anemia doubles the risk of preterm delivery and low birth weight [10,11]. Iron endowment at birth depends on iron stored during gestation, tightly connected to maternal iron status, and iron received perinatally as Hb, depending on the time of cord clamping [12]. Adequate iron stores at birth are necessary to satisfy requirements in the first 6–9 months of age, when the neonatal gut is not fully developed to properly regulate iron intake and breast milk cannot meet the recommended needs [2]. Poor levels of iron at birth, on the contrary, predict future ID and/or IDA during infancy [12].

In the same way, iron homeostasis can be deeply influenced by prematurity. Iron is mostly (>66%) transferred during the third trimester of pregnancy [10] so that total iron stores are inversely related to gestational age. Moreover, many pregnancy complications, such as multiple pregnancies, obesity, gestational diabetes, and hypertension with intrauterine growth restriction (IUGR) [13], can also induce impaired iron endowment due to chronic placental insufficiency [10,14]. Iron demand, as with all nutrients, increases during fetal and neonatal development [15]. In premature infants, the early onset of erythropoiesis and the fast catch-up growth occurring in the first 6–8 weeks of life require additional iron, especially in the most immature neonates [16]. Moreover, premature infants' iron stores can be further depleted by recurrent phlebotomy and administration of recombinant human erythropoietin (rHuEPO) in the absence of adequate iron supplementation.

Low iron reserves and increased iron requirement explain why preterm infants are at high risk of ID/IDA and need iron supplementation [1,14]. It is estimated that between 25% and 85% of premature newborns develop iron deficiency, usually in the first six months of life [16]. In preterm neonates, ID can affect the majority of organs, causing poor growth, temperature instability, thyroid dysfunction, decreased cell-mediated immune response and impaired DNA and collagen synthesis, even before microcytic and hypochromic anemia appears [16,17]. However, the main concern is the impact of ID on brain development [9,18].

On the other hand, premature infants are vulnerable to oxidative stress caused by non-transferrin-bound iron (NTBI) overload due to the immature antioxidant system and the high transferrin saturation [1,6,19,20]. NTBI can derive from high doses of oral or parental iron supplementation and recurrent erythrocyte transfusions [14]. The latter is relevant if we consider that around 40% of very low birth weight (VLBW) and more than 90% of extremely low birth weight (ELBW) infants receive at least one blood transfusion during hospitalization [21]. Birth, itself, is an oxidative challenge since there is a rapid increase in the oxygen concentrations compared to the hypoxic intrauterine environment [22]. Indeed, plasma NTBI concentrations appear to be higher in the neonatal period if compared to the following ages [19,20]. Iron excess cannot be removed by physiological pathways and can accumulate and generate free radicals resulting in cellular toxicity. The same toxic reaction can be produced when the iron is delocalized from its binding protein, as it happens in the setting of hypoxia [6,23]. As a result, the sickest premature neonates are prone to develop complications that may share the same etiology, grouped under the expression coined by Saugstad, "the oxygen radical disease of neonatology" [24]: bronchopulmonary dysplasia (BPD), retinopathy of prematurity (ROP), necrotizing enterocolitis (NEC), intraventricular hemorrhage (IVH), periventricular leukomalacia (PVL), and punctate white matter lesions (PWM) [1,21,25].

2. Iron and Brain Development

Iron is critical for brain development in the fetal and early neonatal period, and major issues are related to the long-lasting effect of ID on neurodevelopment. Biologically, in the case of negative iron balance, iron is redistributed following a hierarchical strategy and primarily used by red cells to the detriment of other tissues: firstly liver, followed by the heart, skeletal muscle and. finally. brain [4,26]. It results that ID can injure the brain even in the absence of IDA [9,27,28]. Indeed, ID can impact brain functions because several iron-dependent enzymes are essential for neurotransmitter synthesis, myelination, synaptogenesis, gene expression and neuronal energy production [4,26].

The American Academy of Pediatrics (AAP) has highlighted the relevance of ID and IDA screening during infancy [2], due to both short- and long-term negative consequences of IDA on motor, cognitive, social, and behavioral development [3,29,30].

Both timing and duration of ID are critical because the brain's affected areas are in a crucial developing phase at the time of ID [9]. In particular, ID during gestation and lactation carries the most severe effects, as it occurs during the brain's growth spurt, [9]. Rodent models have shown that early (from the late fetal period to 24 months of postnatal age) ID can affect the dopaminergic system in the striatum, and alter gene expression and dendritogenesis in the hippocampus, leading to motor and memory life-long alterations, respectively [9]. In the same way, the composition of myelin lipids persists irreversibly altered in adulthood despite iron treatment [9].

Intrauterine ID, as well, can have life-long consequences as proved by the association between cord ferritin levels below the lowest quartile (<76 mg/L), a marker of in-utero fetal iron status [31], and language and fine motor skills delay at five years of age [2,32].

Scarce data evaluated the relationship between in-utero ID and long-term neurobehavioral effects in preterm infants. Premature infants suffering from fetal ID have abnormal auditory brainstem-evoked responses (ABR), a marker of brain maturation, with longer latencies in the perinatal period [31]. Moreover, anemic preterm infants show altered neurological reflexes at 37 weeks, probably suggesting impaired myelination or neurotransmitters synthesis [33]. Interestingly, ID in premature infants tends to express through motor deficits, while cognitive impairment prevails in term infants [16].

Based on preclinical evidence [34], limited benefits were reported for the promotion of mental or motor development in infants with IDA [35,36]. This result could be explained by the late timing of the onset of supplementation: ID begins prenatally, and interventions targeting infancy or early childhood were too late [37]. On the other hand, various studies showed that iron supplementation in infants at risk of ID had positive effects on motor and cognitive development [38–40]. Similarly, early (<61 days of life) iron supplementation in premature infants improves neurocognitive outcome VLBW neonates [41].

The main core of the debate is related to the fact that not only ID can be troublesome, but also iron excess, as mentioned above, may induce oxidative stress, which contributes to the pathophysiology of several prematurity-related diseases [25].

Indeed, preterm infants often experience repeated episodes of hyperoxia, hypoxia, and ischemia resulting in free radicals and reactive oxygen species (ROS) production that these patients cannot cope with, due to an ineffective anti-oxidant system [25]. Specifically, several antioxidant enzymes, such as the superoxide dismutase, catalase, and glutathione peroxidase, show a decreased activity in the immature brain [42].

Iron becomes toxic when not bound to proteins [43,44]. Neonates, particularly if born prematurely, are prone to generate NTBI as a result of repeated episodes of hypoxia, acidosis, and ischemia in the perinatal period, when plasma transferrin, ceruloplasmin and total iron bind capacity (TIBC) are constitutionally low [42]. Indeed, amoeboid microglial cells of the periventricular white matter show increased intracellular iron concentration after a hypoxic insult that can lead to oligodendrocyte cell death and axonal swelling [45].

Growing evidence suggests a role for iron in hypoxic-ischemic encephalopathy (HIE). Indeed, high amounts of NTBI were found in the cerebrospinal fluid (CSF) and the serum of newborns after a hypoxic-ischemic injury [23,46]. NTBI concentrations are directly related to the severity of brain injury [23], and blood NTBI has been considered an early predictive marker of long-term neurodevelopmental outcomes [20,46]. Iron-mediated radical factors disrupt the blood-brain barrier and cause endothelial necrosis following a hypoxic-ischemic injury [42].

Similarly, iron-induced neuronal toxicity is a determinant of IVH pathophysiology in the preterm brain as the free iron released from heme destruction after intracerebral hemorrhage (ICH) contributes to secondary brain injury and post-hemorrhagic ventricular dilatation [43]. Indeed, while the primary hit lies in the presence of the hematoma itself, the secondary injury refers to the subsequent release of neurotoxic iron-related compounds from the hematoma. Specifically, heme oxygenase catabolizes heme into carbon monoxide, biliverdin, and free iron. The free iron accumulation increases the risk of oxidative damage to lipids, protein and DNA, by inducing the free radical production by means of the Fenton reaction [43]. In both HIE and IVH, the potential mechanism by which iron can damage the neonatal brain has been recently studied and has been named "ferroptosis", a non-apoptotic iron-dependent pathway of cell death (Figure 1) [43].

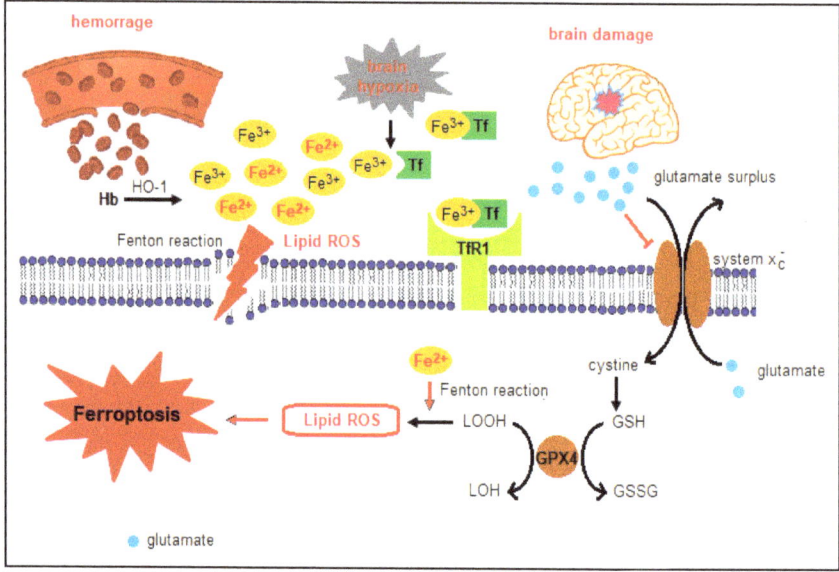

Figure 1. Presumptive molecular pathways of ferroptosis following brain injury in the developing brain. Excess free iron in the brain may be the result of Hb degradation by HO-1 after intracerebral hemorrhage. Similarly, a hypoxic-ischemic insult enhances iron liberation from its binding proteins. Fe^{2+}, the reactive form of iron, promotes ROS production via the Fenton reaction leading to lipid peroxidation and membrane damage while the damaged brain releases glutamate. High extracellular glutamate concentrations inhibit the cystine/glutamate antiporter system xc- thus reducing cellular cystine levels, necessary for GSH synthesis. Reduced intracellular cystine concentration indirectly inactivates GPX4, the enzyme responsible for lipid hydroperoxide reduction and GSH consumption. The accumulation of lipid hydroperoxides in an enriched Fe^{2+} environment leads to significant lipid ROS formation that induces membrane permeabilization and ferroptosis [6,47]. Fe^{2+}: ferrous cation; GPX4: glutathione peroxidase 4; GSSG: oxidized GSH; GSH: reduced glutathione; Hb: hemoglobin; HO-1: heme oxygenase 1; LOOH: lipid hydroperoxides; LOH: lipid alcohols; ROS: reactive oxygen species; TF: transferrin; TfR1: transferrin receptor 1. Adapted from Wang et al. [6].

NTBI can trigger ferroptosis, inducing a process mediated by lipid peroxidation and glutathione consumption with subsequent hydroxyl radical production via Fenton and Haber–Weiss reactions.

Free radicals and nitric oxide generated during brain reperfusion following hypoxic events activate a series of chain reactions that mobilize an increasing amount of iron from its binding proteins and red cells [48], thus amplifying cell death and brain injury [6]. To support this theory, high concentrations of malondialdehyde, a product of lipid peroxidation, have been found in CSF of infants with HIE [23]. This pathogenetic mechanism is relevant in the neonatal brain if we consider the large amount of iron and polyunsaturated fatty acids that constitute the lipidic membrane in the white matter, readily susceptible to free radical attack [46]. Additionally, CSF is characterized by a low TIBC that can bind NTBI and an unbalanced relationship between ceruloplasmin and vitamin C that favors the latter and results in iron oxidation in the active ferrous form [20,49]. Even orally-administered iron can damage brain: preclinical studies demonstrated Parkinson-like neurodegeneration in adults that have been fed with great amounts of enteral iron during breastfeeding [16].

Iron chelators have shown a neuroprotective effect in animal studies [23]. rHuEPO likewise protects against inflammation, apoptosis, and oxidation and decreases unbound iron by stimulating erythropoiesis [43]. In preclinical models of neonatal brain damage, rHuEPO acts as a neuroprotector, promoting neurogenesis and neural regeneration after an insult [50]. In clinical practice, rHuEPO is administered at the dose of 300–500 U/kg for the prevention and treatment of the anemia of prematurity [51]. Low-doses of rHuEPO has been previously associated with better short-term and long-term neurological outcomes in both full-term and preterm infants [50,51]. However, the results from a recent randomized trial, enrolling extremely preterm infants to receive high-dose of rHuEPO (1000 U/kg) in the first weeks of life, did not improve neurodevelopmental at two years of age [52], if compared to the placebo group.

3. Iron Status Measurement

Even if bone marrow aspiration is considered the gold standard for ID diagnosis, it has been replaced in clinical practice by other less invasive laboratory parameters [53], classified in hematological and non-hematological tests. The former includes Hb, mean corpuscular volume (MCV), reticulocyte count, and hemoglobin reticulocytes content, designated as the mean cellular hemoglobin content of reticulocytes (CHr) or reticulocyte hemoglobin equivalent (RET-He). The latter include serum ferritin (SF), transferrin saturation, soluble transferrin receptor (STfR1), zinc protoporphyrin to heme ratio (ZnPP/H).

The changes in iron status tests in response to ID, IDA, or iron overload are reported in Table 1. [14,54,55].

Table 1. Iron status parameters: their response to ID, IDA and iron overload [14,54,55].

Parameter	ID	IDA	Iron Overload
Hb	Normal	Reduced	Normal
MCV	Normal	Reduced	Normal
RET-He/CHr	Reduced	Reduced	Normal
SF	Reduced	Reduced	Increased
Transferrin saturation	Reduced	Reduced	Increased
sTfR1	Increased	Increased	Reduced
ZnPP/H ratio	Increased	Increased	Reduced

ID, iron deficiency; IDA, iron deficiency anemia; Hb, hemoglobin; MCV, mean corpuscular volume; RET-HE, reticulocyte hemoglobin equivalent; CHr, mean cellular hemoglobin content of reticulocytes; SF, serum ferritin; sTfR1, serum transferrin receptor; ZnPP/He ratio, zinc protoporphyrin to heme ratio.

The assessment of neonatal iron status is a challenging task as neonatal blood sampling requires a well-trained phlebotomist and is not routinely performed among healthy newborns. For this reason, neonatologists, instead of "normal values" established from healthy neonates, use "reference ranges" that include values between the 5th and the 95th percentile derived from newborns with minor pathology [56].

Moreover, most hematological parameters are influenced by gestational age and postnatal developmental changes [56]. As a result, gestational age-specific laboratory markers are needed. The site of blood collection (venous, arterial, capillary) and the use of different reagents can further impact on values [57]. Reference ranges for the main iron status parameters in term and preterm neonates are listed in Table 2.

Table 2. Reference ranges for the main iron status parameters in term and preterm neonates.

	Cord Blood		Capillary Blood (within 72 h from Birth)		
	Preterm	Term	Preterm	Term	
Hb (g/dL)	12.4–19.2	13.3–18.4		14.5–22.5	Lorenz et al. 2013 [57]
MCV (fL)	103–133	97.8–118.5		95–121	Lorenz et al. 2013 [57]
Serum ferritin (µg/L)	35–267	40–309			Siddappa et al. 2007 [28]
STfR1 (mg/L)	6.1–13.7	6.4–10.6			Sweet e al. 2001 [58]
ZnPP/H ratio (µmol/mol)	55–135.5	49.6–108.4			Juul et al. 2003 [59]
RET-He (pg)		27.4–36	24.3–36.2	25.5–37.6	Löfving et al. 2018 [60] Lorenz et al. 2017 [61]

Hb, hemoglobin; MCV, mean corpuscular volume; sTfR1, serum transferrin receptor; ZnPP/He ratio, zinc protoporphyrin to heme ratio; RET-HE, reticulocyte hemoglobin equivalent. All are central 95% reference intervals, except for SF that is central 90% and STfR1 that is the interquartile range.

Given the relevance of iron homeostasis in neonates, especially among premature ones, and the potential reversibility of pathologic conditions with prompt treatment, the reliable measurement of iron status is pivotal [57]. However, normative values of the main parameters used for the diagnosis of ID and IDA in premature infants are still lacking [62].

The iron reduction can be summarized through three stages of increasing severity:

1. Iron depletion: decrease of total iron storage, as reflected by SF, the first laboratory index to decline in ID;
2. Iron deficient erythropoiesis: initial reduction of Hb concentration due to complete depletion of iron stores; and
3. Iron deficiency anemia: ID associated with anemia, defined by WHO as Hb level two standard deviations below the median of a healthy population of the same age and sex [5,14].

Hb is the most frequently used hematologic parameter to screen for ID in infants. In clinical practice, the terms "anemia" and "IDA" have been interchangeably used as if the ID is the only cause of anemia [14,63]. However, Hb alone lacks sensibility and specificity since low Hb levels can derive from several conditions other than ID, such as hemolysis, chronic infections, genetic disease, or other less common nutrient deficiencies, particularly folate or vitamin B12 [14]. For this reason, to establish IDA, Hb measurement should be associated with: (1) SF and C reactive protein (CRP), or (2) CHr, based on AAP recommendations [14].

However, anemia suggests a severe depletion of iron stores. Indeed Hb is a late marker of ID and is not a reliable indicator of neonatal iron status, especially if measured in newborns suffering from chronic hypoxia, where stored iron is prioritized to preserve erythropoiesis to the detriment of other tissues [13].

Since ID alone, even without anemia, may impair neurodevelopment, prompt diagnosis and treatment of ID are essential. The AAP suggests to screen ID through the measurements of (1) SF and CRP, or (2) CHr [14].

Serum ferritin estimates total iron body stores; its cord blood concentration steadily increases throughout gestation [62]. Recently, ferritin concentration has been measured in cord blood in neonates from 23 to 41 gestational age [28]. Specifically, SF values below 35 µg/L indicate ID in preterm infants and correlates with complete depletion of liver iron stores [28]. On the other hand, SF concentrations >300 µg/L depict iron overload [64]. However, SF is an acute phase reactant and can reach high concentration during inflammation and infection [2]. As an increase in SF during co-existing inflammatory processes can mask ID, the AAP suggests the simultaneous measurement of SF and CRP [2]:

- low SF concentrations regardless of CRP level confirm ID;
- increased or normal SF levels associated with normal CRP concentrations rule out ID; and
- when high or normal SF concentrations are associated with increased CRP levels, iron status cannot be assessed [14].

Serum ferritin concentrations increase in the early postnatal period due to hemolysis and delivery itself, so that cord ferritin levels are approximately 1/3 of those in the first 72 h of life [58]. The opposite happens to serum iron concentration, increased in the umbilical vein, as a result of iron transport from the mother to the fetus [58].

RET-He and CHr quantify iron concentration inside reticulocytes and, therefore, by providing a real-time assessment of bone marrow iron status, may represent a preventive screening test for ID [63]. Indeed, their detection may anticipate ID diagnosis, if compared to Hb, which is a late marker of ID, since Hb evaluates the whole red blood cell population. Recent studies suggest a role for CHr in predicting future IDA even among infants; however, its measurement is not readily available in a laboratory setting [63]. A linear correlation has been reported between RET-He and CHr [65].

Similarly, STfR1 concentration is related to intracellular iron stores. High STfR1 concentrations are found in term and preterm neonates as a result of maternal ID, reflecting a poor iron endowment [28]. They are not directly influenced by gestational age [58]. Neonatal reference ranges should be established to improve its use in clinical practice.

ZnPP/H detects zinc incorporation into protoporphyrin IX in erythrocytes [66]. In case of insufficient iron delivery to bone marrow and reduced erythropoiesis [62], iron is replaced by zinc, thus increasing ZnPP/H ratio. Nevertheless, it cannot distinguish whether it is caused by body iron stores depletion or enhanced rate of erythropoiesis, as it happens in premature infants during the first weeks of life. ZnPP/H ratio is inversely correlated with gestational age [59,62]. Higher ZnPP/H ratios are detected in those born to mothers affected by gestational diabetes and IUGR or with chorioamnionitis, suggesting a potential association with inflammatory or infectious processes [28,59,62].

Brain iron concentrations are hardly measurable and can be quantified only at autopsy. Differently, serum ferritin can be used as an indirect index of brain ID while cord ferritin as a marker of in-utero fetal iron status [31]. Neurobehavioral tests are used to investigate multiple brain functions that can indicate the injured brain area, such as the Bayley Scales for Infant Development, Griffith Development Scale, Wechsler Preschool and Primary Scale of Intelligence (WPPSI), and the Wechsler Intelligence Scale for Children (WISC). Nevertheless, they show a low specificity for ID, since other nutrients deficiencies (e.g., zinc, copper, iodine) can lead to similar neurobehavioral abnormalities [6].

4. Iron Deficiency and Supplementation

4.1. Risk Factors

4.1.1. Maternal Iron Status

In the past, it has been assumed that a poor maternal iron status during pregnancy, unless determining severe IDA, does not affect fetal or neonatal iron endowment, as testified by the absence of association between maternal and cord blood Hb level [11]. Placental transferrin receptors increase in the case of maternal ID to transfer more iron to the fetus [11]. Conversely, it is known that maternal IDA is associated with preterm delivery and low birth weight, both of which lead to decreased neonatal iron stores [11].

However, a direct relationship between cord blood ferritin concentration, maternal Hb, and SF concentration has been found [11]. These observations may indicate that, even if cord blood Hb concentrations are within normal values, those born from mother with ID have reduced iron stores and are more likely to be anemic during infancy [67].

Iron supplementation during pregnancy is beneficial for both the mothers and their infants. The improvement of maternal iron status, even in women with satisfactory iron stores, prevents ID in the subsequent pregnancy [11] and reduces maternal fatigue with a positive impact on mental health, thus producing indirect postnatal benefits on neonatal development [37]. Moreover, iron intake is associated with higher blood ferritin concentration and better neurodevelopmental outcomes in their infants [27].

4.1.2. Maternal Comorbidities

Up to 10% of pregnancies in the developed countries are complicated by IUGR, secondary to placental insufficiency, and structural abnormalities of the placental vessels. These conditions may impair iron transport to the fetus, while chronic fetal hypoxia induces erythropoietin synthesis and subsequent iron use for Hb production [13]. Low cord blood ferritin has been found in about 50% of IUGR infants (<60 ng/mL). Similarly, maternal diabetes mellitus increases fetal metabolism and oxygen consumption by approximately 30% [62]. Hypoxia stimulates Hb synthesis, which requires 3.47 mg of iron for 1 g of Hb [4]. This increased demand depletes heart, liver, and brain iron stores with a severity that is inversely related to maternal glycemic control [4]. Furthermore, the physiological regulatory mechanism of the placenta seems to be lost. Despite fetal hypoxia, placental transferrin receptor (TfR1) concentration is low, indicating a decreased receptor response capacity [68].

As a result, IUGR infants and those born to a diabetic mother are at higher risk of brain ID. At autopsy, the most severe cases showed total iron brain content reduced by 30–40%, and more than half of them have low ferritin in cord blood [9].

4.1.3. Prematurity

Around 25–85% of premature newborns develop ID, associated or not with IDA, during infancy [16], usually with earlier onset than in full-term neonates. Indeed, at birth, total body iron concentration is, on average, 75 mg/kg in term neonates versus 64 mg/kg in preterm neonates [66]. Similarly, in the latter group, serum iron concentrations and cord SF are lower with higher sTfR1 levels at birth, when compared to term neonates [62].

Many factors contribute to the negative iron imbalance and can explain why premature infants are so vulnerable to ID and IDA. Firstly, even if placental iron transfer begins in the first trimester of pregnancy, approximately 80% of iron accumulates during the last one [68]. Therefore, the more premature the infant is, the poorer its iron status will be. Postnatally, low iron stores are further reduced by the rapid "catch up" growth with rapid blood volume expansion and increased Hb demand, which requires further iron [62]. Moreover, recurrent phlebotomies for diagnostic purposes cause an extra iron loss in VLBW neonates equal to 6 mg/kg/week, on average [64].

In the past, additional iron was supplied with red blood cells (RBC) transfusions to prevent the anemia of prematurity. In the last years, more restrictive RBC transfusion policies are encouraged, particularly among the sickest extremely preterm neonates, because of the associations between early exposure to RBC transfusions, and increased mortality and short-term morbidities [21,69–71].

4.1.4. Low Birth Weight

SGA neonates show lower iron stores when compared to gestation-matched appropriate-for-gestational-age (AGA) neonates in cord blood and at four weeks postnatally [72].

4.1.5. Gender

Gender may influence iron endowment at birth: males have a smaller iron supply at birth reflected by a significantly lower concentration of Hb, MCV, SF, and higher ZnPP and sTfR1 levels at four, six, and nine months when compared with females [73]. These features place male infants at increased risk of ID during infancy. Therefore, to exclude physiological sex-related differences, the construction of gender-specific reference intervals may be beneficial.

4.1.6. Breastfeeding

As human breast milk contains a very low quantity of iron (0.2–0.4 mg/L), exclusively breastfed infants are prone to develop ID [26,74]. The incidence of ID in the first six months of life is 6–15% and 12–37% in industrialized and developing countries, respectively [68]. The iron content in human milk satisfies full-term neonates' iron demand in the first 4–6 months of life, whereas iron stores of preterm neonates are depleted within 1–4 months after birth [16]. Despite the low iron content in human milk, its bioavailability is around 50%, much higher than in formula milk. Indeed lactoferrin, which is an iron-binding protein contained in breast milk, facilitates iron absorption. In contrast, casein and other cow milk's proteins in cow milk-based formula have an inhibitory effect on iron absorption [26].

4.2. Prevention

Recently, placental transfusion techniques, such as delayed cord clamping (DCC) and umbilical cord milking (UCM), have been implemented in routine neonatal care. DCC consists of delaying umbilical cord clamping for at least 30–60 s after delivery in both term and preterm infants not requiring immediate resuscitation [75]. This practice allows the transfer of 25–35 mL/kg of placental blood to the newborn, thus increasing iron stores by approximately 30% after three minutes of DCC [26]. Indeed, DCC, compared to immediate cord clamping, is associated with higher hemoglobin concentration in first weeks after birth in both term and preterm newborns, and lower rates of RBC transfusions in preterm newborns [75–77]. In the long term, DCC maintains its benefits, as evidenced by the higher ferritin levels and the lower incidence of ID at six months of age in term neonates [2,75,78]. Indeed, the amount of blood transferred via DCC is crucial in defining iron endowment at birth [12]. As largely illustrated above, ID and brain development are closely linked. DCC has been associated with improved neurodevelopmental outcome at four years in full-term infants and two years in very preterm newborns [79,80].

UCM consists of a gentle squeezing of the umbilical cord towards the baby two to five times before clamping. Similarly to DCC, UCM enhances iron stores in the first weeks after birth in premature infants as compared to early cord clamping [81]. However, results from a recent randomized clinical trial comparing UCM vs. DCC in preterm infants born before 32 weeks' gestation have shown a significantly higher rate of severe IVH in the UCM group [82].

Phlebotomy is the first cause of anemia in the first weeks of life [83], especially in the most premature newborns. Therefore, there is increasing attention to minimize blood loss in these patients. To this goal, the use of low blood volume point-of-care testing, non-invasive monitoring and the reduction of unnecessary blood sampling are mainstays of prevention [84].

Furthermore, otherwise discarded placental blood has been endorsed as an alternative source for Neonatal Intensive Care Unit (NICU) admission laboratory tests (complete blood count, blood culture, blood type, antibody screen, and metabolic screening) [85,86]. Of note, umbilical cord blood seems not suitable to assess neonatal hemostatic profile, as placental specimens show a procoagulant imbalance if compared to the neonatal counterparts [87]. Drawing blood directly from the umbilical vessels avoids invasive and painful neonatal procedures and results, especially in VLBW infants, in higher hemoglobin concentration, lower rates of RBC transfusions, and need for vasopressors in the first week of life [88]. Additionally, it appears to be a complementary procedure to DCC to maximize circulating blood volume.

4.3. Supplementation

4.3.1. Enteral Iron Supplementation

Enteral supplementation is the preferred route of iron administration. It can be provided through iron fortified-human milk, iron-fortified formula, or medicinal elemental iron, in the form of ferrous sulfate or ferrous fumarate. The former has been associated with better absorption, while the latter produced less oxidative stress in vitro. To our knowledge, no studies have compared the two preparations in premature infants [89].

Iron gut absorption has a high inter-individual variability ranging from 10% to 50% of the dose administered and is increased when given with breast milk or with vitamin C [16,57]. Iron intake depends on:

1. Local factors, such as gastric pH and intestinal mucosal function; and
2. General drivers, such as the source of enteral iron (human or formula milk) and the iron stores of the infant [90].

It has been hypothesized that iron absorption and release may be impaired due to enterocytes' immaturity, thus explaining inadequate iron intakes in orally supplemented neonates [91].

The position paper by the European Society for Pediatric Gastroenterology, Hepatology, and Nutrition (ESPGHAN) recommend an elemental iron intake of 1–2 mg/kg/day for all premature infants with a birth weight less than 2500 g and of 2–3 mg/kg/day for those weighing less than 2000 g [92]. Similarly, the Committee on Nutrition of the AAP suggests a daily iron supplementation of 2 mg/kg for all breastfed preterm infants, from 1 to 12 months of age [93]. An enteral iron dosage >5 mg/kg/day should be avoided in these patients [94].

Iron content in infant formula is 14.6 mg/L and 12 mg/L in standard preterm and term formula, respectively. Based on a standard daily milk intake of 150 mL/kg, formula-fed neonates receive around 1.8–2.2 mg/kg/day of iron [14]. Although being fed with iron-enriched formula, up to 14% of preterm infants develop ID in the first year of life. Thus, iron status should be monitored to individualize iron supplementation of preterm neonates [14].

In case of IDA in preterm newborns, elemental enteral iron supplementation is increased to 3–6 mg/kg per day for three months [93].

The current recommendation may not be adequate to meet the needs of all premature infants. The most immature neonates, such as ELBW, have a poor iron endowment and may require extra iron due to the catch-up growth and increased erythropoiesis. Indeed, 15% of infants with birth-weight <1301 g are iron deficient at two months of age even if supplemented with 4–6 mg/kg of iron since the second week of age [95]. Nevertheless, the majority of ELBW infants receive 3–5 RBC transfusions during their hospital stay that improve their iron stores [16]. For these reasons, the iron status of ELBW infants should be monitored to tailor iron administration.

No gastrointestinal adverse effects have been described after the administration of iron-rich formula or elemental iron. Hematochezia has been reported in 17% of premature infants exposed to high doses of medical iron (8–16 mg/kg/day) [90]. However, a causal link with oral iron administration was not established, and iron supplementation can be resumed after the resolution of symptoms [16].

Concerns were raised regarding the possible interaction in absorption between iron and other divalent cations since they share the same gut transport mechanism (divalent metal transporter 1, DMT1). However, iron supplementation at the recommended doses does not interfere with zinc or selenium uptake, and zinc supplementation does not compromise iron absorption [16,96]. Conversely, it is known that oral iron alters copper metabolism, although further research is needed [97].

Iron supplementation may induce oxidative stress by promoting ROS production as a result of increased intra- and extra-cellular free iron concentrations [98], whose underlying mechanism has been previously mentioned (cfr paragraph 2, Figure 1).

4.3.2. Parenteral Iron Supplementation

In addition to the oral route, iron can be administered parenterally. Intramuscular administration is not recommended because it is painful and prone to complications, while intravenous (i.v.) iron appears to be safe [99]. Although the daily iron intake during the third trimester is about 1.6–2 mg/kg/day, a dose of 120 µg/kg/day is adequate and, since there is no physiologic regulatory mechanism for iron excretion, almost the totality of it gets stored in tissues [16]. When compared with the enteral route, i.v. supplementation is associated with higher SF levels, while inconclusive results are related to its efficacy in supporting erythropoiesis [99]. Besides, the need for i.v. line in a full enterally-fed infant makes the i.v. route unreasonable in clinical practice. Moreover, a transient rise of malondialdehyde (MDA), indicating lipid peroxidation, has been reported after iron infusions, thus suggesting a risk of oxidative stress [16].

4.4. Risk Groups Requiring Tailored Iron Supplementation

Preterm infants treated with rHuEPO require higher doses of iron because rHuEPO improves growth, stimulates erythropoiesis, and decreases the number of RBC transfusions at the expense of tissues iron stores, as reflected by the decrease in SF after the initiation of rHuEPO therapy [90,100]. The AAP recommends an oral iron supplementation of 6 mg/kg/day during rHuEPO therapy [93]. This dose is appropriate to sustain erythropoiesis; however, it may be inadequate to preserve body iron stores. No differences have been found in the SF levels nor in the hematological response after an oral iron supplementation at a high dose (16 mg/kg/day) or low dose (8 mg/kg/day) in infants treated with rHuEPO, as reported by Bader et al. [90].

Ferritin concentration higher than 100 µg/L should be considered the threshold to guide iron administration during rHuEPO therapy [16].

Despite the lack of specific recommendations, infants with increased SF concentrations (>350 µg/L) might require personalized iron supplementation. This condition can indicate two different states:

1. Iron overload (e.g., after recurrent erythrocyte transfusions); or
2. Iron sequestration (e.g., in the setting of an inflammatory process).

While the former group is at risk of iron overload associated insults, and should not be supplemented, the latter can suffer from bone marrow ID and subsequent insufficient erythropoiesis and thus could benefit from iron administration. Assessing bone marrow iron status by measuring reticulocyte count and ZnPP/H ratio can support decision making [16].

Nevertheless, one out of four premature neonates with SF levels >95th percentile at hospital discharge will manifest ID at 6–12 months of age if iron supplementation is discontinued [16].

4.5. Timing of Iron Supplementation and Screening of ID

Iron supplementation should start from four to six weeks of age [16] when serum iron and ferritin concentration start reducing and iron incorporation in RBC occurs more efficiently [16]. The AAP does not recommend iron supplementation before the second week of age, due to the immature antioxidant capacity before that age [4]. In contrast, iron supplementation, by two weeks of age, as suggested by ESPGHAN [94], is associated with decreased rates of RBC transfusions and incidence of ID at 2–6 months of age when compared with later onset. Only one study evaluated the long-term effect of early (started at a median age of 14 days) versus late (eight weeks) iron supplementation reporting better cognitive and motor outcomes at five years of age following the earlier start [41]. However, this study was underpowered to evaluate improvements in neurocognitive development [41,101]. Therefore, in the absence of consistent data, considering the potential risk of iron administration in the first month of life due to iron overload and immaturity of the gastrointestinal function, caution is required, especially in ELBW infants.

Iron supplementation should be provided at least up to six months of age when weaning with iron-rich foods begins [94]. The AAP recommends prolonging iron supplementation until the end of the first year of life [93].

The iron status of premature infants should be monitored periodically. The frequency and timing of follow up controls should be scheduled, taking into account the iron status at discharge, iron supplementation, and type of feeding [16].

5. Iron Overload and Toxicity

5.1. Risk Factors

5.1.1. RBC Transfusions

Transfusion-derived iron is the main cause of iron overload in premature infants. Around 80% of VLBW and 95% of ELBW infants require at least one RBC transfusion during hospitalization, with 0.5–1 mg of iron intake for each mL of packed RBC transfused. [16].

Biologically, the exceeding iron cannot be actively excreted by humans. Consequently, after multiple transfusions, higher serum and ferritin concentrations and liver iron storage can be found in preterm infants [16].

The pathogenesis of prematurity-related comorbidities is multifactorial. The association between the rate of erythrocyte transfusions and the incidence of NEC, IVH, ROP, and BPD has been suggested [21,102–104]. In this context, iron (excess) has been hypothesized to play a causative role due to its impact on the immune system [105], nitric oxide-induced vasoregulation [106], and oxidative stress [107]. Specifically, both the preparation and storage of pediatric packed RBCs may predispose to redox unbalance. Indeed, pediatric RBCs are prepared from adult blood, by replacing most of the plasma with additive solutions, thus reducing the net amount of iron-binding proteins and antioxidants [108].

During storage, the exposure of blood to shear stress, plastic bags, anticoagulants, and additives contributes to the increase of extracellular iron and NTBI [109], leading to a rise in MDA [110].

In adults, the storage duration of transfused RBCs does not impact on mortality [111]. In pediatrics, there is a low level of evidence stemming from observational studies of the association between longer storage duration of transfused RBCs and worse outcomes [112]. However, data from clinical trials do not support the use of fresh blood [113,114]. Donor exposure is another relevant issue, especially when it comes to the smallest and sickest premature infants, requiring multiple transfusions in the early days of life. The use of satellite bags (small-volume aliquots from the same unit of donor blood) may limit the donor exposure rate [115,116].

Finally, procedures that require massive blood products exposure, as in the case of exchange transfusion or extracorporeal membrane oxygenation, further increases the neonatal exposure to hemolysis, oxidative stress and, hence, the risk of mortality [117,118].

5.1.2. Excessive Iron Supplementation

At routinely-used dosage, parenteral or enteral iron does not produce oxidative stress injury, even if a transient peak of serum iron level can be registered after administration [16]. It is reported that even an enteral supplementation at higher doses (up to 18 mg/kg/day) [119] does not cause oxidative stress damage but, instead, stimulate erythropoiesis, as low ZnPP/H ratio testify [66]. In VLBW infants, a one-week course of high doses of oral iron (18 mg/kg/day) did not result in a change in oxidative stress biomarkers nor anti-oxidants levels [89].

However, lower doses (3–6 mg/kg/day) for a longer period (up to nine months of age) produce an increase in glutathione peroxidase concentrations, a marker of oxidative stress [120]. Moreover, large doses of enteral iron administration have been linked to hemolysis in preterm infants with vitamin E deficiency [16].

5.2. Iron Toxicity

Iron excess has been associated with poor growth and interference with zinc and copper metabolism [26]. The relationship between iron and infection is widely recognized [121]. Previous studies reported an increased incidence of respiratory tract infections in neonates supplemented with high iron doses (formula fortified with 20.7 mg iron/L) [120]. Certainly, NTBI acts as a potent pro-oxidant agent through the generation of ROS.

Recently, a trial showed that iron-fortified foods modulate the intestinal microbiota, with overgrowth of pathogenic enterobacteria, thus triggering gut inflammation [122]. The consequences of this process are not yet known and deserve to be explored.

Premature infants are vulnerable to iron toxicity due to low TIBC levels and immature anti-oxidant defenses that facilitates iron oxidation of the ferrous state with the increase of ROS production [16]. Vitamin E and vitamin C are radical-scavenging antioxidants, which are poorly adsorbed until the 34th week of gestation and low activity in the first two weeks of life [4]. Finally, superoxide dismutase (SOD), which is an enzyme with a key antioxidant role, is lacking in preterm neonates [4,25].

A recent study involving 95 premature neonates found no association between moderate iron overload, as defined by SF >400 ng/mL but <1000 ng/mL at 34–35 weeks of corrected age and neurodevelopmental impairment at 8–12 months [119]. However, preterm newborns in the first weeks of life are prone to develop oxidative stress, due to concomitant predisposing risk factors. Therefore even modest SF levels may damage the brain [119].

The early identification of biomarkers of oxidative stress could prevent future sequelae and allow new therapeutic strategies. To date, serum and urinary prostanoids, particularly urinary 8-isoprostane, and visfatin, an adipocytokine involved in inflammation, have been identified as potential markers of oxidative stress in premature newborns [25,89,123].

Additionally, the dosage of plasma antioxidants, such as glutathione, vitamin E, and vitamin C (ascorbic acid), particularly oxidized to total ascorbic acid ratio (DHAA/TAA), has been proposed to prevent oxidative stress [89]. Recently, serum gamma-glutamyltransferase (GGT) has been found to have a role in ROS production and glutathione synthesis, and it might be used as a cheap and reliable marker of oxidative stress [124]. Plasma adenosine appears as a promising biomarker to predict brain damage; however, its role in the neonatal setting has yet to be demonstrated [25].

6. Concluding Remarks and Future Perspectives

Many preventive measures have already been implemented in clinical practice to tackle ID, and iron supplementation is recommended for all preterm neonates. However, since iron levels are influenced by several perinatal factors, a tailored-supplementation based on laboratory iron status parameters should be encouraged.

For this reason, gestational age-related reference ranges for the main iron-related diagnostic indices should be established, especially for the most immature neonates. Attention should be paid to the new ID markers, such as RET-He and CHr, which could anticipate ID diagnosis, thus allowing a prompt therapy.

Beyond ID and IDA, which have been widely addressed, iron overload is emerging as a 'new' issue in the management of sick preterm infants. Future efforts should focus on the early identification of biomarkers of oxidative stress, which could improve patients' care by paving the way for innovative therapeutic targets.

The main risk factors, prevention strategies, and therapies for iron deficiency and overload are summarized in Figure 2.

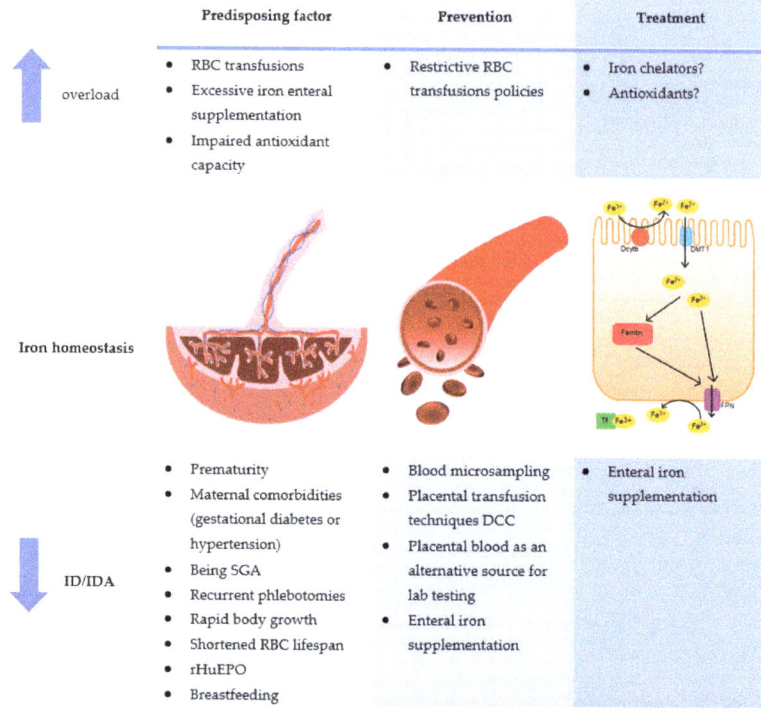

Figure 2. Iron homeostasis in preterm newborns: risk factors, prevention strategies and treatment.

DCC: delayed cord clamping; Dcytb: duodenal cytochrome b; DMT1: divalent metal transporter; Fe^{2+}: ferrous cation; Fe^{3+}: ferric cation; FPN: ferroportin; RBC: red blood cell; rHuEPO: recombinant human erythropoietin; SGA: small for gestational age; TF: transferrin.

Author Contributions: Conceptualization: G.R., G.C., F.M. (Fabio Mosca), and S.G.; methodology: G.R., F.M. (Francesca Manzoni), V.C., G.C., F.M. (Fabio Mosca), and S.G.; supervision: G.C., F.M. (Fabio Mosca), and S.G.; visualization: G.R., F.M. (Francesca Manzoni), and V.C.; writing—original draft preparation: G.R. and F.M. (Francesca Manzoni); writing—review and editing: V.C., G.C., F.M. (Fabio Mosca), and S.G. All authors have read and agreed to the published version of the manuscript.

Funding: This research received no external funding.

Conflicts of Interest: The authors declare no conflict of interest.

List of Abbreviation

AAP	American Academy of Pediatrics
ABR	Auditory brainstem-evoked response
AGA	Appropriate-for-gestational-age
BPD	Bronchopulmonary dysplasia
CHr	Reticulocyte hemoglobin content
CRP	C reactive protein
CSF	Cerebrospinal fluid
DCC	Delayed cord clamping
DHAA/TAA	Oxidized to total ascorbic acid ratio

DMT1	Divalent metal transporter 1
ELBW	Extremely low birth weight
ESPGHAN	The European Society for Pediatric Gastroenterology, Hepatology, and Nutrition
GGT	Gamma-glutamyltransferase
Hb	Hemoglobin
HIE	Hypoxic-ischemic encephalopathy
ICH	Intracerebral hemorrhage
ID	Iron deficiency
IDA	Iron deficiency anemia
IUGR	Intrauterine growth restriction
i.v.	Intravenous
IVH	Intraventricular hemorrhage
MDA	Malondialdehyde
MCV	Mean corpuscular volume
NEC	Necrotizing enterocolitis
NICU	Neonatal Intensive Care Unit
NTBI	Non-transferrin-bound iron
PVL	Periventricular leukomalacia
PWM	Punctate white matter lesions
RBC	Red blood cells
RET-He	Reticulocyte hemoglobin equivalent
rHuEPO	Recombinant human erythropoietin
ROP	Retinopathy of prematurity
ROS	Reactive oxygen species
SF	Serum ferritin
SGA	Small-for-gestational-age
STfR1	Soluble transferrin receptor
TACO	Transfusion-associated circulatory overload
TfR1	Transferrin receptor
TIBC	Total iron bind capacity
TRALI	Transfusion-related acute lung injury
UCM	Umbilical cord milking
VLBW	Very low birth weight
ZnPP/H	Zinc protoporphyrin to heme ratio

References

1. Moreno-Fernández, J.; Ochoa, J.J.; Latunde-Dada, G.O.; Diaz-Castro, J. Iron deficiency and iron homeostasis in low birth weight preterm infants: A systematic review. *Nutrients* **2019**, *11*, 1090. [CrossRef] [PubMed]
2. Cao, C.; O'Brien, K.O. Pregnancy and iron homeostasis: An update. *Nutr. Rev.* **2013**, *71*, 35–51. [CrossRef]
3. Lozoff, B.; Beard, J.; Connor, J.; Felt, B.; Georgieff, M.; Schallert, T. Long-lasting neural and behavioral effects of iron deficiency in infancy. *Nutr. Rev.* **2006**, *64*, S34–S91. [CrossRef] [PubMed]
4. Georgieff, M.K. Iron. In *Neonatal Nutrition and Metabolism*; Cambridge University Press (CUP): Cambridge, UK, 2009; pp. 291–298.
5. United Nations Administrative Committee on Coordination/Sub-Committee on Nutririon; International Food Policy Research Institute. *Fourth Report of the World Nutrition Situation*; United Nations Administrative Committee on Coordination/Sub-Committee on Nutrition: Geneva, Switzerland, 2000.
6. Wang, Y.; Wu, Y.; Li, T.; Wang, X.; Zhu, C. Iron metabolism and brain development in premature infants. *Front. Physiol.* **2019**, *10*, 463. [CrossRef] [PubMed]
7. Gkouvatsos, K.; Papanikolaou, G.; Pantopoulos, K. Regulation of iron transport and the role of transferrin. *Biochim. Biophys. Acta* **2012**, *1820*, 188–202. [CrossRef] [PubMed]
8. Bastian, T.W.; Von Hohenberg, W.C.; Mickelson, D.J.; Lanier, L.M.; Georgieff, M.K. Iron deficiency impairs developing hippocampal neuron gene expression, energy metabolism and dendrite complexity. *Dev. Neurosci.* **2016**, *38*, 264–276. [CrossRef]

9. Lozoff, B.; Georgieff, M.K. Iron deficiency and brain development. *Semin. Pediatr. Neurol.* **2006**, *13*, 158–165. [CrossRef]
10. Scholl, T.O. Maternal iron status: Relation to fetal growth, length of gestation and the neonate's iron endowment. *Nutr. Rev.* **2011**, *69*, S23–S29. [CrossRef]
11. Allen, L.H. Anemia and iron deficiency: Effects on pregnancy outcome. *Am. J. Clin. Nutr.* **2000**, *71*, 1280S–1284S. [CrossRef]
12. Chaparro, C.M. Timing of umbilical cord clamping: Effect on iron endowment of the newborn and later iron status. *Nutr. Rev.* **2011**, *69*, S30–S36. [CrossRef]
13. Mukhopadhyay, K.; Yadav, R.K.; Kishore, S.S.; Garewal, G.; Jain, V.; Narang, A. Iron status at birth and at 4 weeks in term small-for-gestation infants in comparison with appropriate-for-gestation infants. *J. Matern. Neonatal Med.* **2010**, *24*, 886–890. [CrossRef] [PubMed]
14. Baker, R.D.; Greer, F.R. Diagnosis and prevention of iron deficiency and iron-deficiency anemia in infants and young children (0–3 years of age). *Pediatrics* **2010**, *126*, 1040–1050. [CrossRef] [PubMed]
15. Collard, K.J.; Anderson, B.; Storfer-Isser, A.; Taylor, H.G.; Rosen, C.L.; Redline, S. Iron homeostasis in the neonate. *Pediatrics* **2009**, *123*, 1208–1216. [CrossRef] [PubMed]
16. Rao, R.B.; Georgieff, M.K. Iron therapy for preterm infants. *Clin. Perinatol.* **2009**, *36*, 27–42. [CrossRef]
17. Aggett, P.J. Trace elements of the micropremie. *Clin. Perinatol.* **2000**, *27*, 119–129. [CrossRef]
18. Georgieff, M.K. Long-term brain and behavioral consequences of early iron deficiency. *Nutr. Rev.* **2011**, *69*, S43–S48. [CrossRef]
19. Buonocore, G.; Perrone, S.; Longini, M.; Vezzosi, P. Oxidative stress in preterm neonates at birth and on the seventh day of life. *Pediatr. Res.* **2002**, *52*, 46–49. [CrossRef]
20. Buonocore, G.; Perrone, S.; Longini, M.; Paffetti, P.; Vezzosi, P.; Gatti, M.G.; Bracci, R. Non protein bound iron as early predictive marker of neonatal brain damage. *Brain* **2003**, *126*, 1224–1230. [CrossRef]
21. Dusi, E.; Cortinovis, I.; Villa, S.; Fumagalli, M.; Agosti, M.; Milani, S.; Mosca, F.; Ghirardello, S. Effects of red blood cell transfusions on the risk of developing complications or death: An observational study of a cohort of very low birth weight infants. *Am. J. Perinatol.* **2016**, *34*, 88–95. [CrossRef]
22. Chen, J.; Smith, L.E. Retinopathy of prematurity. *Angiogenesis* **2007**, *10*, 133–140. [CrossRef]
23. Shouman, B.O.; Mesbah, A.; Aly, H. Iron metabolism and lipid peroxidation products in infants with hypoxic ischemic encephalopathy. *J. Perinatol.* **2008**, *28*, 487–491. [CrossRef] [PubMed]
24. Saugstad, O.D. The oxygen radical disease in neonatology. *Indian J. Pediatr.* **1989**, *56*, 585–593. [CrossRef] [PubMed]
25. Panfoli, I.; Candiano, G.; Malova, M.; De Angelis, L.; Cardiello, V.; Buonocore, G.; Ramenghi, L.A. Oxidative stress as a primary risk factor for brain damage in preterm newborns. *Front. Pediatr.* **2018**, *6*. [CrossRef] [PubMed]
26. Lönnerdal, B.; Georgieff, M.K.; Hernell, O. Developmental physiology of iron absorption, homeostasis, and metabolism in the healthy term infant. *J. Pediatr.* **2015**, *167*, S8–S14. [CrossRef]
27. Beard, J.L.; Connor, J.R. Iron status and neural functioning. *Annu. Rev. Nutr.* **2003**, *23*, 41–58. [CrossRef]
28. Siddappa, A.M.; Rao, R.B.; Long, J.D.; Widness, J.A.; Georgieff, M.K. The assessment of newborn iron stores at birth: A review of the literature and standards for ferritin concentrations. *Neonatology* **2007**, *92*, 73–82. [CrossRef]
29. Walker, S.; Wachs, T.D.; Gardner, J.M.; Lozoff, B.; Wasserman, G.A.; Pollitt, E.; Carter, J.A. Child development: Risk factors for adverse outcomes in developing countries. *Lancet* **2007**, *369*, 145–157. [CrossRef]
30. Grantham-McGregor, S.M.; Ani, C. A review of studies on the effect of iron deficiency on cognitive development in children. *J. Nutr.* **2001**, *131*, 649S–668S. [CrossRef]
31. Amin, S.B.; Orlando, M.; Eddins, A.; Macdonald, M.; Monczynski, C.; Wang, H. In utero iron status and auditory neural maturation in premature infants as evaluated by auditory brainstem response. *J. Pediatr.* **2009**, *156*, 377–381. [CrossRef]
32. Tamura, T.; Goldenberg, R.L.; Hou, J.; Johnston, K.E.; Cliver, S.P.; Ramey, S.L.; Nelson, K.G. Cord serum ferritin concentrations and mental and psychomotor development of children at five years of age. *J. Pediatr.* **2002**, *140*, 165–170. [CrossRef]
33. Armony-Sivan, R.; Eidelman, A.I.; Lanir, A.; Sredni, D.; Yehuda, S. Iron status and neurobehavioral development of premature infants. *J. Perinatol.* **2004**, *24*, 757–762. [CrossRef] [PubMed]

34. Felt, B.T.; Lozoff, B. Brain iron and behavior of rats are not normalized by treatment of iron deficiency anemia during early development. *J. Nutr.* **1996**, *126*, 693–701. [CrossRef] [PubMed]
35. Pasricha, S.-R.; Hayes, E.; Kalumba, K.; Biggs, B.-A. Effect of daily iron supplementation on health in children aged 4–23 months: A systematic review and meta-analysis of randomised controlled trials. *Lancet Glob. Health* **2013**, *1*, e77–e86. [CrossRef]
36. Wang, B.; Zhan, S.; Gong, T.; Lee, L. Iron therapy for improving psychomotor development and cognitive function in children under the age of three with iron deficiency anaemia. *Cochrane Database Syst. Rev.* **2013**, *2013*, CD001444. [CrossRef] [PubMed]
37. Christian, P.; Mullany, L.C.; Hurley, K.M.; Katz, J.; Black, R.E. Nutrition and maternal, neonatal, and child health. *Semin. Perinatol.* **2015**, *39*, 361–372. [CrossRef]
38. Friel, J.K.; Aziz, K.; Andrews, W.L.; Harding, S.; Courage, M.L.; Adams, R.J. A double-masked, randomized control trial of iron supplementation in early infancy in healthy term breast-fed infants. *J. Pediatr.* **2003**, *143*, 582–586. [CrossRef]
39. Lozoff, B.; De Andraca, I.; Castillo, M.; Smith, J.B.; Walter, T.; Pino, P. Behavioral and developmental effects of preventing irondeficiency anemia in healthy full-term infants. *Pediatrics* **2003**, *112*, 846–854.
40. Szajewska, H.; Ruszczyński, M.; Chmielewska, A. Effects of iron supplementation in nonanemic pregnant women, infants, and young children on the mental performance and psychomotor development of children: A systematic review of randomized controlled trials. *Am. J. Clin. Nutr.* **2010**, *91*, 1684–1690. [CrossRef]
41. Steinmacher, J.; Pohlandt, F.; Bode, H.; Sander, S.; Kron, M.; Franz, A.R. Randomized trial of early versus late enteral iron supplementation in infants with a birth weight of less than 1301 grams: Neurocognitive development at 5.3 years' corrected age. *Pediatrics* **2007**, *120*, 538–546. [CrossRef]
42. Perrone, S.; Tataranno, L.M.; Stazzoni, G.; Ramenghi, L.A.; Buonocore, G. Brain susceptibility to oxidative stress in the perinatal period. *J. Matern. Neonatal Med.* **2013**, *28*, 2291–2295. [CrossRef] [PubMed]
43. Wu, Y.; Song, J.; Wang, Y.; Wang, X.; Culmsee, C.; Zhu, C. The potential role of ferroptosis in neonatal brain injury. *Front. Mol. Neurosci.* **2019**, *13*, 115. [CrossRef]
44. Buonocore, G.; Zani, S.; Sargentini, I.; Gioia, D.; Signorini, C.; Bracci, R. Hypoxia-induced free iron release in the red cells of newborn infants. *Acta Paediatr.* **1998**, *87*, 77–81. [CrossRef] [PubMed]
45. Rathnasamy, G.; Ling, E.-A.; Kaur, C. Iron and iron regulatory proteins in amoeboid microglial cells are linked to oligodendrocyte death in hypoxic neonatal rat periventricular white matter through production of proinflammatory cytokines and reactive oxygen/nitrogen species. *J. Neurosci.* **2011**, *31*, 17982–17995. [CrossRef] [PubMed]
46. Dorrepaal, C.A.; Berger, H.M.; Benders, M.J.; Van Zoeren-Grobben, D.; Van De Bor, M.; Van Bel, F. Nonprotein-bound iron in postasphyxial reperfusion injury of the newborn. *Pediatrics* **1996**, *98*, 883–889. [PubMed]
47. Magtanong, L.; Dixon, S.J. Ferroptosis and brain injury. *Dev. Neurosci.* **2018**, *40*, 382–395. [CrossRef]
48. Ciccoli, L.; Rossi, V.; Leoncini, S.; Signorini, C.; Blanco-Garcia, J. Iron release in newborn and adult erythrocytes exposed to hypoxia-reoxygenation. *Biochim. Biophys. Acta* **2004**, *1672*, 203–213. [CrossRef]
49. Halliwell, B. Reactive oxygen species and the central nervous system. *J. Neurochem.* **1992**, *59*, 1609–1623. [CrossRef]
50. Song, J.; Sun, H.; Xu, F.; Kang, W.; Gao, L.; Guo, J.; Zhang, Y.; Xia, L.; Wang, X.; Zhu, C. Recombinant human erythropoietin improves neurological outcomes in very preterm infants. *Ann. Neurol.* **2016**, *80*, 24–34. [CrossRef]
51. Zhu, C.; Kang, W.; Xu, F.; Cheng, X.; Zhang, Z.; Jia, L.; Ji, L.; Guo, X.; Xiong, H.; Simbruner, G.; et al. Erythropoietin improved neurologic outcomes in newborns with hypoxic-ischemic encephalopathy. *Pediatrics* **2009**, *124*, e218–e226. [CrossRef]
52. Juul, S.E.; Comstock, B.A.; Wadhawan, R.; Mayock, D.E.; Courtney, S.E.; Robinson, T.; Ahmad, K.A.; Bendel-Stenzel, E.; Baserga, M.; LaGamma, E.F.; et al. A randomized trial of erythropoietin for neuroprotection in preterm infants. *N. Engl. J. Med.* **2020**, *382*, 233–243. [CrossRef]
53. Lorenz, L.; Arand, J.; Büchner, K.; Wacker-Gussmann, A.; Peter, A.; Poets, C.F.; Franz, A.R. Reticulocyte haemoglobin content as a marker of iron deficiency. *Arch. Dis. Child. Fetal Neonatal Ed.* **2014**, *100*, F198–F202. [CrossRef] [PubMed]

54. Uçar, M.A.; Falay, M.; Dağdas, S.; Ceran, F.; Urlu, S.M.; Özet, G. The importance of RET-He in the diagnosis of iron deficiency and iron deficiency anemia and the evaluation of response to oral iron therapy. *J. Med. Biochem.* **2019**, *38*, 496–502. [CrossRef] [PubMed]
55. Al, R. Zinc protoporphyrin/heme ratio for diagnosis of preanemic iron deficiency. *Pediatrics* **1999**, *104*, e37.
56. Christensen, R.D.; Henry, E.; Jopling, J.; Wiedmeier, S.E. The CBC: Reference ranges for neonates. *Semin. Perinatol.* **2009**, *33*, 3–11. [CrossRef] [PubMed]
57. Lorenz, L.; Peter, A.; Poets, C.F.; Franz, A.R. A review of cord blood concentrations of iron status parameters to define reference ranges for preterm infants. *Neonatology* **2013**, *104*, 194–202. [CrossRef]
58. Sweet, D.G.; Savage, G.; Tubman, R.; Lappin, T.R.J.; Halliday, H.L. Cord blood transferrin receptors to assess fetal iron status. *Arch. Dis. Child. Fetal Neonatal Ed.* **2001**, *85*, F46–F48. [CrossRef]
59. Juul, S.; Zerzan, J.C.; Strandjord, T.P.; Woodrum, D.E. Zinc protoporphyrin/heme as an indicator of iron status in NICU patients. *J. Pediatr.* **2003**, *142*, 273–278. [CrossRef]
60. Löfving, A.; Domellöf, M.; Hellström-Westas, L.; Andersson, O. Reference intervals for reticulocyte hemoglobin content in healthy infants. *Pediatr. Res.* **2018**, *84*, 657–661. [CrossRef]
61. Lorenz, L.; Peter, A.; Arand, J.; Springer, F.; Poets, C.F.; Franz, A.R. Reference ranges of reticulocyte haemoglobin content in preterm and term infants: A retrospective analysis. *Neonatology* **2016**, *111*, 189–194. [CrossRef]
62. Beard, J.; DeRegnier, R.; Shaw, M.D.; Rao, R.; Georgieff, M. Diagnosis of iron deficiency in infants. *Lab. Med.* **2007**, *38*, 103–108. [CrossRef]
63. Ullrich, C.; Wu, A.; Armsby, C.; Rieber, S.; Wingerter, S.; Brugnara, C.; Shapiro, D.; Bernstein, H. Screening healthy infants for iron deficiency using reticulocyte hemoglobin content. *JAMA* **2005**, *294*, 924. [CrossRef] [PubMed]
64. Domellöf, M. Meeting the iron needs of low and very low birth weight infants. *Ann. Nutr. Metab.* **2017**, *71*, 16–23. [CrossRef] [PubMed]
65. Peerschke, E.; Pessin, M.; Maslak, P. Using the hemoglobin content of reticulocytes (RET-He) to evaluate anemia in patients with cancer. *Am. J. Clin. Pathol.* **2014**, *142*, 506–512. [CrossRef]
66. Miller, S.M.; McPherson, R.J.; Juul, S.E. Iron sulfate supplementation decreases zinc protoporphyrin to heme ratio in premature infants. *J. Pediatr.* **2006**, *148*, 44–48. [CrossRef] [PubMed]
67. Colomer, J.; Colomer, C.; Gutierrez, D.; Jubert, A.; Nolasco, A.; Donat, J.; Fernández-Delgado, R.; Donat, F.; Álvarez-Dardet, C. Anaemia during pregnancy as a risk factor for infant iron deficiency: Report from the Valencia Infant Anaemia Cohort (VIAC) study. *Paediatr. Périnat. Epidemiol.* **1990**, *4*, 196–204. [CrossRef] [PubMed]
68. Cao, C.; Fleming, M.D. The placenta: The forgotten essential organ of iron transport. *Nutr. Rev.* **2016**, *74*, 421–431. [CrossRef]
69. Lust, C.; Vesoulis, Z.A.; Jackups, R.; Liao, S.; Rao, R.; Mathur, A.M. Early red cell transfusion is associated with development of severe retinopathy of prematurity. *J. Perinatol.* **2018**, *39*, 393–400. [CrossRef]
70. Rashid, N.; Al-Sufayan, F.; Seshia, M.M.K.; Baier, R.J. Post transfusion lung injury in the neonatal population. *J. Perinatol.* **2012**, *33*, 292–296. [CrossRef]
71. Kelly, A.M.; Williamson, L.M. Neonatal transfusion. *Early Hum. Dev.* **2013**, *89*, 855–860. [CrossRef]
72. Mukhopadhyay, K.; Yadav, R.K.; Kishore, S.S.; Garewal, G.; Jain, V.; Narang, A. Iron status at birth and at 4 weeks in preterm-SGA infants in comparison with preterm and term-AGA infants. *J. Matern. Neonatal Med.* **2012**, *25*, 1474–1478. [CrossRef]
73. Ziegler, E.E.; Nelson, S.E.; Jeter, J.M. Iron stores of breastfed infants during the first year of life. *Nutrients* **2014**, *6*, 2023–2034. [CrossRef]
74. Friel, J.K.; Qasem, W.; Cai, C. Iron and the breastfed infant. *Antioxidants* **2018**, *7*, 54. [CrossRef] [PubMed]
75. Ghirardello, S.; Di Tommaso, M.; Fiocchi, S.; Locatelli, A.; Perrone, B.; Pratesi, S.; Saracco, P. Italian recommendations for placental transfusion strategies. *Front. Pediatr.* **2018**, *6*. [CrossRef]
76. Qian, Y.; Ying, X.; Wang, P.; Lu, Z.; Hua, Y. Early versus delayed umbilical cord clamping on maternal and neonatal outcomes. *Arch. Gynecol. Obstet.* **2019**, *300*, 531–543. [CrossRef] [PubMed]
77. Mercer, J.S.; Erickson-Owens, D. Delayed cord clamping increases infants' iron stores. *Lancet* **2006**, *367*, 1956–1958. [CrossRef]

78. Chaparro, C.M.; Neufeld, L.M.; Alavez, G.T.; Cedillo, R.E.-L.; Dewey, K.G. Effect of timing of umbilical cord clamping on iron status in Mexican infants: A randomised controlled trial. *Lancet* **2006**, *367*, 1997–2004. [CrossRef]
79. Armstrong-Buisseret, L.; Powers, K.; Dorling, J.; Bradshaw, L.; Johnson, S.; Mitchell, E.; Duley, L. Randomised trial of cord clamping at very preterm birth: Outcomes at 2 years. *Arch. Dis. Child. Fetal Neonatal Ed.* **2019**, *105*, 292–298. [CrossRef]
80. Andersson, O.; Lindquist, B.; Lindgren, M.; Stjernqvist, K.; Domellöf, M.; Hellström-Westas, L. Effect of delayed cord clamping on neurodevelopment at 4 years of age. *JAMA Pediatr.* **2015**, *169*, 631. [CrossRef]
81. Kumar, B.; Upadhyay, A.; Gothwal, S.; Jaiswal, V.; Joshi, P.; Dubey, K. Umbilical cord milking and hematological parameters in moderate to late preterm neonates: A randomized controlled trial. *Indian Pediatr.* **2015**, *52*, 753–757. [CrossRef]
82. Katheria, A.; Reister, F.; Essers, J.; Mendler, M.; Hummler, H.; Subramaniam, A.; Carlo, W.; Tita, A.; Truong, G.; Davis-Nelson, S.; et al. Association of umbilical cord milking vs delayed umbilical cord clamping with death or severe intraventricular hemorrhage among preterm infants. *JAMA* **2019**, *322*, 1877–1886. [CrossRef]
83. Akkermans, M.D.; Uijterschout, L.; Abbink, M.; Vos, P.; Rövekamp-Abels, L.; Boersma, B.; Van Goudoever, J.B.; Brus, F. Predictive factors of iron depletion in late preterm infants at the postnatal age of 6 weeks. *Eur. J. Clin. Nutr.* **2016**, *70*, 941–946. [CrossRef] [PubMed]
84. Lemyre, B.; Sample, M.; Lacaze-Masmonteil, T. Minimizing blood loss and the need for transfusions in very premature infants. *Paediatr. Child Health* **2016**, *20*, 451–456. [CrossRef]
85. Carroll, P.; Christensen, R.D. New and underutilized uses of umbilical cord blood in neonatal care. *Matern. Health Neonatol. Perinatol.* **2015**, *1*, 16. [CrossRef] [PubMed]
86. Carroll, P. Umbilical cord blood—An untapped resource. *Clin. Perinatol.* **2015**, *42*, 541–556. [CrossRef] [PubMed]
87. Raffaeli, G.; Tripodi, A.; Manzoni, F.; Scalambrino, E.; Pesenti, N.; Amodeo, I.; Cavallaro, G.; Villamor, E.; Peyvandi, F.; Mosca, F.; et al. Is placental blood a reliable source for the evaluation of neonatal hemostasis at birth? *Transfusion* **2020**. [CrossRef] [PubMed]
88. Baer, V.L.; Lambert, D.K.; Carroll, P.; Gerday, E.; Christensen, R.D. Using umbilical cord blood for the initial blood tests of VLBW neonates results in higher hemoglobin and fewer RBC transfusions. *J. Perinatol.* **2012**, *33*, 363–365. [CrossRef]
89. Braekke, K.; Bechensteen, A.G.; Halvorsen, B.L.; Blomhoff, R.; Haaland, K.; Staff, A.C. Oxidative stress markers and antioxidant status after oral iron supplementation to very low birth weight infants. *J. Pediatr.* **2007**, *151*, 23–28. [CrossRef]
90. Bader, D.; Kugelman, A.; Maor-Rogin, N.; Weinger-Abend, M.; Hershkowitz, S.; Tamir, A.; Lanir, A.; Attias, J.; Barak, M. The role of high-dose oral iron supplementation during erythropoietin therapy for anemia of prematurity. *J. Perinatol.* **2001**, *21*, 215–220. [CrossRef]
91. Brozovic, B.; Burland, W.; Simpson, K.; Lord, J. Iron status of preterm low birth weight infants and their response to oral iron. *Arch. Dis. Child.* **1974**, *49*, 386–389. [CrossRef]
92. Lapillonne, A.; Bronsky, J.; Campoy, C.; Embleton, N.; Fewtrell, M.; Mis, N.F.; Gerasimidis, K.; Hojsak, I.; Hulst, J.; Indrio, F.; et al. Feeding the late and moderately preterm infant. *J. Pediatr. Gastroenterol. Nutr.* **2019**, *69*, 259–270. [CrossRef]
93. American academy of pediatrics. Nutrition committee of the canadian paediatric society and the committee on nutrition of the american academy of pediatrics. Breast-feeding. A commentary in celebration of the international year of the child, 1979. *Pediatrics* **1978**, *62*, 23–54.
94. Agostoni, C.; Buonocore, G.; Carnielli, V.; De Curtis, M.; Darmaun, D.; Decsi, T.; Domellöf, M.; Embleton, N.; Fusch, C.; Genzel-Boroviczeny, O.; et al. Enteral nutrient supply for preterm infants: Commentary from the European society of paediatric gastroenterology, hepatology and nutrition committee on nutrition. *J. Pediatr. Gastroenterol. Nutr.* **2010**, *50*, 85–91. [CrossRef] [PubMed]
95. Franz, A.R.; Mihatsch, W.A.; Sander, S.; Kron, M.; Pohlandt, F. Prospective randomized trial of early versus late enteral iron supplementation in infants with a birth weight of less than 1301 grams. *Pediatrics* **2000**, *106*, 700–706. [CrossRef] [PubMed]
96. Friel, J.K.; Serfass, R.E.; Fennessey, P.V.; Miller, L.V.; Andrews, W.L.; Simmons, B.S.; Downton, G.F.; Kwa, P.G. Elevated intakes of zinc in infant formulas do not interfere with iron absorption in premature infants. *J. Pediatr. Gastroenterol. Nutr.* **1998**, *27*, 312–316. [CrossRef]

97. Lönnerdal, B.; Kelleher, S.L. Iron metabolism in infants and children. *Food Nutr. Bull.* **2007**, *28*, S491–S499. [CrossRef]
98. Fusch, G.; Mitra, S.; Topp, H.; Agarwal, A.; Yiu, S.H.; Bruhs, J.; Rochow, N.; Lange, A.; Heckmann, M.; Fusch, C. Source and quality of enteral nutrition influences oxidative stress in preterm infants: A prospective cohort study. *J. Parenter. Enter. Nutr.* **2018**, *42*, 1288–1294. [CrossRef]
99. Meyer, M.; Haworth, C.; Meyer, J.; Commerford, A. A comparison of oral and intravenous iron supplementation in preterm infants receiving recombinant erythropoietin. *J. Pediatr.* **1996**, *129*, 258–263. [CrossRef]
100. Aher, S.M.; Ohlsson, A. Late erythropoiesis-stimulating agents to prevent red blood cell transfusion in preterm or low birth weight infants. *Cochrane Database Syst. Rev.* **2019**, *2*, CD004868. [CrossRef]
101. Jin, H.-X.; Wang, R.-S.; Chen, S.-J.; Wang, A.-P.; Liu, X.-Y. Early and late Iron supplementation for low birth weight infants: A meta-analysis. *Ital. J. Pediatr.* **2015**, *41*, 16. [CrossRef]
102. Cooke, R.W.; Drury, J.A.; Yoxall, C.W.; James, C. Blood transfusion and chronic lung disease in preterm infants. *Eur. J. Pediatr.* **1997**, *156*, 47–50. [CrossRef]
103. Dani, C.; Reali, M.; Bertini, G.; Martelli, E.; Pezzati, M.; Rubaltelli, F.F. The role of blood transfusions and iron intake on retinopathy of prematurity. *Early Hum. Dev.* **2001**, *62*, 57–63. [CrossRef]
104. Patel, R.M.; Knezevic, A.; Yang, J.; Shenvi, N.; Hinkes, M.; Roback, J.D.; Easley, K.A.; Josephson, C.D. Enteral iron supplementation, red blood cell transfusion, and risk of bronchopulmonary dysplasia in very-low-birth-weight infants. *Transfusion* **2019**, *59*, 1675–1682. [CrossRef] [PubMed]
105. Blau, J.; Calo, J.M.; Dozor, D.; Sutton, M.; Alpan, G.; La Gamma, E.F. Transfusion-related acute gut injury: Necrotizing enterocolitis in very low birth weight neonates after packed red blood cell transfusion. *J. Pediatr.* **2011**, *158*, 403–409. [CrossRef] [PubMed]
106. Alexander, J.T.; El-Ali, A.M.; Newman, J.L.; Karatela, S.; Predmore, B.L.; Lefer, D.J.; Sutliff, R.L.; Roback, J.D. Red blood cells stored for increasing periods produce progressive impairments in nitric oxide-mediated vasodilation. *Transfusion* **2013**, *53*, 2619–2628. [CrossRef]
107. Collard, K.J. Is there a causal relationship between the receipt of blood transfusions and the development of chronic lung disease of prematurity? *Med. Hypotheses* **2006**, *66*, 355–364. [CrossRef]
108. Collard, K.J. Transfusion related morbidity in premature babies: Possible mechanisms and implications for practice. *World J. Clin. Pediatr.* **2014**, *3*, 19–29. [CrossRef]
109. Ozment, C.P.; Turi, J.L. Iron overload following red blood cell transfusion and its impact on disease severity. *Biochim. Biophys. Acta* **2009**, *1790*, 694–701. [CrossRef]
110. Collard, K.J.; White, D.; Copplestone, A. The influence of storage age on iron status, oxidative stress and antioxidant protection in paediatric packed cell units. *High Speed Blood Transfus. Equip.* **2013**, *12*, 210–219.
111. Shah, A.; Brunskill, S.; Desborough, M.; Doree, C.; Trivella, M.; Stanworth, S.J. Transfusion of red blood cells stored for shorter versus longer duration for all conditions. *Cochrane Database Syst. Rev.* **2018**, *12*, CD010801. [CrossRef]
112. Karam, O.; Tucci, M.; Bateman, S.T.; Ducruet, T.; Spinella, P.C.; Randolph, A.G.; Lacroix, J. Association between length of storage of red blood cell units and outcome of critically ill children: A prospective observational study. *Crit. Care* **2010**, *14*, R57. [CrossRef]
113. Fergusson, D.; Hebert, P.; Hogan, D.L.; Lebel, L.; Rouvinez-Bouali, N.; Smyth, J.A.; Sankaran, K.; Tinmouth, A.; Blajchman, M.A.; Kovacs, L.; et al. Effect of fresh red blood cell transfusions on clinical outcomes in premature, very low-birth-weight infants. *JAMA* **2012**, *308*, 1443–1451. [CrossRef]
114. Spinella, P.C.; Tucci, M.; Fergusson, D.A.; Lacroix, J.; Hébert, P.C.; Leteurtre, S.; Schechtman, K.B.; Doctor, A.; Berg, R.A.; Bockelmann, T.; et al. Effect of fresh vs standard-issue red blood cell transfusions on multiple organ dysfunction syndrome in critically ill pediatric patients: A randomized clinical trial. *JAMA* **2019**, *322*, 2179–2190. [CrossRef] [PubMed]
115. Valentine, S.L.; Bembea, M.M.; Muszynski, J.A.; Cholette, J.M.; Doctor, A.; Spinella, P.C.; Steiner, M.E.; Tucci, M.; Hassan, N.E.; Parker, R.I.; et al. Consensus recommendations for red blood cell transfusion practice in critically ill children from the pediatric critical care transfusion and anemia expertise initiative. *Pediatr. Crit. Care Med.* **2018**, *19*, 884–898. [CrossRef] [PubMed]
116. Howarth, C.; Banerjee, J.; Aladangady, N. Red blood cell transfusion in preterm infants: Current evidence and controversies. *Neonatology* **2018**, *114*, 7–16. [CrossRef]

117. Raffaeli, G.; Ghirardello, S.; Passera, S.; Mosca, F.; Cavallaro, G. Oxidative stress and neonatal respiratory extracorporeal membrane oxygenation. *Front. Physiol.* **2018**, *9*, 1739. [CrossRef] [PubMed]
118. Keene, S.D.; Patel, R.M.; Stansfield, B.K.; Davis, J.; Josephson, C.D.; Winkler, A.M. Blood product transfusion and mortality in neonatal extracorporeal membrane oxygenation. *Transfusion* **2019**, *60*, 262–268. [CrossRef]
119. Amin, S.B.; Myers, G.; Wang, H. Association between neonatal iron overload and early human brain development in premature infants. *Early Hum. Dev.* **2012**, *88*, 583–587. [CrossRef]
120. Friel, J.K.; Andrews, W.L.; Aziz, K.; Kwa, P.G.; Lepage, G.; L'Abbe, M.R. A randomized trial of two levels of iron supplementation and developmental outcome in low birth weight infants. *J. Pediatr.* **2001**, *139*, 254–260. [CrossRef]
121. Patruta, S.; Horl, W. Iron and infection. *Kidney Int. Suppl.* **1999**, *69*, S125–S130. [CrossRef]
122. Jaeggi, T.; Kortman, G.A.M.; Moretti, D.; Chassard, C.; Holding, P.; Dostal, A.; Boekhorst, J.; Timmerman, H.M.; Swinkels, R.W.; Tjalsma, H.; et al. Iron fortification adversely affects the gut microbiome, increases pathogen abundance and induces intestinal inflammation in Kenyan infants. *Gut* **2014**, *64*, 731–742. [CrossRef]
123. Marseglia, L.; D'Angelo, G.; Manti, M.; Aversa, S.; Fiamingo, C.; Arrigo, T.; Barberi, I.; Mamì, C.; Gitto, E. Visfatin: New marker of oxidative stress in preterm newborns. *Int. J. Immunopathol. Pharmacol.* **2015**, *29*, 23–29. [CrossRef] [PubMed]
124. Lee, D.; Blomhoff, R.; Jacobs, D.R. ReviewIs serum gamma glutamyltransferase a marker of oxidative stress? *Free Radic. Res.* **2004**, *38*, 535–539. [CrossRef] [PubMed]

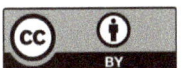

© 2020 by the authors. Licensee MDPI, Basel, Switzerland. This article is an open access article distributed under the terms and conditions of the Creative Commons Attribution (CC BY) license (http://creativecommons.org/licenses/by/4.0/).

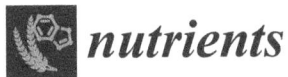

Review

Multifactorial Etiology of Anemia in Celiac Disease and Effect of Gluten-Free Diet: A Comprehensive Review

Rafael Martín-Masot [1], Maria Teresa Nestares [2,*], Javier Diaz-Castro [2], Inmaculada López-Aliaga [2], Maria Jose Muñoz Alférez [2], Jorge Moreno-Fernandez [2] and José Maldonado [3,4,5,6]

1. Pediatric Clinical Management Unit, Málaga Regional University Hospital, 29010 Málaga, Spain; rafammgr@gmail.com
2. Department of Physiology and Institute of Nutrition and Food Technology "José MataixVerdú", University of Granada, 18071 Granada, Spain; javierdc@ugr.es (J.D.-C.); milopez@ugr.es (I.L.-A.); malferez@ugr.es (M.J.M.A.); jorgemf@ugr.es (J.M.-F.)
3. Department of Pediatrics, University of Granada, 18071 Granada, Spain; jmaldon@ugr.es
4. Biosanitary Research Institute, 18012 Granada, Spain
5. Maternal and Child Health Network, Institute Carlos III, 28020 Madrid, Spain
6. Pediatric Clinical Management Unit. Virgen de las Nieves University Hospital, 18014 Granada, Spain
* Correspondence: nestares@ugr.es; Tel.: +34-6-9698-9989

Received: 6 September 2019; Accepted: 15 October 2019; Published: 23 October 2019

Abstract: Celiac disease (CD) is a multisystemic disorder with different clinical expressions, from malabsorption with diarrhea, anemia, and nutritional compromise to extraintestinal manifestations. Anemia might be the only clinical expression of the disease, and iron deficiency anemia is considered one of the most frequent extraintestinal clinical manifestations of CD. Therefore, CD should be suspected in the presence of anemia without a known etiology. Assessment of tissue anti-transglutaminase and anti-endomysial antibodies are indicated in these cases and, if positive, digestive endoscopy and intestinal biopsy should be performed. Anemia in CD has a multifactorial pathogenesis and, although it is frequently a consequence of iron deficiency, it can be caused by deficiencies of folate or vitamin B_{12}, or by blood loss or by its association with inflammatory bowel disease (IBD) or other associated diseases. The association between CD and IBD should be considered during anemia treatment in patients with IBD, because the similarity of symptoms could delay the diagnosis. Vitamin B_{12} deficiency is common in CD and may be responsible for anemia and peripheral myeloneuropathy. Folate deficiency is a well-known cause of anemia in adults, but there is little information in children with CD; it is still unknown if anemia is a symptom of the most typical CD in adult patients either by predisposition due to the fact of age or because biochemical and clinical manifestations take longer to appear.

Keywords: celiac disease; gluten-free diet; iron deficiency; anemia; micronutrient deficiencies

1. Introduction

Celiac disease (CD) is one of the most frequent genetic diseases, affecting 1% of the world population. Diagnosed cases are increasing and it seems to be due to the actual increase in the incidence rather than due to the advancement of diagnostic methods or to the larger awareness of the disease among the lay population [1,2].

Celiac disease is a systemic disorder, caused by an immune reaction activated by the ingestion of gluten and related proteins occurring in individuals carrying haplotypes of major histocompatibility antigen (HLA) class II: more than 90% of celiac patients are HLA-DQ2 haplotype positive, and almost all of the remaining patients carry HLA-DQ8. Exposure to gluten has a double effect, triggering both innate and adaptive immune responses, with symptoms at the intestinal and extra-intestinal levels [3]. The contact of the intestinal mucosa with gluten leads to a characteristic histological lesion, although not pathognomonic. Their typical histological features are an increase in intraepithelial lymphocytes, villous atrophy, crypt hyperplasia, and infiltration of inflammatory cells in the lamina propria.

Diagnosis of CD is conducted by combining serological screening tests (anti-tissue-transglutaminase and anti-endomysial IgA antibodies) and an intestinal biopsy [4]. The duodenal biopsy can be avoided [5] in adolescents and children with symptoms or signs of CD and with high anti-tissue-transglutaminase antibody levels, positivity for anti-endomysial antibodies, and presence of HLA DQ21 or HLA-DQ8 heterodimer.

Recent reports have demonstrated that specific miRNAs are modulated in duodenal mucosa affected by CD. The miRNAs dysregulated during the development of CD could be potentially involved in the pathogenesis of CD [6]. Overexpression or downregulation of several miRNAs could potentially stimulate or inhibit pathways related to the pathogenesis of CD. A study has demonstrated the regulation of circulating miRNA-21 and miRNA-31 expression levels in children with CD and showed that miR-21 expression level was positively correlated with the anti-tissue-transglutaminase IgA antibodies [7]. This correlation may indicate that the altered expression of the circulating miRNAs could be used as potential non-invasive diagnostic and prognostic biomarkers for CD patients. In addition, Vaira et al. [8] have shown the downregulation of miR-194-5p and the overexpression of miR-638 in celiac patients with anemia compared with celiac patients with classical symptoms.

Patients with CD could feature various deficiency states, leading to anemia and bone mass loss and a wide range of digestive and extra-digestive symptoms. Upon diagnosis, nutritional deficiencies were found in vitamins and minerals; patients should be tested for micronutrient deficiencies, in particular iron, folic acid, vitamin B_{12}, vitamin D, copper, and zinc. Celiac disease is a cause of anemia, usually due to the malabsorption of iron, folic acid, and vitamin B_{12} [9]. Anemia is mainly due to the fact of iron deficiency as a consequence of iron malabsorption. Iron malabsorption is usually observed in CD, being considered a clinical diagnostic feature of CD even in subjects not presenting the classic digestive symptoms. Iron deficiency anemia (IDA) is a frequent finding in patients with overt CD (10–20% of cases) [10], despite the fact that they are consuming iron supplements. A recent meta-analysis found that more than 3% of patients with IDA have histological evidence of CD. This high percentage of subjects with IDA who are celiac, reinforces the need for screening CD in patients with IDA [11]. Folate and vitamin B_{12} malabsorption, nutritional deficiencies, blood loss, inflammation, development of refractory CD or concomitant *Helicobacter pylori* infection are other causes of anemia in such patients [12] (Table 1).

Table 1. Etiology of anemia in celiac disease.

Cause	Incidence
Iron deficiency	12–69% (adults) 10–20% (children)
Folic acid deficiency	20–30%
Vitamin B_{12} deficiency	8–41%
Copper deficiency	Very low
Zinc deficiency	Very low *
Bad response to the gluten-free diet	23%
Medullary aplasia	Very low (12 cases)
Chronic disease	4–17%

* It has been reported that 50% of celiac patients have low serum levels at diagnosis, but it has not been related to celiac disease (CD).

The mainstay of treatment for CD remains adherence to a gluten-free diet (GFD). In the vast majority of cases, strict monitoring of GFD leads to the disappearance of clinical symptoms and serological signs, the recovery of normal histology in the duodenum and the prevention of complications derived from CD [13]. However, in approximately 20% of celiac patients, symptoms persist despite excluding gluten from their diet [14].

The aim was to perform a review of recent literature data regarding causes of anemia in CD patients. For this purpose, we performed a literature search on two databases—PubMed and Embase—using the Medical Subject Headings (MESH) term "celiac disease" and several keywords referring to the associated hematological features and nutritional imbalances. Articles identified from this search strategy were evaluated for relevance to the topic. Clinically significant full-text articles were selected for their inclusion in this review.

2. Micronutrient Deficiencies and Celiac Disease

2.1. Iron Deficiency

Iron is an essential micronutrient, it is required for adequate erythropoietic function, oxidative metabolism, enzymatic activities, and cellular immune responses [15]. IDA is a major public health problem. Iron deficiency anemia occurs when iron loss and body's requirement for iron are not met by dietary sources, therefore the iron storage of the organism is depleted. This pathological process is characterized by the production of smaller red cells because the concentration of hemoglobin (Hb) is abnormally low [15]. Iron deficiency anemia results in fatigue and diminished muscular oxygenation, which may affect muscle strength and quality and, subsequently, physical performance [16]. Celiac disease constitutes one of the groups at highest risk of iron deficiency (ID) [17]. Iron requirements exceed iron intake at some time points throughout life: the first 6–18 months of life and then, for women, during adolescence and all fertile period. Iron deficiency during the first year of life occurs at a time point of rapid neural development and when morphological, biochemical, and bioenergetic alterations may all influence future functioning [18]. The brain is the most vulnerable organ during critical periods of development [19]. Iron is present in the brain from very early in life, when it participates in the neural myelination processes [20], learning, and interacting behaviors, and iron is needed by enzymes involved in the synthesis of serotonin and dopamine neurotransmitters [21].

The most common causes of ID are blood loss and failure of the enterocytes of the proximal intestine to uptake iron from the diet in patients who have enough dietary iron. Celiac disease leads to an abnormal immune response, which is followed by a chronic inflammation of the small intestinal mucosa with progressive disappearance of intestinal villi [22] leading to a decrease in absorption of many nutrients, including iron [23,24]. Unfortunately, this interesting association between CD and IDA has been poorly appreciated [25] in spite of the great interest of micronutrient deficiency as a diagnostic clue in asymptomatic CD, especially for iron and IDA [26].

Celiac disease is an increasingly recognized disorder in Caucasian populations of European origin. Murray et al. [27] analyzed HLA genotypes and frequencies of CD between Caucasians and non-Caucasians with ID. The results showed that CD is associated with ID in Caucasians, but CD is rare among non-Caucasians—even among individuals with features of CD, such as ID. Pirán Arce et al. [28] evaluated the nutritional status of iron in 44 celiac children by determining biochemical parameters and their relationship with the intake of this mineral and adherence to the GFD. These authors concluded that under conditions of adequate iron consumption, iron status is related to the degree of adherence to the GFD. Although GFD is an effective treatment for CD, IDA remains an occasional finding during follow-up and correlates to inadequate gluten exclusion [10].

Malabsorption causes should be considered especially in refractory IDA; this malabsorption can be the only manifestation in subclinical and silent CD [29,30]. The study of Shahriari et al. [11] suggests serologic screening for CD in patients with refractory IDA to minimize the complications of CD and repeated iron treatment. A study [31] revealed a significant association between *H. pylori* infection and

IDA in patients with CD, and Samasca et al. [32] recommend performing the screening for *H. pylori* infection in patients with CD and ID, but currently there is no evidence to support this recommendation.

Elli et al. [33] evaluated the role of the *TMPRSS6* variant *rs855791* in GFD treated CD patients with IDA persistence against non-IDA CD and non-CD subjects. The authors found a significantly higher percentage of *TMPTSS6* mutation in CD patients than in non-CD controls, while no differences were found between IDA and non-IDA CD patients. Conversely, De Falco et al. [34] investigated the role of HFE *C282Y, H63D,* and *TMPRSS6 A736V* gene variants in the pathogenesis of IDA in CD patients, at diagnosis and after 1 year of GFD. This study suggests a protective role of HFE in IDA CD patients and confirms the role of *TMPRSS6* in predicting oral iron response modulating hepcidin action on iron absorption. Iron supplementation therapeutic management in CD could depend on *TMPRSS6* genotype that could predict persistent IDA despite iron supplementation and GFD.

Iron enters the enterocytes through an apical divalent metal transporter (DMT-1) (Figure 1). Sharma et al. [35] have evaluated iron regulatory proteins in celiac patients compared to controls and iron deficient patients using duodenal biopsies. The results showed that DMT-1, ferroportin, hephaestin, and transferrin receptor protein mRNA increased, primarily due to the fact of iron deficiency, while body iron stores were reduced in CD. In contrast, these authors [35] showed that expression of DMT1 and ferroportin are increased in CD patients with or without ID. In this study, ferritin expression was also found to be increased in CD, but only in those with ID.

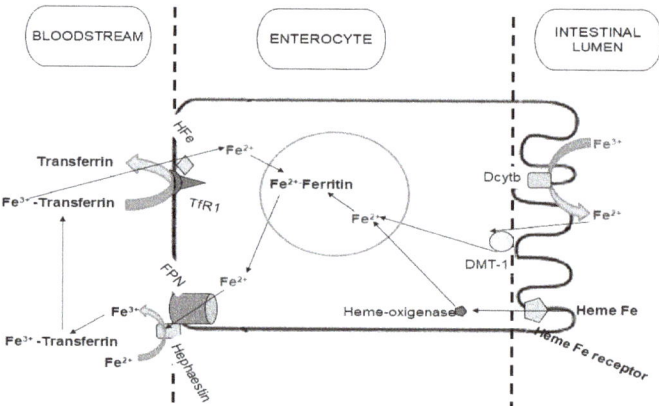

Figure 1. Iron absorption metabolism. Non-heme iron is ultimately taken up from the lumen by divalent metal transporter (DMT-1) on the microvillus membrane, before joining the labile iron pool in the cell. Ferric iron has to be reduced to the ferrous form by duodenal cytochrome b (Dcytb) before the uptake. Ferrous iron in the labile iron pool is then transferred to the circulation by ferroportin (FPN), which requires hephaestin for oxidation to the ferric form to bind transferrin. Heme iron is taken up by a specific receptor. Internalized heme iron is degraded by heme-oxygenase, releasing non-heme iron. The non-heme iron is then transported to the cytoplasm, joining the labile iron pool and is then transferred to the bloodstream by FPN in the same manner as non-heme iron.

Tolone et al. [36] reported the link between DMT-1 *IVS4+44C-AA* and anemia in 387 Italian celiac children and the functional role of the polymorphism. They found that the DMT-1 *IVS4+44-AA* genotype confers a four-fold risk of developing anemia, despite the atrophy degree. Anemia in patients with CD is multifactorial.

Patients with CD may benefit from iron supplementation (iron sulfate), but intolerance to iron sulfate could reduce the efficacy of this supplementation. Sucrosomial iron, a presentation of ferric pyrophosphate covered by a phospholipid and sucrester membrane, can be effective in providing iron supplementation in difficult-to-treat patients with CD and intolerance to iron sulfate, allowing good intestinal absorption independently of the DMT-1 carrier [37]. A study provides evidence that

Feralgine[TM], a solution of ferrous bisglycinate chelate and sodium alginate, is well absorbed in celiac patients [38]. Furthermore, it might by suggested that the iron complex might be absorbed regardless of the presence of DMT-1.

The prevalence of CD in subjects presenting IDA has been described by other authors [39–41] with different results, due to the probable differences in the study of the designs. Lasa et al. [40] designed a study to avoid the abovementioned bias. They decided to evaluate all patients diagnosed with IDA by performing upper endoscopy and duodenal biopsies, and not only those with positive antibodies or with IDA of unknown origin (after an extensive work-up). Patients with IDA have an increased risk for CD, up to 25% of these patients may not present any endoscopic sign suggesting villous atrophy [39]. This finding makes routine duodenal biopsy necessary when performing upper endoscopy on IDA patients. In a systematic review and meta-analysis, Mahadev et al. [3] found that approximately 1 out of 31 patients with IDA have histologic evidence of CD; this prevalence value justifies the screening of patients with IDA for CD (Figure 2).

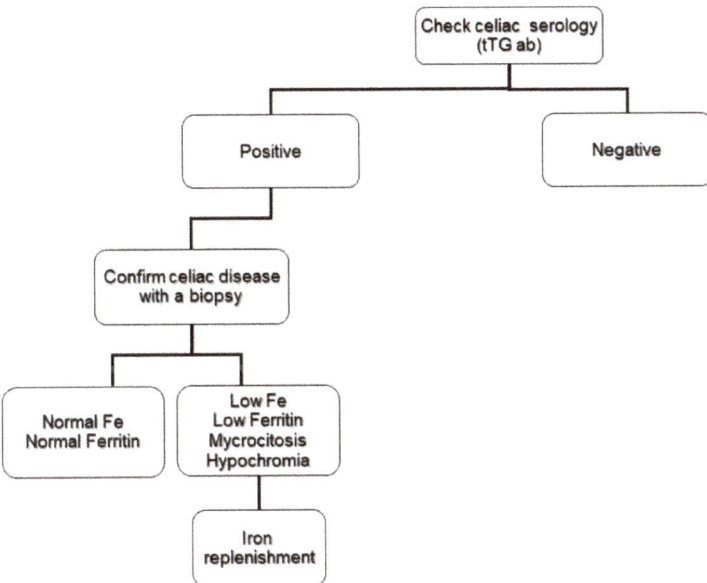

Figure 2. Abbreviated flow chart of the investigation of iron deficiency anemia in celiac disease patients.

2.2. Folate and Vitamin B_{12} Deficiency

Usually, people suffering from CD can develop folate and vitamin B_{12} deficiencies as a result of generalized malabsorption linked to villi atrophy. Both vitamins are essential for normal hematopoiesis and neurologic function.

Folate absorption occurs primarily in the jejunum, which is commonly affected by CD [10,42]. Several studies in adult celiac patients have shown an increased risk of folate deficiency, which can reach up to 20–30% of newly diagnosed patients [43,44]. Prior to uptake, folate must be deconjugated by a brush border membrane peptidase and the intestinal mucosa damage in CD may affect enzyme activity leading to a folate deficiency. Serum and red cell folate measurements are usually used for the diagnosis of folate deficiency. Serum folate levels reflect largely folate intake and it is common for levels to be high in patients with a vitamin B_{12} deficiency. Red cell folate is not a specific indicator for folate deficiency, as it can be decreased in patients with vitamin B_{12}, but red cell folate levels are less influenced by variations in folate intake. Patients with CD commonly have elevated levels of homocysteine which may serve as an important clue for the diagnosis. However, the sensitivity of this measurement is somewhat less for vitamin B_{12} deficiency [45].

Vitamin B_{12} requires formation of a primary complex with intrinsic factor to be absorbed in the proximal small intestine, and small amounts may also be absorbed by passive transport throughout the entire intestine. Deficiency of vitamin B_{12} is common in CD and frequently results in anemia. Though the terminal ileum is the primary site of absorption of vitamin B_{12}, García-Manzanares and Lucendo [44] reported a prevalence of vitamin B_{12} deficiency between 8% and 41% in patients with newly diagnosed CD.

The causes of B_{12} deficiency in CD are still not clear, but they may be related to complications of small intestinal injury including a decreased gastric acidity, cobalamin intake due to the frequent finding of bacterial overgrowth, autoimmune gastritis, and decreased efficiency of the intrinsic factor or even dysfunction of the distal small intestine. Abnormalities in the absorption of folate or vitamin B_{12} may result in anemia in children with untreated CD. The range of low folate and low vitamin B_{12} prevalence were 15.7–18.3% and 4.3–8%, respectively [42,46].

Both folate and vitamin B_{12} deficiencies can lead to a macrocytic anemia with low values for hemoglobin or hematocrit, and high mean corpuscular volume levels. Vitamin B_{12} deficiency should be considered in patients with CD and hematological and neurological disorders [47]. Vitamin B_{12} levels measured within the lower range of normal or if they coexist with folic acid deficiency can be misleading and difficult to interpret. Under these circumstances, high serum levels of methylmalonic acid may improve the diagnostic accuracy of vitamin B_{12} deficiency [48].

2.3. Copper and Zinc Deficiency

Micronutrient deficiencies are common in celiac patients. In addition to the abovementioned deficiencies (i.e., iron, folic acid, and vitamin B_{12}), at the time of diagnosis there may be deficiencies for other vitamins and minerals, in particular copper and zinc [22].

Copper deficiency is a rare complication in CD and its prevalence remains unknown. This deficiency can lead to anemia, thrombocytopenia, neutropenia, and peripheral neuronal involvement. In adult celiac patients, peripheral myeloneuropathy has been described along with hypocupremia with a good clinical response to copper supplementation [49,50]. Halfdanarion et al. [51] reported five cases of adult celiac patients with copper deficiency; all of them presented neurological complications and three of them presented hematological abnormalities. Cavallieri et al. [52] recently described a rare case of myelopathy induced by copper deficiency secondary to undiagnosed CD, and they have suggested that patients with hypocupremia should be tested for CD.

Likewise, the presence of clinical alterations as a consequence of zinc deficiency is also uncommon in celiac patients. Fractional zinc absorption is no different between celiac patients and controls, but the rapid zinc exchange body compartment is lower in CD than in control patients [49]. The mechanism of zinc depletion and its possible implications are unknown [53].

3. Aplastic Anemia and Celiac Disease

Celiac disease has been linked to various hematological abnormalities [54], such as anemia, thrombopenia or thrombocytosis, leukopenia, splenic dysfunction, immunoglobulin A deficiency or lymphoma. Anemia is the most frequent cause of CD. In addition to the various etiologies of anemia in CD (iron deficiency, due to the micronutrient deficiency or chronic disorders), various cases of aplastic anemia associated with CD have been described in the literature [55–60], both in pediatric age and in adulthood. Despite the underlying mechanism of this association being still unknown [55], it has been suggested that both conditions might share a similar underlying pathophysiological mechanism, mediated by autoreactive T cells involved in tissue destruction [56] (Table 2). In all cases, the patient presented with pancytopenia and the diagnosis was achieved by bone marrow biopsy. Pancytopenia was resolved with the GFD only in some cases [57], while in other cases, the response was only partial and immunosuppressive treatment was required or even hematopoietic progenitor transplantation.

Although infrequent, aplastic anemia may be an underdiagnosed entity [56], so it will be necessary to have the diagnostic suspicion both in the case of pancytopenia without apparent cause and in CD with pancytopenia. The etiology of anemia may be due to the presence of several factors, such as autoimmunity or chronic inflammation caused by the CD [60]. Based on the cases reported to date, it seems that the GFD is not enough to improve pancytopenia; therefore, most patients require other treatments. Some authors have suggested that the prognosis is better at pediatric age, possibly because the duration of exposure to chronic inflammation is shorter, and the GFD may probably reverse the process [57].

Table 2. Characteristics of patients with aplastic anemia and celiac disease.

Study Reported	Grey-Davies [51]	Salmeron [53]	Maheswari [52]	Basu [54]	Badyal [55]	Omar [50]
Number of cases	3	5	1	1	1	1
Anemia diagnosis	Bone marrow biopsy	Bone marrow biopsy	Bone marrow biopsy	Bone marrow biopsy	Bone marrow biopsy	Bone marrow biopsy
Age (years)	23, 37, 43	Not reported	13	40	9	6
Intestinal biopsy	Villus atrophy	Villus atrophy	Villus atrophy	Villus atrophy	Not available	Villus atrophy
Treatment	GFD, corticotherapy, antithymocyte globulin, cyclosporine	GFD, antithymocyte globulin, cyclosporine. hematopoietic cell transplantation	GFD	GFD, corticotherapy, cyclosporine	GFD, corticotherapy, antithymocyte globulin	GFD

GFD; Gluten Free Diet.

4. Anemia of Chronic Disease

Anemia of chronic disease (ACD) is an old concept in the scientific literature, but current research on the role of pro-inflammatory cytokines and iron metabolism has yielded more information about the pathophysiology of this disease. This type of anemia is linked to the deterioration of the production of erythrocytes associated with chronic inflammatory conditions including cancer, infections or autoimmune diseases. In addition, recent epidemiological studies have linked ACD with obesity, aging, and kidney failure. This type of anemia responds to a multifactorial pathogenesis including four fundamental mechanisms. These mechanisms consist of abnormalities in iron utilization, decrease in half-life of red blood cells, direct inhibition of hematopoiesis, and relative deficiency of erythropoietin [61].

Hospitalized patients feature acute or chronic inflammation caused by immune activation and occurring associated with anemia, ACD being the most common form found in these patients [62]. Under these conditions, erythropoiesis can be directly inhibited by an increase in the production of inflammatory cytokines inducing changes in iron homeostasis which could be characterized by reductions in both iron absorption and macrophage iron release [63]. Iron is a fundamental component of all living cells because iron is a cofactor for mitochondrial respiratory chain enzymes, the citric acid cycle, DNA synthesis, as well as an essential component for the transport of O_2 through the hemoglobin and myoglobin. In addition, a sufficient amount of iron is important for immune preservation due to the fact of its role in promoting the growth of immune system cells, as the immune function and iron metabolism are widely linked.

Anemia of chronic disease is not considered a frequent cause of anemia in celiac patients; in fact, systemic inflammation, based on the increase in serum levels of acute phase proteins, is rare in CD patients, although gliadin-dependent activation of mononuclear cells of the mucous lamina propria causes an overproduction of proinflammatory cytokines such as interferon-γ (IFN-γ) and interleukin-6 (IL-6) [64,65]; both cytokines are mediators of ACD [66,67]. These proinflammatory cytokines are key factors in iron metabolism and in the development of ACD in celiac patients.

Thus, IL-6 inhibits the expression of the transferrin receptor mRNA, stimulates the synthesis of DMT-1, and is a mediator of hypoferremia in inflammation, which induces the synthesis of the hepcidin hormone regulating the iron export. An increase in hepcidin synthesis causes an increase in the degradation of ferroportin and the inhibition of iron release by the enterocyte, which leads to the alteration in the iron homeostasis associated with ACD [10,68]. IFN-γ stimulates ferritin transcription but at the same time inhibits its translation. IFN-γ also inhibits the transferrin receptor mRNA expression, which blocks the incorporation of iron mediated by the transferrin receptor, but increases the expression of DMT-1, thereby increasing the uptake and storage of ferrous iron. IFN-γ also decreases the mRNA of the transmembrane protein ferroportin, which exports iron to the outside of the cells. Therefore, IFN-γ favors iron retention within monocytes [52].

In this sense, some cytokines such as TNF-alpha, IL-1, and IL-10 are also released into circulation due to the inflammatory process [69]. These cytokines act on the liver and they contribute to the increase of hepcidin production, inhibiting the duodenal absorption of dietary iron. DMT-1 expression can also be induced by these cytokines. The net effect is the uptake of circulating iron in the reticuloendothelial system. In addition, IL-15 also seems to contribute to this pathway [70]. IL-15 is involved in the pathophysiology of CD and is partly responsible for sustained inflammation in active disease [71]. Taking into account all the above mentioned inflammatory pathways, CD could contribute to the development of de novo ACD. GFD is capable of reducing the oxidative state of patients with CD, although chronic inflammation persists even after two years of GFD. These patients showed a persistent high level of IFN-γ, IL-1α, interferon-inducible protein 10 (IP-10), and tumor necrosis factor beta (TNF-β) [23].

Bergamaschi et al. [72] studied anemia in patients with CD, reporting that ACD affected 17% of the subjects (11 out of 65 patients). Iron status parameters are similar in patients with ACD and those usually found during inflammatory processes, and an isolated iron deficiency or other pathogenic mechanisms could not be the explanation for their anemia. Their results reported a defective production of endogenous erythropoietin, in addition to changes in iron homeostasis, as a pathogenic mechanism of ACD. Other study conducted by Harper et al. [23] also confirmed that ACD can affect patients with CD and this fact is not completely unexpected, although these patients generally lack signs of systemic inflammation. Even though, the mean serum levels of inflammatory cytokines contributing to ACD (including IL-1β, IL-6, TNF-α, and IFN-γ) increased during active CD [73–76]. Although with a lower prevalence (3.9%), Berry et al. [77] also reported the presence of ACD in patients with CD.

In light of the observed studies and although ACD is not the most prevalent hematological disorder in patients with CD, it is necessary to take into account the pathogenesis of CD influence on its pathogenesis, given the role of iron in inflammatory signaling and in the turnover of epithelial cells.

5. Refractory Anemia to the Gluten-Free Diet

The etiology of persistent refractory anemia is multiple, and it must first be ruled out that it is due to the poor adherence to a GFD. Other causes of refractory anemia are chronic inflammation or anemia of chronic disorders, refractory celiac disease (RCD), the higher prevalence of the disease than expected by the involvement of other intestinal sections or the appearance of other comorbidities [77].

The first suggested finding is that it is a false refractoriness or persistence of anemia because the adherence to the treatment is not being conducted correctly. GFD is not easy to comply with nor is it generally well performed [78]. The traditional methods used to monitor the disease have poor performance, because, for example, with the serological method, for every six examinations we would detect the transgression in only one of them [79], besides presenting little correlation with villus atrophy [80]. The immunogenic gluten peptide in feces is postulated as a better tool for assessing diet adherence [81].

Celiac disease responds in the majority of patients on a GFD in a few weeks [13]. However, despite the correct adherence to a GFD, villous atrophy, malabsorption, and chronic intestinal inflammation persist in some patients for 12 months, which defines the RCD [82–84]. This can lead to persistence of symptoms and signs, including anemia. RCD is considered a rarity in pediatric age and, although its exact prevalence and incidence in adulthood is unknown, it is an uncommon condition [85]. Due to the poor response of the disease to treatment at this stage and its prognosis, it is important to correctly make the diagnosis [86], which is considered exclusion. The complete histological evaluation of the entire small intestine is needed for the diagnosis of refractoriness or complications [87].

In a recent study [88], mucosal involvement in patients with RCD was compared to patients with uncomplicated CD, showing that the involvement was greater in patients' refractory to treatment, which may indicate that one of the causes of the persistence of symptoms is precisely the greatest extent of the disease. In a study [89] conducted in adult patients with CD and persistent IDA, 23% of patients showed lesions that were detected by video capsule endoscopy (VCE) of the small intestine. In another recent study conducted in pediatric CD patients [90], patients with anemia at diagnosis showed significantly larger histological lesions than CD patients without anemia; 92% of the patients recovered from the anemia after one year of adherence to a GFD. In patients with suspected RCD, especially type II, the performance of VCE is recommended [91]. Video capsule endoscopy is a relatively safe method with high sensitivity (approximately 89%) and specificity (approximately 95%) [92] to detect villus atrophy, and this could help differentiate RCD type I and II [88].

Furthermore, it is important to distinguish patients with uncomplicated CD from those with RCD, due to the risk of developing complications such as enteropathy associated with T-cell lymphoma (EATL), adenocarcinoma, jejunoileitis or B-cell lymphoma [93,94]. If left untreated, CD presents an increased risk of developing long-term tumors, especially of EATL and small bowel adenocarcinoma [95] compared to the general population. Enteropathy associated with T-cell lymphoma is sometimes diagnosed due to the signs and symptoms such as perforation, intestinal occlusion or bleeding, and persistent anemia, which may be an indicator of it. Likewise, ulcerative jejunoileitis is one of the phenotypic expressions of RCD. The characteristic symptom of this complication is abdominal pain, in relation to sub-occlusive symptoms, although the disease may present with hemorrhagic symptoms, perforation or protein-losing enteropathy due to the presence of inflammatory ulcers and strictures in the entire small intestine. In addition, it is associated with an increased risk of EATL [96].

The presence of other comorbidities, not always associated with CD itself, are linked to persistent symptoms once adherence to the GFD has been verified, such as microscopic colitis, irritable bowel syndrome, food allergies, motility disorders or collagen sprinkles [85]. The sprue collagen manifests itself in the form of refractoriness, and its occasional association with EATL has also been described [97]. The diagnosis is performed by biopsy and pathological analysis.

6. Conclusions and Future Perspectives

Celiac disease is a multisystemic disorder with different forms of clinical expression, from malabsorption with diarrhea, anemia, and growth retardation in children, to extraintestinal manifestations, such as those due to the fact of malabsorption and micronutrient deficiencies, including iron, folic acid, and vitamin B_{12}. In fact, anemia may be the only clinical expression of the disease, and IDA is considered one of the most frequent extraintestinal clinical manifestations of CD. Celiac disease should be suspected in the presence of anemia without known etiology. Therefore, the determination of tissue anti-transglutaminase antibodies and anti-endomysial antibodies are indicated in these cases and, if positive, the performance of digestive endoscopy and intestinal biopsy is recommended.

Anemia in CD has a multifactorial pathogenesis and, although it is more frequently a consequence of iron deficiency, anemia can also be caused by deficiencies of folate or vitamin B_{12}, as well as by blood loss or by its association with inflammatory bowel disease (IBD) or other associated diseases. The association between CD and IBD should be considered because the similarity of the symptoms could delay the diagnosis; the possibility of association among both pathologies should always be taken into account during the treatment of anemia in patients with IBD.

Vitamin B_{12} deficiency is common in CD and may be responsible for anemia and peripheral myeloneuropathy. Folate deficiency is a well-known cause of anemia in adults, but there is little information in children with CD. To date, it is still unknown if anemia is a symptom of the most typical

CD in adult patients either by predisposition due to the age or because the biochemical and clinical manifestations take longer to appear.

Iron is a critical micronutrient whose deficiency in CD, in most cases, is a consequence of malabsorption secondary to the damage of the villi of the intestinal mucosa. However, iron deficiency in CD may also be a consequence of the reduced expression of different regulatory proteins. Alterations of iron absorption that could explain the inappropriate response to a GFD. It is known that the iron transporter DMT1 is positively regulated in CD to counteract iron malabsorption by villus atrophy, and that the risk of anemia in CD is related to the DMT-1 IVS + 44 AA genotype. A variant of this genotype can limit the overexpression of the transporter occurring normally prior to iron deficiency, being ineffective to counteract iron deficiency in the severe stage of the disease. Furthermore, the evaluation of the TMPRSS6 genotype, which influences iron metabolism through its effects on hepcidin, could be of clinical importance for the therapeutic management of iron supplementation, because a mutation can induce a poor response to iron therapy and predict the persistence of IDA despite iron treatment and GFD.

Author Contributions: Conceptualization, R.M.-M. and M.T.N.; Methodology, R.M.-M.; Resources, R.M.-M., M.T.N., J.D.-C., I.L.-A., M.J.M.A., J.M.-F. and J.M.; Writing-Original Draft Preparation, R.M.-M.; Resources, R.M.-M., M.T.N., J.D.-C., I.L.-A., M.J.M.A., J.M.-F. and J.M.; Writing-Review & Editing, R.M.-M. and M.T.N.; Supervision, J.M.

Funding: This research received no external funding.

Acknowledgments: Jorge Moreno-Fernandez is supported by a fellowship from the Ministry of Education, Culture and Sport (Spain) and is grateful to the Excellence Ph.D. Program "Nutrición y Ciencias de los Alimentos" from the University of Granada. The authors also thank Susan Stevenson for her efficient support in the revision of the English language. We acknowledge Nutraceutical Translations for English-language editing of this review.

Conflicts of Interest: The authors declare no conflict of interest.

References

1. Rubio-Tapia, A.; Ludvigsson, J.F.; Brantner, T.L.; Murray, J.A.; Everhart, J.E. The Prevalence of Celiac Disease in the United States. *Am. J. Gastroenterol.* **2012**, *107*, 1538–1544. [CrossRef] [PubMed]
2. Larson, S.A.; Khaleghi, S.; Rubio-Tapia, A.; Ovsyannikova, I.G.; King, K.S.; Larson, J.J.; Lahr, B.D.; Poland, G.A.; Camilleri, M.J.; Murray, J.A. Prevalence and Morbidity of Undiagnosed Celiac Disease from a Community-Based Study. *Gastroenterology* **2017**, *152*, 830–839.
3. Mahadev, S.; Laszkowska, M.; Sundström, J.; Björkholm, M.; Lebwohl, B.; Green, P.H.; Ludvigsson, J.F. Prevalence of Celiac Disease in Patients With Iron Deficiency Anemia—A Systematic Review with Meta-analysis. *Gastroenterology* **2018**, *155*, 374–382. [CrossRef] [PubMed]
4. Guandalini, S.; Assiri, A. Celiac disease: A review. *JAMA Pediatr.* **2014**, *168*, 272–278. [CrossRef] [PubMed]
5. Husby, S.; Koletzko, S.; Korponay-Szabo, I.R.; Mearin, M.L.; Phillips, A.; Shamir, R.; Troncone, R.; Giersiepen, K.; Branski, D.; Catassi, C.; et al. European Society for Pediatric Gastroenterology, Hepatology, and Nutrition guidelines for the diagnosis of coeliac disease. *J. Pediatr. Gastroenterol. Nutr.* **2012**, *54*, 136–160. [CrossRef]
6. Felli, C.; Balsassarre, A.; Masoptti, A. Intestinal and circulating microRNAs in coeliac disease. *Int. J. Mol. Sci.* **2017**, *18*, 1907. [CrossRef]
7. Amr, K.S.; Bayoumi, F.S.; Eissa, E.; Abu-Zekry, M. Circulating microRNAs as potential non-invasive biomarkers in pediatric patients with celiac disease. *Eur. Ann. Allergy Clin. Immunol.* **2019**, *51*, 159–164. [CrossRef]
8. Vaira, V.; Roncoroni, L.; Barisani, D.; Gaudioso, G.; Bosari, S.; Bulfamante, G.; Doneda, L.; Conte, D.; Tomba, C.; Bardella, M.T.; et al. MicroRNA profiles in coeliac patients distinguish different clinical phenotypes and are modulated by gliadin peptides in primary duodenal fibroblast. *Clin. Sci.* **2014**, *126*, 417–423. [CrossRef]
9. Bledsoe, A.C.; King, K.S.; Larson, J.J.; Snyder, M.; Absah, I.; Murray, J.A. Micronutrient Deficiencies Are Common in Contemporary Celiac Disease Despite Lack of Overt Malabsorption Symptoms. *Mayo Clin. Proc.* **2019**, *94*, 1253–1260. [CrossRef]

10. Halfdanarson, T.R.; Litzow, M.R.; Murray, J.A. Hematologic manifestations of celiac disease. *Blood* **2007**, *109*, 412–421. [CrossRef]
11. Shahriari, M.; Honar, N.; Yousefi, A.; Javaherizadeh, H. Association of potential celiac disease and refractory iron deficiency anemia in children and adolescents. *Arq. Gastroenterol.* **2018**, *55*, 78–81. [CrossRef] [PubMed]
12. Elli, L.; Norsa, L.; Zullo, A.; Carroccio, A.; Girelli, C.; Oliva, S.; Romano, C.; Leandro, G.; Bellini, M.; Marmo, R.; et al. Diagnosis of chronic anaemia in gastrointestinal disorders: A guideline by the Italian Association of Hospital Gastroenterologist and Endoscopist (AIGO) and the Italian Society of Pardiatric Gastroenterology Hepatology and Nutrition (SIGENP). *Dig. Liver Dis.* **2019**, *51*, 471–483. [CrossRef] [PubMed]
13. Murray, J.A.; Watson, T.; Clearman, B.; Mitros, F. Effect of a gluten-free diet on gastrointestinal symptoms in celiac disease. *Am. J. Clin. Nutr.* **2004**, *79*, 669–673. [CrossRef] [PubMed]
14. Leffler, D.A.; Dennis, M.; Hyett, B.; Kelly, E.; Schuppan, D.; Kelly, C.P. Etiologies and Predictors of Diagnosis in Nonresponsive Celiac Disease. *Clin. Gastroenterol. Hepatol.* **2007**, *5*, 445–450. [CrossRef] [PubMed]
15. Muñoz, M.; Villar, I.; García-Erce, J.A. An update on iron physiology. *World J. Gastroenterol.* **2009**, *15*, 4617. [CrossRef] [PubMed]
16. DeLoughery, T.G. Microcytic anemia. *N. Engl. J. Med.* **2014**, *371*, 1324–1331. [CrossRef]
17. Leung, A.K.; Chan, K.W. Iron deficiency anemia. *Adv. Pediatr.* **2001**, *48*, 385–408.
18. Rao, R.; Georgieff, M.K. Iron in fetal and neonatal nutrition. *Semin. Fetal Neonatal Med.* **2007**, *12*, 54–63. [CrossRef]
19. Beard, J. Iron Deficiency Alters Brain Development and Functioning. *J. Nutr.* **2003**, *133*, 1468S–1472S. [CrossRef]
20. Beard, J.L.; Wiesinger, J.A.; Connor, J.R. Pre- and Postweaning Iron Deficiency Alters Myelination in Sprague-Dawley Rats. *Dev. Neurosci.* **2003**, *25*, 308–315. [CrossRef]
21. Beard, J.L.; Connor, J.R. Iron status and neural functioning. *Annu. Rev. Nutr.* **2003**, *23*, 41–58. [CrossRef] [PubMed]
22. Rubio-Tapia, A.; Hill, I.D.; Kelly, C.P.; Calderwood, A.H.; Murray, J.A. ACG Clinical Guidelines: Diagnosis and Management of Celiac Disease. *Am. J. Gastroenterol.* **2013**, *108*, 656–676. [CrossRef] [PubMed]
23. Harper, J.W.; Holleran, S.F.; Ramakrishnan, R.; Bhagat, G.; Green, P.H.R. Anemia in celiac disease is multifactorial in etiology. *Am. J. Hematol.* **2007**, *82*, 996–1000. [CrossRef] [PubMed]
24. Annibale, B.; Severi, C.; Chistolini, A.; Antonelli, G.; Lahner, E.; Marcheggiano, A.; Iannoni, C.; Monarca, B.; Delle Fave, G. Efficacy of gluten-free diet alone on recovery from iron deficiency anemia in adult celiac patients. *Am. J. Gastroenterol.* **2001**, *96*, 132–137. [CrossRef] [PubMed]
25. Smukalla, S.; Lebwohl, B.; Mears, J.G.; Leslie, L.A.; Green, P.H. How often do hematologists consider celiac disease in iron-deficiency anemia? Results of a national survey. *Clin. Adv. Hematol. Oncol.* **2014**, *12*, 100–105.
26. Oxentenko, A.S.; Murray, J.A. Celiac Disease: Ten Things That Every Gastroenterologist Should Know. *Clin. Gastroenterol. Hepatol.* **2015**, *13*, 1396–1404. [CrossRef]
27. Murray, J.A.; McLachlan, S.; Adams, P.C.; Eckfeldt, J.H.; Garner, C.P.; Vulpe, C.D.; Gordeuk, V.R.; Brantner, T.; Leiendecker–Foster, C.; Killeen, A.A.; et al. Association between celiac disease and iron deficiency in caucasians, but not non-caucasians. *Clin. Gastroenterol. Hepatol.* **2013**, *11*, 808–814. [CrossRef]
28. Pirán Arce, M.F.; Aballay, L.R.; Leporati, J.L.; Navarro, A.; Forneris, M. Blood iron levels in accordance with adherence to a gluten-free diet in celiac school aged children. *Nutr. Hosp.* **2018**, *35*, 25–32.
29. Brandimarte, G.; Tursi, A.; Giorgetti, G.M. Changing trends in clinical form of celiac disease. Which is now the main form of celiac disease in clinical practice? *Minerva Gastroenterol. Dietol.* **2002**, *48*, 121–130.
30. Sharma, M.; Singh, P.; Agnihotri, A.; Das, P.; Mishra, A.; Verma, A.K.; Ahuja, A.; Sreenivas, V.; Khadgawat, R.; Gupta, S.D.; et al. Celiac disease: A disease with varied manifestations in adults and adolescents. *J. Dig. Dis.* **2013**, *14*, 518–525. [CrossRef]
31. Rostami-Nejad, M.; Aldulaimi, D.; Livett, H.; Rostami, K.H. pylori associated with iron deficiency anemia even in celiac disease patients; strongly evidence based but weakly reflected in practice. *Gastroenterol. Hepatol. Bed Bench.* **2015**, *8*, 178. [PubMed]
32. Samasca, G.; Deleanu, D.; Sur, G.; Lupan, I.; Giulia, A.; Carpa, R. Is it necessary to screen Helicobacter pylori infection in patients with celiac disease and iron deficiency? *Gastroenterol. Hepatol.* **2016**, *9*, 345.

33. Elli, L.; Poggiali, E.; Tomba, C.; Andreozzi, F.; Nava, I.; Bardella, M.T.; Campostrini, N.; Girelli, D.; Conte, D.; Cappellini, M.D. Does TMPRSS6 RS855791 polymorphism contribute to iron defiociency in treated celiac disease? *Am. J. Gastroenterol.* **2015**, *110*, 200–202. [CrossRef] [PubMed]
34. De Falco, L.; Tortora, R.; Imperatore, G.; Bruno, M.; Capasso, M.; Girelli, D.; Castagna, A.; Caporaso, N.; Iolascon, A.; Rispo, A. The role of *TMPRSS6* and *HFE* variants in iron deficiency anemia in celiac disease. *Am. J. Hematol.* **2018**, *93*, 383–393. [CrossRef] [PubMed]
35. Sharma, N.; Begum, J.; Eksteen, B.; Elagib, A.; Brookes, M.; Cooper, B.T.; Tselepis, C.; Iqbal, T.H. Differential ferritin expression is associated with iron defficiency in coeliac disease. *Eur. J. Gastroenterol. Hepatol.* **2009**, *21*, 794–804. [CrossRef] [PubMed]
36. Tolone, C.; Bellini, G.; Punzo, F.; Papparella, A.; Miele, E.; Vitale, A.; Nobili, B.; Strisciuglio, C.; Rossi, F. The DMT1 IVS4+44C> A polymorphism and the risk of iron deficiency anemia in children with celiac disease. *PLoS ONE* **2017**, *12*, e0185822. [CrossRef]
37. Elli, L.; Ferretti, F.; Branchi, F.; Tomba, C.; Lombardo, V.; Scricciolo, A.; Doneda, L.; Roncoroni, L. Sucrosomial iron supplementation in anemic patients with celiac disease not tolerating oral ferrous sulfate: A prospective study. *Nutrients* **2018**, *10*, 330. [CrossRef]
38. Giancotti, L.; Talarico, V.; Mazza, G.A.; Marrazzo, S.; Gangemi, P.; Miniero, R.; Bertini, M. Feralgine^{TM} a new approach for iron defficiency anemia in celiac patients. *Nutrients* **2019**, *11*, 887. [CrossRef]
39. Zamani, F.; Mohamadnejad, M.; Shakeri, R.; Amiri, A.; Najafi, S.; Alimohamadi, S.M.; Tavangar, S.M.; Ghavamzadeh, A.; Malekzadeh, R. Gluten sensitive enteropathy in patients with iron deficiency anemia of unknown origin. *World J. Gastroenterol.* **2008**, *14*, 7381. [CrossRef]
40. Lasa, J.S.; Olivera, P.; Soifer, L.; Moore, R. La anemia ferropénica como presentación de enfermedad celíaca subclínica en una población argentina. *Rev. Gastroenterol. Méx.* **2017**, *82*, 270–273. [CrossRef]
41. Repo, M.; Lindfors, K.; Mäki, M.; Huhtala, H.; Laurila, K.; Lähdeaho, M.L.; Saavalainen, P.; Kaukinen, K.; Kurppa, K. Anemia and iron deficiency in children with potential celiac disease. *J. Pediatr. Gastroenterol. Nutr.* **2017**, *64*, 56–62. [CrossRef] [PubMed]
42. Dinler, G.; Atalay, E.; Kalayci, A.G. Celiac disease in 87 children with typical and atypical symptoms in Black Sea region of Turkey. *World J. Pediatr.* **2009**, *5*, 282–286. [CrossRef] [PubMed]
43. Wierdsma, N.; van Bokhorst-de van der Schueren, M.; Berkenpas, M.; Mulder, C.; van Bodegraven, A. Vitamin and Mineral Deficiencies Are Highly Prevalent in Newly Diagnosed Celiac Disease Patients. *Nutrients* **2013**, *5*, 3975–3992. [CrossRef] [PubMed]
44. García-Manzanares, Á.; Lucendo, A.J. Review: Nutritional and Dietary Aspects of Celiac Disease. *Nutr. Clin. Pract.* **2011**, *26*, 163–173. [CrossRef]
45. Carmel, R. *Megaloblastic Anemias: Disorders Of impaired DNA Synthesis*, 1st ed.; Wintrobe's Clinical Hematology; Williams & Wilkins: Baltimore, MD, USA, 2004.
46. Kuloğlu, Z.; Kirsaçlioğlu, C.T.; Kansu, A.; Ensari, A.; Girgin, N. Celiac disease: Presentation of 109 children. *Yonsei Med. J.* **2009**, *50*, 617–623. [CrossRef]
47. Ward, P.C.J. Modern approaches to the investigation of vitamin B12 deficiency. *Clin. Lab. Med.* **2002**, *22*, 435–445. [CrossRef]
48. Klee, G.G. Cobalamin and folate evaluation: Measurement of methylmalonic acid and homocysteine vs vitamin B(12) and folate. *Clin. Chem.* **2000**, *46*, 1277–1283.
49. Guevara Pacheco, G.; Chávez Cortés, E.; Castillo-Durán, C. Deficiencia de micronutrientes y enfermedad celíaca. *Arch. Argent Pediatr.* **2014**, *112*, 457–463.
50. Freeman, H.J. Neurological disorders in adult celiac disease. *Can. J. Gastroenterol.* **2008**, *22*, 909–911. [CrossRef]
51. Halfdanarion, T.R.; Kumar, N.; Hogan, W.J.; Murray, J.A. Copper deficiency in celiac disease. *J. Clin. Gastroenterol.* **2009**, *43*, 162–164. [CrossRef]
52. Cavallieri, F.; Fin, N.; Contardi, S.; Fiorini, M.; Corradini, E.; Valzania, F. Subacute copper-deficiency myelopathy in as patient with occult celiac disease. *J. Spinal Cord Med.* **2017**, *40*, 489–491. [CrossRef] [PubMed]

53. Tran, C.D.; Katsikeros, R.; Manton, N.; Krebs, N.F.; Hambidge, K.M.; Butler, R.N.; Davidson, G.P. Zinc homeostasis and gut function in children with celiac disease. *Am. J. Clin. Nutr.* **2011**, *94*, 1026–1032. [CrossRef] [PubMed]
54. Baydoun, A.; Maakaron, J.E.; Halawi, H.; Abou Rahal, J.; Taher, A.T. Hematological manifestations of celiac disease. *Scand. J. Gastroenterol.* **2012**, *47*, 1401–1411. [CrossRef] [PubMed]
55. Irfan, O.; Mahmood, S.; Nand, H.; Billoo, G. Celiac disease associated with aplastic anemia in a 6-year-old girl: A case report and review of the literature. *J. Med. Case Rep.* **2018**, *12*, 16. [CrossRef] [PubMed]
56. Grey-Davies, E.; Hows, J.M.; Marsh, J.C.W. Aplastic anaemia in association with coeliac disease: A series of three cases. *Br. J. Haematol.* **2008**, *143*, 258–260. [CrossRef]
57. Maheshwari, A.; Nirupam, N.; Aneja, S.; Meena, R.; Chandra, J.; Kumar, P. Association of Celiac Disease with Aplastic Anemia. *Indian J. Pediatr.* **2012**, *79*, 1372–1373. [CrossRef]
58. Salmeron, G.; Patey, N.; De Latour, R.P.; Raffoux, E.; Gluckman, E.; Brousse, N.; Socié, G.; Robin, M. Coeliac disease and aplastic anaemia: A specific entity? *Br. J. Haematol.* **2009**, *146*, 122–124. [CrossRef]
59. Basu, A.; Ray, Y.; Bowmik, P.; Rahman, M.; Dikshit, N.; Goswami, R.P. Rare association of coeliac disease with aplastic anaemia: Report of a case from India. *Indian J. Hematol. Blood Transfus.* **2014**, *30*, 208–211. [CrossRef]
60. Badyal, R.K.; Sachdeva, M.U.S.; Varma, N.; Thapa, B.R. A Rare Association of Celiac Disease and Aplastic Anemia: Case Report of a Child and Review of Literature. *Pediatr. Dev. Pathol.* **2014**, *17*, 470–473. [CrossRef]
61. Garrdner, L.; Benz, E. *Hematology. Basic Principles and Practice*, 3rd ed.; Churchill Livinstone: London, UK, 2000.
62. Weiss, G.; Goodnough, L.T. Anemia of Chronic Disease. *N. Engl. J. Med.* **2005**, *352*, 1011–1023. [CrossRef]
63. Ciccocioppo, R.; Di Sabatino, A.; Bauer, M.; Della Riccia, D.N.; Bizzini, F.; Biagi, F.; Cifone, M.G.; Corazza, G.R.; Schuppan, D. Matrix metalloproteinase pattern in celiac duodenal mucosa. *Lab. Investig.* **2005**, *85*, 397–407. [CrossRef] [PubMed]
64. Di Sabatino, A.; Ciccocioppo, R.; Cupelli, F.; Cinque, B.; Millimaggi, D.; Clarkson, M.M.; Paulli, M.; Cifone, M.G.; Corazza, G.R. Epithelium derived interleukin 15 regulates intraepithelial lymphocyte Th1 cytokine production, cytotoxicity, and survival in coeliac disease. *Gut* **2006**, *55*, 469–477. [CrossRef] [PubMed]
65. Wang, C.Q.; Udupa, K.B.; Lipschitz, D.A. Interferon-γ exerts its negative regulatory effect primarily on the earliest stages of murine erythroid progenitor cell development. *J. Cell. Physiol.* **1995**, *162*, 134–138. [CrossRef] [PubMed]
66. Ludwiczek, S.; Aigner, E.; Theurl, I.; Weiss, G. Cytokine-mediated regulation of iron transport in human monocytic cells. *Blood* **2003**, *101*, 4148–4154. [CrossRef] [PubMed]
67. Högberg, L.; Danielsson, L.; Jarleman, S.; Sundqvist, T.; Stenhammar, L. Serum zinc in small children with coeliac disease. *Acta Paediatr.* **2008**, *98*, 343–345. [CrossRef] [PubMed]
68. Zerga, M. Anemia de los trastornos crónicos. *Hematologia* **2004**, *8*, 45–55.
69. Mullarky, I.K.; Szaba, F.M.; Kummer, L.W.; Wilhelm, L.B.; Parent, M.A.; Johnson, L.L.; Smiley, S.T. Gamma interferon suppresses erythropoiesis via interleukin-15. *Infect. Immun.* **2007**, *75*, 2630–2633. [CrossRef]
70. Benahmed, M.; Meresse, B.; Arnulf, B.; Barbe, U.; Mention, J.J.; Verkarre, V.; Allez, M.; Cellier, C.; Hermine, O.; Cerf–Bensussan, N. Inhibition of TGF-β Signaling by IL-15: A New Role for IL-15 in the Loss of Immune Homeostasis in Celiac Disease. *Gastroenterology* **2007**, *132*, 994–1008. [CrossRef]
71. Diaz-Castro, J.; Muriel-Neyra, C.; Martin-Masot, R.; Moreno-Fernandez, J.; Maldonado, J.; Nestares, T. Oxidative stress, DNA stability and evoked inflammatory signaling in young celiac patients consuming a gluten-free diet. *Eur. J. Nutr.* **2019**, 1–8. [CrossRef]
72. Bergamaschi, G.; Markopoulos, K.; Albertini, R.; Di Sabatino, A.; Biagi, F.; Ciccocioppo, R.; Arbustini, E.; Corazza, G.R. Anemia of chronic disease and defective erythropoietin production in patients with celiac disease. *Haematologica* **2008**, *93*, 1785–1791. [CrossRef]
73. Cataldo, F.; Lio, D.; Marino, V.; Scola, L.; Crivello, A.; Corazza, G.R.; Working Groups of the SIGEP and 'Club del Tenue'. Plasma cytokine profiles in patients with celiac disease and selective IgA deficiency. *Pediatr. Allergy Immunol.* **2003**, *14*, 320–324. [CrossRef] [PubMed]
74. Fornari, M.C.; Pedreira, S.; Niveloni, S.; González, D.; Diez, R.A.; Vázquez, H.; Mazure, R.; Sugai, E.; Smecuol, E.; Boerr, L.; et al. Pre- and Post-Treatment Serum Levels of Cytokines IL-1β, IL-6, and IL-1 Receptor Antagonist in Celiac Disease. Are They Related to the Associated Osteopenia? *Am. J. Gastroenterol.* **1998**, *93*, 413–418. [CrossRef] [PubMed]

75. Romaldini, C.C.; Barbieri, D.; Okay, T.S.; Raiz, R.; Cançado, E.L.R. Serum soluble interleukin-2 receptor, interleukin-6, and tumor necrosis factor-alpha levels in children with celiac disease: Response to treatment. *J. Pediatr. Gastroenterol. Nutr.* **2002**, *35*, 513–517. [CrossRef] [PubMed]
76. Merendino, R.A.; Di Pasquale, G.; Sturniolo, G.C.; Ruello, A.; Albanese, V.; Minciullo, P.L.; Di Mauro, S.; Gangemi, S. Relationship between IL-18 and sICAM-1 serum levels in patients affected by coeliac disease: Preliminary considerations. *Immunol. Lett.* **2003**, *85*, 257–260. [CrossRef]
77. Berry, N.; Basha, J.; Varma, N.; Varma, S.; Prasad, K.K.; Vaiphei, K.; Dhaka, N.; Sinha, S.K.; Kochhar, R. Anemia in celiac disease is multifactorial in etiology: A prospective study from India. *JGH Open* **2018**, *2*, 196–200. [CrossRef] [PubMed]
78. Elli, L.; Ferretti, F.; Orlando, S.; Vecchi, M.; Monguzzi, E.; Roncoroni, L.; Schuppan, D. Management of celiac disease in daily clinical practice. *Eur. J. Intern. Med.* **2019**, *61*, 15–24. [CrossRef]
79. Barratt, S.M.; Leeds, J.S.; Sanders, D.S. Quality of life in Coeliac Disease is determined by perceived degree of difficulty adhering to a gluten-free diet, not the level of dietary adherence ultimately achieved. *J. Gastrointestin Liver Dis.* **2011**, *20*, 241–245.
80. Martín Masot, R.; Ortega Páez, E. El péptido del gluten en heces puede ser útil en el seguimiento de la enfermedad celíaca. *Evid. Pediatr.* **2018**, *14*, 37.
81. Silvester, J.A.; Kurada, S.; Szwajcer, A.; Kelly, C.P.; Leffler, D.A.; Duerksen, D.R. Tests for Serum Transglutaminase and Endomysial Antibodies Do Not Detect Most Patients with Celiac Disease and Persistent Villous Atrophy on Gluten-free Diets: A Meta-analysis. *Gastroenterology* **2017**, *153*, 689–701. [CrossRef]
82. Gerasimidis, K.; Zafeiropoulou, K.; Mackinder, M.; Ijaz, U.Z.; Duncan, H.; Buchanan, E.; Cardigan, T.; Edwards, C.A.; McGrogan, P.; Russell, R.K. Comparison of Clinical Methods With the Faecal Gluten Immunogenic Peptide to Assess Gluten Intake in Coeliac Disease. *J. Pediatr. Gastroenterol. Nutr.* **2018**, *67*, 356–360. [CrossRef]
83. Rubio-Tapia, A.; Murray, J.A. Classification and management of refractory coeliac disease. *Gut* **2010**, *59*, 547–557. [CrossRef] [PubMed]
84. van Gils, T.; Nijeboer, P.; van Wanrooij, R.L.; Bouma, G.; Mulder, C.J.J. Mechanisms and management of refractory coeliac disease. *Nat. Rev. Gastroenterol. Hepatol.* **2015**, *12*, 572–579. [CrossRef] [PubMed]
85. Ryan, B.M.; Kelleher, D. Refractory celiac disease. *Gastroenterology* **2000**, *119*, 243–251. [CrossRef] [PubMed]
86. Rishi, A.R.; Rubio-Tapia, A.; Murray, J.A. Refractory celiac disease. *Expert Rev. Gastroenterol. Hepatol.* **2016**, *10*, 537–546. [CrossRef]
87. Mooney, P.D.; Evans, K.E.; Singh, S.; Sanders, D.S. Treatment failure in coeliac disease: A practical guide to investigation and treatment of non-responsive and refractory coeliac disease. *J. Gastrointestin Liver Dis.* **2012**, *21*, 197–203.
88. Branchi, F.; Locatelli, M.; Tomba, C.; Conte, D.; Ferretti, F.; Elli, L. Enteroscopy and radiology for the management of celiac disease complications: Time for a pragmatic roadmap. *Dig. Liver Dis.* **2016**, *48*, 578–586. [CrossRef]
89. Chetcuti Zammit, S.; Sanders, D.S.; Sidhu, R. Capsule endoscopy for patients with coeliac disease. *Expert Rev. Gastroenterol. Hepatol.* **2018**, *12*, 779–790. [CrossRef]
90. Efthymakis, K.; Milano, A.; Laterza, F.; Serio, M.; Neri, M. Iron deficiency anemia despite effective gluten-free diet in celiac disease: Diagnostic role of small bowel capsule endoscopy. *Dig. Liver Dis.* **2017**, *49*, 412–416. [CrossRef]
91. Rajalahti, T.; Repo, M.; Kivelä, L.; Huhtala, H.; Mäki, M.; Kaukinen, K.; Lindfors, K.; Kurppa, K. Anemia in Pediatric Celiac Disease. *J. Pediatr. Gastroenterol. Nutr.* **2017**, *64*, e1–e6. [CrossRef]
92. Lewis, S.K.; Semrad, C.E. Capsule Endoscopy and Enteroscopy in Celiac Disease. *Gastroenterol. Clin.* **2019**, *48*, 73–84. [CrossRef]
93. Rokkas, T.; Niv, Y. The role of video capsule endoscopy in the diagnosis of celiac disease. *Eur. J. Gastroenterol. Hepatol.* **2012**, *24*, 303–308. [CrossRef] [PubMed]
94. Eigner, W.; Bashir, K.; Primas, C.; Kazemi-Shirazi, L.; Wrba, F.; Trauner, M.; Vogelsang, H. Dynamics of occurrence of refractory coeliac disease and associated complications over 25 years. *Aliment. Pharmacol. Ther.* **2017**, *45*, 364–372. [CrossRef] [PubMed]

95. Oruc, N.; Ozütemız, O.; Tekın, F.; Sezak, M.; Tunçyürek, M.; Krasinskas, A.M.; Tombuloğlu, M. Celiac disease associated with B-cell lymphoma. *Turk. J. Gastroenterol.* **2010**, *21*, 168–171. [CrossRef] [PubMed]
96. Ilus, T.; Kaukinen, K.; Virta, L.J.; Pukkala, E.; Collin, P. Incidence of Malignancies in Diagnosed Celiac Patients: A Population-based Estimate. *Am. J. Gastroenterol.* **2014**, *109*, 1471–1477. [CrossRef]
97. Delabie, J.; Holte, H.; Vose, J.M.; Ullrich, F.; Jaffe, E.S.; Savage, K.J.; Connors, J.M.; Rimsza, L.; Harris, N.L.; Müller-Hermelink, K.; et al. Enteropathy-associated T-cell lymphoma: Clinical and histological findings from the international peripheral T-cell lymphoma project. *Blood* **2011**, *118*, 148–155. [CrossRef]

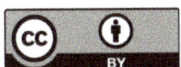

© 2019 by the authors. Licensee MDPI, Basel, Switzerland. This article is an open access article distributed under the terms and conditions of the Creative Commons Attribution (CC BY) license (http://creativecommons.org/licenses/by/4.0/).

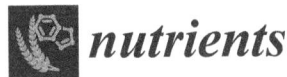

Review

Anemia of Inflammation with An Emphasis on Chronic Kidney Disease

Sajidah Begum [1] and Gladys O. Latunde-Dada [2,*]

1. Faculty of Life Sciences and Medicine, Henriette Raphael House Guy's Campus King's College London, London SE1 1UL, UK; sajidah.begum@kcl.ac.uk
2. Department of Nutritional Sciences, School of Life Course Sciences, King's College London. Franklin-Wilkins-Building, 150 Stamford Street, London SE1 9NH, UK
* Correspondence: yemisi.latunde-dada@kcl.ac.uk; Tel.: +44-20-7848-4256

Received: 28 August 2019; Accepted: 30 September 2019; Published: 11 October 2019

Abstract: Iron is vital for a vast variety of cellular processes and its homeostasis is strictly controlled and regulated. Nevertheless, disorders of iron metabolism are diverse and can be caused by insufficiency, overload or iron mal-distribution in tissues. Iron deficiency (ID) progresses to iron-deficiency anemia (IDA) after iron stores are depleted. Inflammation is of diverse etiology in anemia of chronic disease (ACD). It results in serum hypoferremia and tissue hyperferritinemia, which are caused by elevated serum hepcidin levels, and this underlies the onset of functional iron-deficiency anemia. Inflammation is also inhibitory to erythropoietin function and may directly increase hepcidin level, which influences iron metabolism. Consequently, immune responses orchestrate iron metabolism, aggravate iron sequestration and, ultimately, impair the processes of erythropoiesis. Hence, functional iron-deficiency anemia is a risk factor for several ailments, disorders and diseases. Therefore, therapeutic strategies depend on the symptoms, severity, comorbidities and the associated risk factors of anemia. Oral iron supplements can be employed to treat ID and mild anemia particularly, when gastrointestinal intolerance is minimal. Intravenous (IV) iron is the option in moderate and severe anemic conditions, for patients with compromised intestinal integrity, or when oral iron is refractory. Erythropoietin (EPO) is used to treat functional iron deficiency, and blood transfusion is restricted to refractory patients or in life-threatening emergency situations. Despite these interventions, many patients remain anemic and do not respond to conventional treatment approaches. However, various novel therapies are being developed to treat persistent anemia in patients.

Keywords: iron; anemia; kidney; hepcidin; erythropoietin

1. Introduction

Iron is an essential micronutrient required for a number of cellular processes. It is involved in the structure and function of hemoglobin and myoglobin, as well as in the formation of heme enzymes and other iron-containing enzymes of the electron transport chain. Iron is necessary for many biological functions, however, when in excess, toxicity results due to the production of reactive oxygen species and this leads to the malfunctioning of organs [1]. Iron deficiency (ID) describes a condition in which the iron stores in the body are reduced but not sufficiently to limit erythropoiesis. If iron deficiency is severe enough to reduce erythropoiesis, iron-deficiency anemia (IDA) results [2]. In 2016, a systematic analysis for the Global Burden of Disease Study stated that IDA is one of the five leading causes of years lived with disability, particularly in women, and thereby highlighted the prevention and treatment of IDA as a major public health goal [3]. IDA is estimated to affect 1.24 billion people in the world, comprising mostly children and reproductive women, and particularly, in less-developed economies [4]. Iron deficiency (ID) in the absence of anemia has been suggested to be twice the incidence of IDA [5]. Substantive evidence has revealed that both ID and IDA have deleterious consequences on cognition, mental function, work performance, and pregnancy outcomes [6,7]. Furthermore, functional iron deficiency occurs when iron is sequestered in storage organs during inflammation and infections or in situations such as increased erythropoiesis either naturally, due to increased Erythropoietin (EPO) release in response to anemia, or, pharmacologically by erythropoietin-stimulating agents (ESA's) [8,9].

Anemia describes a state in which there is a reduced erythrocyte count or a reduced level of hemoglobin within erythrocytes [10]. Anemia can be classified in several ways; which can be based on etiological factors, such as nutritional, aplastic, hemorrhagic or hemolytic. However, in clinical practice, classification could be based on the morphology of erythrocytes such as the mean corpuscular volume (MCV). Based on the MCV, anemia can be described as microcytic (MCV< 82 fL), normocytic (MCV = 82–98 fL) or macrocytic (MCV >98 fL). The limitation of this classification is that red cell morphology during hematopoiesis is often not influenced during the early stages of iron deficiency and a class of anemia type could transverse 2 classification groups. Broadly, however, typical examples of microcytic anemia are iron deficiency, thalassemic and sideroblastic anemia. Normocytic anemia includes hemolytic and anemia of chronic disease and folic and vitamin-B12-deficiency anemia are macrocytic.

2. Causes of Iron-Deficiency Anemia

Several factors contribute to the development of iron-deficiency anemia and these are presented in a recent review [5]. Physiologically, an increased demand for iron which cannot be met from dietary sources will lead to iron deficiency. This occurs during rapid growth of infants and adolescents, menstrual blood loss, post blood donation and during the first and second trimesters of pregnancy. Nutritionally, inadequate iron intake, malnutrition or poor dietary absorption can lead to iron-deficiency anemia. Pathological causes include decreased absorption and chronic blood loss. Causes of decreased absorption include gastrectomy, bariatric surgery, duodenal bypass, inflammatory bowel disease and atrophic gastritis. Causes of chronic blood loss include bleeding of the gastrointestinal tract (oesophagitis, peptic ulcer, diverticulitis, benign and malignant tumour, hookworm infestation and hemorrhoids), genitourinary system (heavy menses, menorrhagia, intravascular haemolysis (paroxysmal nocturnal haemoglobinuria) and systemic bleeding (trauma, hemorragic telangiectasia and chronic schistosomiasis). Certain classes of drugs have also been implicated in the development of iron-deficiency anemia and these include glucocorticoids, salicylates, non-steroidal anti-inflammatory drugs and proton pump inhibitors. Iron-refractory iron-deficiency anemia is an inherited cause of iron-deficiency anemia. Finally, the availability of iron can be restricted, leading to functional iron deficiency that is associated with anemia of chronic inflammatory conditions [2,5,11,12]. This is a literature review on a few other types of anemia that are associated or concomitant with chronic disease inflammatory conditions. It evaluates the variations in phenotypes, management and discusses the differences in the therapeutic approaches employed.

3. Anemia of Inflammation or Anemia of Chronic Disease

Inflammation is an immune response to injury and infection. The inflammatory process causes hypoferremia as an acute-phase response to fight against infection. It involves the secretion of cytokines to regulate iron redistribution, creating hypoferremia that delays pathogen growth, thereby causing the invaders to be engulfed by phagocytes. The orchestrated defense system mounted by the host to fight and fence off pathogens culminates sequentially in tissue iron sequestration, serum iron deficiency, and anemia. This epitomizes the essentiality of life preservation and survival in a competitive hostile environment as normal tissue functions (oxygen delivery) are partially or transiently sacrificed to combat infection [13]. Concomitant with the survival response is the marshalling of the armoury of the erythropoietic drive to override and inhibit both inflammatory and iron-sensing pathways in order to attenuate the downregulation of iron absorption by hepcidin [14–16]. Anemia of Chronic Disease (ACD) thus has a multifactorial etiology and has been estimated to afflict over a billion individuals globally [4]. It is prevalent in chronic diseases and disorders, such as heart disease, cancer, inflammatory bowel disease and chronic kidney disease, in which inflammation causes anemia due to increased levels of hepcidin in circulation [4]. The manifestation of the proinflammatory process in a spectrum results in variation in hepcidin levels and the magnitudes of anemia phenotype. ACD, therefore, is caused by a complex interplay of proinflammatory cytokines which induce dysregulation in iron homeostasis, erythroid progenitor cell differentiation, erythropoietin synthesis and red cell longevity, all culminating in the pathogenesis of anemia [17].

Systemic inflammation induced by infection, trauma, dialysis, malignancy or autoimmune disorders activate immune cells to produce cytokines such as Interleukins, (IL) IL1, IL6, IL10, interferon γ (IFNγ) and tumor necrosis factor α (TNFα). Erythropoiesis is impaired by iron restriction, suppression of EPO production and shortened life-span of erythroid progenitors, all culminating in iron-deficiency anemia [17] (Table 1). Thus, ACD is an underlying secondary disorder that is deleterious to the survival of erythrocytes and erythropoiesis.

Table 1. Features of anemia of inflammation [17].

Cells/Tissue	Cytokine	Effector Function
Hepatocytes	IL6 and lipopolysaccharide (LPS)	Induction of hepcidin expression in the liver. Hepcidin inhibits iron efflux from the macrophages and the duodenum by blocking or degrading ferroportin.
Macrophage		
	Lipopolysaccharide (LPS) and TNFα	Increase DMT1 expression and uptake of ferrous iron(Fe^{2+}).
	TNFα	Promotes damage of erythrocyte membranes and the stimulation of phagocytosis.
	IFNγ and LPS	Decrease expression of ferroportin to inhibit iron efflux and accentuated by hepcidin.
	TNFα-IL1, IL6 and IL10	Induction of ferritin expression, storage and retention of iron within macrophages.
Monocytes	IL10	Enhances TfR1 expression to promote uptake of transferrin-bound iron.
Kidney	TNFα, IFNγ and IL1	Dysregulated erythropoietin receptor EPOR expression and signalling via blunted expression of Scribble (Scb) and inhibition of erythropoietin (EPO) and erythroferrone (ERFE) which production. The cytokines also directly inhibit the differentiation and proliferation of erythroid progenitor cells.

TNFα, tumor necrosis factor α; TfR1: Erythropoietin receptor 1; IFNγ, interferon γ; DMT1, divalent metal transporter 1.

4. Anemia of Cancer

Anemia is prevalent in various types of cancer and iron deficiency accounts for a significant proportion of this comorbidity [18]. The etiology of different tumor types could be multifactorial and complicated by varying underlying factors, but an overriding cause of anemia is chemotherapy-induced. Persistent blood loss, coupled with nutritional deficiencies, culminate in dysregulated iron homeostasis [19]. Features of ID in cancer range from a spectrum of low to high or elevated serum ferritin, a blend of mild absolute ID and a functional ID (FID) gradient. However, as it is a chronic disease that is akin to an inflammatory condition, most cancer patients suffer from FID [19]. It was reported that the prevalence of anemia is about 50% of non-myeloid tumor patients undergoing systemic therapy in a cohort of Spanish hospitals [20]. Moreover, a Europe-wide study that evaluated routine practice in chemotherapy-induced anemia (CIA) management showed that 74% of patients exhibited Hb ≤10 g/dL, including 15% with severe anemia (Hb <8 g/dL). Furthermore 42% of the cancer patients had low-iron levels (ferritin ≤100 ng/mL) [21]. Anemia thus contributes significantly to disease burden and reduced quality of life in cancer patients undergoing therapy. It is, therefore, imperative to treat anemia in the different malignant forms of cancers. Conventional therapeutic approaches include red blood transfusion, the administration of erythropoietin-stimulating agents (ESA), intravenous iron supplementation (IV) and a combination of ESA and IV [22]. While blood transfusion predisposes patients to thromboembolism and increased mortality [22], ESA administration could be refractory in cancer patients. The adverse consequences of IV on oxidative stress and tumorigenesis in heterogeneous cancers are not yet clarified in clinical trials [23]. Recent guidelines and recommendations on the treatment of cancer-related anemia advocate reduction or avoidance of red blood cells (RBC) transfusions, intravenous (IV) alone or a combinatorial use of IV to enhance low-dosage ESA administration [23]. Novel approaches to the treatment of functional anemia that typify chronic diseases, including cancer, are discussed herein later under anemia of chronic kidney disease (ACKD).

5. Anemia of Heart Failure

Anemia is prevalent in patients with heart failure (HF), correlates with severity of the disease and is responsible for increased morbidity and mortality in patients [24]. It is characterized by decreased exercise capacity (reduced exercise capacity of 5,6 and worse) by the New York Heart Association (NYHA) functional classification. There are different causes of anemia in HF, arising from the heterogeneous manifestations of the disorder [25]. Anemia caused by absolute iron deficiency in HF may be due to nutritional factors, such as low dietary iron, poor appetite loss, decreased iron absorption due to gastrointestinal blood loss caused by gut inflammation and consequences of iatrogenic agents [26]. However, as it is a chronic disease that is akin to an inflammatory condition, most HF patients suffer from FID [26]. Hemodilution and renal insufficiency are also linked with anemia of HF. Incidence of iron deficiency in chronic HF patients in Europe is about 50%, compared with 61% in Asian populations [27]. A study that analysed about 2000 patients in cohorts in Poland, Spain and the Netherlands reported a prevalence of 32% cases of ID, 12% of IDA and a combination of both as 20% [28]. Anemia thus results significantly in disease burden, increased hospitalizations, and reduced quality of life in HF patients, as well as decreased functional capacity. Conventional therapy for numerous clinical trials is intravenous (IV) iron administration, particularly in patients with symptomatic systolic HF. Intravenous iron infusion has been shown to significantly reduce hospitalizations, improve quality of life, increase exercise capacity and decrease mortality in HF patients. Therapy of symptomatic diastolic HF with IV iron has yet to be clarified or confirmed. Recent guidelines and recommendations on the treatment of HF-related anemia advocate IV iron for symptomatic patients (serum ferritin <100 µg/L, or ferritin between 100–299 µg/L and transferrin saturation (TSAT) <20%) to improve exercise capacity and quality of life [29]. Serum ferritin and TSAT mean values could be variable in HD patients due to confounding factors that are influenced by the magnitude of the symptoms [30]. Such confounders, complexities and the multifactorial nature of iron metabolism dysregulation [31] possibly account for the unreliability of serum hepcidin as a clinical marker of iron status in HD patients [32]. The choice of IV administration of iron compounds varies in different countries.

6. Anemia of Surgery

Anemia is prevalent in patients undergoing major surgery and poses an additional independently modifiable risk to patients undergoing blood transfusion [33]. Anemia can range from 7–35% in orthopaedic surgery patients and is associated with high morbidity and mortality [34]. Iron deficiency due to increased requirements, reduced absorption, increased lysis and losses of red blood cells are the main causes of preoperative anemia. Moreover, anemia prior to surgery coupled with increased lysis and losses of red blood cells, iron-sequestration and restricted erythropoiesis lead to over 80% prevalence in postoperative anemia [35]. Perioperative anemia manifests mostly as absolute and functional iron-deficiency anemia that are respectively characterized by scarcity and sequestration of iron in tissues [36]. A chronic inflammatory condition accentuates iron sequestration and FID in the patients. Of note also is that hematinic deficiencies lead insidiously to latent iron deficiency without anemia. A large study of hospital patients of diverse surgical procedures (cardiac, gynecological, colorectal/liver cancer resection) reported the overall prevalence of anemia as 36%. In the anemic patients, 62% had absolute iron deficiency, while FID was 10% [37]. Women accounted for more than twice in number in the cohort. Perioperative and postoperative anemia thus contribute significantly to disease burden and reduced quality of life, the magnitude of which varies with the different disorders. Conventional therapeutic approaches advocate the diagnosis and treatment of anemia before any surgical procedure. Iron deficiency without anemia needs to be treated to replenish iron stores for preoperative requirements and postoperative anemia challenge [38]. Preoperative oral iron could be prescribed for mild-to-moderate anemia patients that are tolerant and do not suffer from adverse gastrointestinal consequences. IV iron supplementation, preferably as a large single dose, is the therapy guideline in moderate to severe postoperative anemic patients. However, a combination of IV and ESA is recommended only in severe anemia that is refractive and resistant over a long period of time.

Red blood cell transfusion (RBCT) may be an acute, inevitable option to correct severe anemia in critically physiologically drained patients after surgery. Guidelines and recommendations for RBCT are restrictive because of the attendant risk of infection, thromboembolic events, high morbidity and mortality in the patients [39,40]. Patient blood management (PBM) that involves evaluation of the hematological status of patients will not only prevent preoperative anemia, but also reduce intraoperative transfusion risk and postoperative complications [41]. Recent guidelines and recommendations advocate a preoperative Hb <13 g/dL to be considered as suboptimal in both men and women and treated before any major surgical procedure [38].

7. Anemia of Inflammatory Bowel Disease (IBD)

Anemia is a common comorbidity of inflammatory bowel disease (IBD). The aetiology of IBD is multifactorial and the pathogenesis is complicated by varying underlying factors, such as genetic predisposition, immune dysregulation, loss of mucosal integrity and intestinal microbial composition. This results in a spectrum of chronic relapsing inflammatory disorders that are characterized by ulceration and bleeding of the mucosal epithelium. An inflammatory condition in IBD elevates hepcidin levels in circulation, hence functional iron deficiency ensues; however, chronic intestinal bleeding results also in absolute iron deficiency. Consequently, negative regulators (erythroferrone, growth differentiation factor 15 (GDF-15), platelet-derived growth factor-BB (PDGF-BB) and/or hypoxia-inducible factors (HIFs)) of hepcidin expression dominate to enhance iron absorption from the gastrointestinal tract [42]. Anemia in IBD could arise from several factors that include intestinal blood loss, medications and reduced iron absorption that is also a consequence of reduced appetite during active flaring episodes of the disorder. Moreover, vitamin deficiencies such as those of folate and vitamin B12 are common due to decreased absorption from abnormal duodenum. Absolute iron deficiency caused by diminished absorption and depleted iron stores leads to anemia. Other extenuating consequences of pathological conditions promote acute-phase reactants and cytokines that impair erythroid differentiation and proliferation [43]. A retrospective cohort study, of patients diagnosed with Crohn's disease and ulcerative colitis during the period 1963–2010 was randomly selected from the population-based IBD cohort of Örebro University Hospital in Sweden and revealed a mean annual incidence rate of anemia as 15.9 per 100 person-years and a prevalence of 22.6%. Of this, anemia was 19.3 per 100 person-years and the prevalence was 28.7% in Crohn's compared with 12.9% and 16.5%, respectively, for ulcerative colitis [44]. In earlier reports, however, anemia incidence correlated with the disease activity rather than type, although anemia was higher in women [45]. Apart from the consequences of anemia, such as fatigue, headache, dizziness, shortness of breath, or tachycardia, anemia exerts a significant impact on the quality of life of IBD patients. Disease burden caused by abdominal pain or diarrhoea is compounded by persistently debilitating chronic fatigue that is due to anemia [46].

Conventional management and therapeutic approaches recommend anemia screening every 3 months for outpatients with active disease and 6 to 12 months for those in the mild or remission state [47,48]. The thresholds for diagnosis according to World Health Organization (WHO) guideline in adult males and non-pregnant women, stipulate haemoglobin (Hb) of <13.0 g/dL, <12.0 g/dL, and

<11.0 g/dL in pregnant women [48]. Specifically, to screen for anemia in IBD patients [49] TfS <20% and a serum ferritin concentration <30 g/L (with a serum CRP level within the normal range or a ferritin concentration of less than 100 g/L with an elevated serum CRP level) are specified. Recommendations for anemia management in IBD patient care are currently conflicting and remain, thereby, an ongoing process because of limited evidence from human studies. However, recommendations for oral iron therapy should be limited to IBD patients with mild anemia and with due considerations given to doses, duration and the types of iron compounds used. This is with the objective to maximize efficiency and efficacy while minimizing side effects. In IBD patients with moderate to severe anemia, oral iron causes gastrointestinal disturbances and is refractory, then, intravenous (IV) iron is the preferred recommendation [50,51]. Inhibition of iron absorption by hepcidin-induced inflammation is by-passed by IV iron to replenish iron stores and replete Hb levels in the patients. ESA, in combination with IV, is prescribed for FID in IBD patients and blood transfusion is an option as an acute measure only in critically anemic patients [50]. Iron therapy and treatment of the other symptoms of IBD will culminate in the reduction of disease burden to improve the quality of life of the patients.

8. Anemia of Rheumatoid Arthritis (RA)

Patients with rheumatoid arthritis (RA) may display IDA and anemia of chronic disease (ACD). IDA could be due to gastrointestinal bleeding, gynaecological blood loss, or urinary bleeding or chemotherapy-induced [51]. As inflammation is a chronic condition in RA, FID is common. ACD in RA arises from several factors, including ineffective erythropoiesis inflammatory markers (e.g., IL-6 and TNF-α), and disordered iron metabolism. Functional iron deficiency in ACD can be due to overexpression of iron-regulatory hormone, hepcidin, leading to sequestration into storage sites from circulation, resulting in hypoferrinemia and iron-restricted erythropoiesis. Although decreased serum hepcidin levels were reported to correlate with the reduction of disease activity [52], this observation was not evident in other studies [53,54]. Hepcidin could be suppressed, independently of inflammation. Therefore, the use of hepcidin as a diagnostic tool in the routine clinical management of this disease still requires further investigation. Prevalence of anemia in RA has been reported to range from 64–70%, while ACD was observed in 50–60% of patients [55,56]. RA patients have been reported to have both physical disability and increased mortality [57,58]. Relief in swollen, painful, tender joints, pain, muscle strength, and energy levels symptoms has been reported because of the resolution of anemia in RA patients [58].

Since anemia in RA is multifactorial and often associated with other malignancies, it is important to diagnose the nature and the types of anemia in order to apply the most appropriate treatment regimen. The safety and the use of EPO in the treatment of ACD in RA are controversial [59]. However, regarding the vital role of IL-6 in ACD, a recent study reported a significant increase in Hb and Hct levels after IL-6 receptor inhibitor tocilizumab (TCZ) therapy in anemic and non-anemic patients with rheumatoid arthritis, compared with other biologic and non-biologic disease-modifying antirheumatic drugs (DMARDs) [60].

9. Anemia of Chronic Kidney Disease

Chronic kidney disease (CKD) is a condition in which renal function deteriorates over time as the glomerular filtration rate (GFR) declines progressively. Anemia in CKD is of clinical concern as it predisposes patients to cardiovascular disease, and is associated with poor quality of life, increased hospitalizations, impaired cognition and mortality [61]. Anemia is a consequence of chronic kidney disease (CKD), principally because of the depreciation of and reduced synthesis of erythropoietin. Hence Glomerular Filtration Rate (GFR) is a predictor of anemia in patients with CKD [62]. The progression of anemia leads to several debilitating symptoms, such as lethargy, muscle fatigue, and deterioration of renal function. These culminate ultimately in a high prevalence of cardiovascular diseases, such as left ventricular hypertrophy and heart failure, which account for a significant number of mortalities in patients with CKD [63,64]. However, the etiology of anemia in CKD is multifactorial. EPO is an anti-apoptotic hormone, produced by the kidneys, which promotes the survival, proliferation and differentiation of erythrocyte precursors [65,66]. As CKD progresses, renal mass declines, which reduces EPO production and EPO-deficiency results [66]. The expression of EPO is regulated by the transcription factor, HIF-2α. EPO is produced by peritubular interstitial fibroblasts in the renal cortex and outer medulla and not by the renal tubular epithelial cells or peritubular endothelial cells [67,68], as previously presumed. The regulation of EPO production is by HIF 2α and is modulated by oxygen pressure in the cells and tissues [69,70]. Ablation of HIF-2α, and not HIF-1α, was shown to cause anemia that was restored by recombinant EPO [71]. The regulation of erythropoietin by HIF-2α is also confirmed by increased erythropoietin levels and the ensuing erythrocytosis when the HIF-2α translation is de-repressed in iron regulatory protein 1 (IRP1) knockout mice [72–75]. Under normoxia, HIF-2α is hydroxylated by O_2-and iron-dependent HIF prolyl-4-hydroxylases (HIF-PHD) and targeted for proteasomal degradation in a E3-ligase complex. However, under hypoxic conditions, HIF-2α is stabilized and is no longer degraded but translocated to the nucleus where it forms a heterodimer with HIF-β or the aryl hydrocarbon receptor nuclear translocator (ARNT). HIF-2α/β heterodimers, together with transcriptional coactivators, such as CREB-binding protein (CBP) and p300, bind to consensus elements in the 5' or 3' regions of the gene for the kidney or liver, respectively, to initiate and increase EPO transcription. Factors such as iron chelators, nitric oxide, ROS or $CoCl_2$ inhibit HIF-PHDs association (increased HIF-2α), which culminates to increase EPO transcription and production [72]. Conversely, excess iron was shown to decrease levels of HIF 2α and EPO expression in an erythropoietin-deficient mouse model [76]. Furthermore, kynurenine, a product of L-tryptophan catabolism is increased in anemia of inflammation and in CKD [77]. Kynurenine activates ARNT and competes with HIF-2α to prevent its binding to HIF-β, thereby decreasing EPO production. Similarly, in CKD, a uremic toxin, indoxyl-sulfate, apart from simulating hepcidin expression [78], may also activate ARNT to suppress EPO production [79]. Consequently, an elevated hepcidin level is caused by a medley of interacting factors, such as inflammation, excess iron, decreased EPO/erythropoiesis or metabolites or products of certain processes or pathways of systemic metabolism (Figure 1). The mechanisms by which each player directly influences EPO production are still not yet clearly defined.

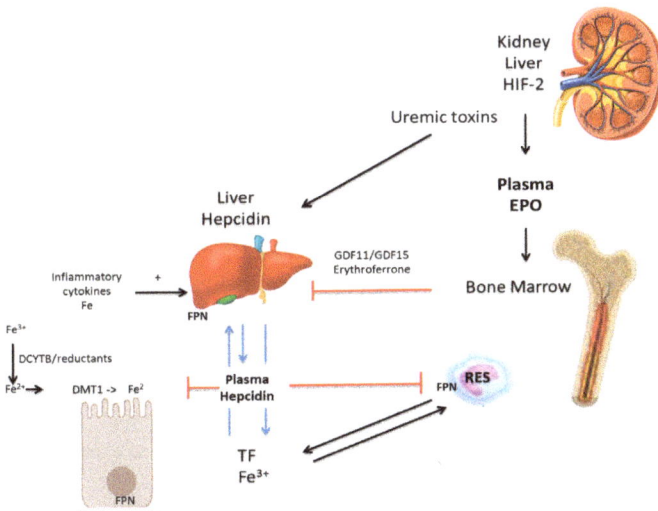

Figure 1. Iron metabolism and the mechanisms of renal anemia. In the enterocyte, duodenal cytochrome b (DCYTB) and other dietary reducing agents reduce ferric iron (Fe^{3+}) to its ferrous (Fe^{2+}) state, via the divalent metal transporter 1 (DMT1). Iron efflux into the circulation occurs via hepcidin-regulated

ferroportin (FPN). In blood, iron is transported bound to transferrin (TF) to the liver, cells of the reticulo-endothelial system (RES) and to other tissues and organs. Inflammatory cytokines suppress erythropoiesis in the bone marrow and stimulate hepcidin production in the liver, which influences iron absorption and efflux negatively. Decreased GDF11/GDF15 or erythroferrone leads to increased hepcidin production. Uremic toxins enhance hepcidin expression and modulate the EPO level via Hif-2α, which also induces the transcription of DCYTB, DMT1, FPN, and TF [72].

In the advanced stages of CKD, regular hemodialysis contributes to absolute iron deficiency. Blood is lost during the hemodialysis process in the tubing and the apparatus and also, through the numerous blood samples taken from the patient [80,81]. Under normal physiological conditions, macrophages engulf senescent erythrocytes and recycle the iron incorporated in hemoglobin [82]. During such blood losses, this opportunity for iron recycling is lost [77,83]. After blood loss, in healthy individuals, EPO aids in the absorption of iron, but this is reduced in CKD patients as they suffer from EPO deficiency as their condition deteriorates. Therefore, in CKD, there is difficulty in replenishing iron stores and consequently, erythropoiesis is limited [84].

Hepcidin Expression and Function in CKD Patients

Iron availability is the rate-limiting step in the maturation of erythroblasts into erythrocytes [9]. EPO increases the synthesis of erythrocytes in the bone marrow and this leads to a depletion of iron stores and the reduced availability of iron contributes to anemia in CKD [66,85]. Replenishing these iron stores in CKD is also more difficult than in healthy subjects, thereby exacerbating the problem [86].

Furthermore, the reduced glomerular filtration rate in CKD results in impaired renal clearance of hepcidin. Dialysis reduces hepcidin level; however, this rapidly rises again in the interval between dialysis sessions [85]. Mobilization of iron from hepatocyte and reticuloendothelial stores is restricted, leading to absolute iron deficiency due to reduced intestinal absorption of iron [87]. This impairs erythropoiesis, which is iron-dependent and contributes to anemia. CKD patients have a greater predisposition to infection as long-term hemodialysis exposes the patients repeatedly to pathogens in the environment [88]. As previously discussed, this inflammatory state promotes increased hepcidin levels, which contributes to impaired iron absorption and mobilisation [89,90]. Hepcidin produces these effects by downregulating FPN function and iron efflux into the blood. [9,87,91].

Hepcidin expression is suppressed by erythropoiesis to meet iron demand to support the process and EPO has been reported to have a direct effect [16,89,92], possibly in conjunction with co-factors, such as twisted gastrulation protein homolog 1 (TWSG 1), growth differentiation factor 15 (GDF15), GDF11, and erythroferrone (ERFE). The functions of TWSG-, GDF11 and GDF15 in the inhibition of erythropoiesis are still controversial. However, erythroblasts synthesise ERFE upon stimulation by EPO and this inhibits the expression of the hepcidin gene [84,93], particularly under stress. As CKD progresses, reduced production of EPO results in dwindling erythrocyte production and consequently, decreased erythroferrone production. This, in turn, leads to increased hepcidin expression, which reduces iron absorption and decreases iron mobilisation from the stores [93,94]. Reduced iron levels limit erythrocyte maturation and exacerbate anemia of CKD even further.

The regulation of hepcidin induction at the cellular level and in the liver is both intricate and complex and involves membrane-bound iron sensors that include the transferrin receptors (TfR) 1 and 2, HFE, and hemojuvelin (HJV). The signal for hepcidin expression is initiated by bone morphogenic protein (BMP) ligands using the glycosylphosphatidylinositol-anchored membrane protein, HJV, as a coreceptor that binds to Type I and Type II BMP serine threonine kinase receptors. This induces a cascade of activation and phosphorylation of the receptors that channel downstream to Suppressor of Mothers Against Decapentaplegic (SMAD) proteins involved in signalling during hepcidin expression. A detailed description of the triggers that regulate the hepcidin expression process is reviewed elsewhere [14,18]. In summary, hepcidin expression is regulated by the BMP6-HJV-SMAD and IL-6-STAT3 signaling cascade. BMP6 binds the BMP receptors and HJV coreceptor, which causes the phosphorylation of SMAD1/5/8. Phosphorylated SMAD proteins associate with SMAD4 and these complexes traverse the nuclear membrane to bind to the promoter region of the hepcidin gene to induce hepcidin expression. The inflammatory stimulus, IL-6, binds the IL-6 receptor and activates Janus kinase 2 (JAK2), which phosphorylates Signal Transducer and Activator of Transcription 3 (STAT3). Phosphorylated STAT3 translocates into the hepatocyte nucleus to bind the STAT3 responsive element at the promoter region of the hepcidin gene to induce hepcidin expression.

10. Treatment of Anemia in CKD

To treat anemia in CKD, it is necessary to enhance the synthesis of erythrocytes, as well as ensure the maintenance of adequate levels of iron for hemoglobin formation [88,95]. The National Institute for Health and Care Excellence (NICE) recommends the use of either iron or erythropoiesis-stimulating agents, or both in combination, for the treatment of anemia of CKD [96]. This is aimed at addressing both absolute and functional iron deficiency that lead to restricted iron access and EPO deficiency [97]. As deficiency in EPO is a major contributory factor to anemia in CKD, recombinant human erythropoietin (rHuEPO), such as epoetin alpha and epoetin beta, are used in the treatment of anemia in CKD patients [98]. This initial therapy was brought into clinical practice in the 1980's and has been found to successfully treat the signs and symptoms of anemic CKD, such as fatigue, weakness and headaches [99]. In addition, these patients also required less frequent blood transfusions, a further benefit from the use of ESAs in anemic CKD [99]. However, large randomized control studies including the Normal Hematocrit Study (NHCT), the Correction of Haemoglobin and Outcomes in Renal Insufficiency (CHOIR) trial, the Cardiovascular Risk Reduction by Early Anemia Treatment (CREATE) trial and the Trial to Reduce Cardiovascular Events with Aranesp Therapy (TREAT), which highlighted the potential harm of high-dose ESA therapy, have challenged these therapeutic claims from utilising ESAs [100]. It has been emphasized that the complete correction of anemia, and indeed raising hemoglobin levels above 11 g/dL was associated with adverse outcomes. These include an increased risk of stroke, cardiovascular incidents, rapid malignant progression in cancer patients and increased mortality in other patients [61]. Moreover, pure red blood cell aplasia can be induced in rare instances through the use of ESAs, which, in turn, promotes severe anemia and results in the patient becoming transfusion-dependent [66]. It was proposed that these adverse outcomes were due to the very high doses of ESA that are administered [61]. Such high doses of ESA are often prescribed to patients that are hyporesponsive to ESA therapy to correct their hemoglobin deficits and higher doses are provided to attain target hemoglobin levels. The results from randomized controlled trials have subsequently influenced KDIGO guidelines, which recommend that non-dialyzed CKD patients are not administered ESA if haemoglobin levels are above 10 g/dL. CKD patients on dialysis should receive ESA therapy when hemoglobin levels lie between 9 g/dL and 10 g/dL. In all adult patients, ESA therapy should be used to maintain haemoglobin levels no higher than 11.5 g/dL [100].

Evidence from large randomized control studies highlighting the negative health effects of high-dose ESA administration was the reason for advocating the use of iron therapy as an adjunct to ESAs. Consequently, iron and lower doses of ESA are currently prescribed to preclude the adverse outcomes associated with high-dose ESA administration [66]. Moreover, as ESA therapy acts to increase erythropoiesis, this results in the depletion of the iron pool, causing a relative iron deficiency for which iron supplementation is recommended as a preventive measure [61]. Inflammation inhibits erythropoiesis, which influences erythropoietin (EPO) hyporesponsiveness [101] and decreases the systemic circulation of iron levels by the production of hepcidin [102,103]. Inflammation in CKD, apart from causing decreases in iron availability via elevated hepcidin levels, also directly aggravates anemia by suppressing EPO production [104]. Inflammation also decreases the enhancing effect of EPO on erythropoiesis [105].

11. Iron Supplementation for the Treatment of Anemia of CKD

CKD patients, as previously explained, suffer from increased blood loss and reduced intestinal absorption of dietary iron and thus, iron supplementation is important to prevent absolute iron deficiency. Iron supplementation may be administered through the oral or IV route, nevertheless, both routes have advantages and disadvantages.

Oral administration using ferrous sulphate is adequate for moderate anemia, and the advantages include its relative low cost [99]. However, the side effects include constipation, nausea and abdominal discomfort, as well as reduced patient compliance [98,106]. Additionally, intestinal iron absorption can be impaired in CKD and the efficacy of oral iron can be variable [99]. Incidentally, sucrosomial iron (SI), a newly developed oral iron preparation, in a randomized trial in CKD patients, has been shown to be comparable to IV iron gluconate in elevating hemoglobin levels [107]. The future of oral iron therapy may involve dietary supplementation with nanoparticles. Nanoparticulate tartrate-modified Fe (III) poly oxo-hydroxide (Nana Fe (III)) has also been shown to be absorbed by a DMT1-independent mechanism for replenishing hemoglobin levels in mice without the side effects associated with oral therapy [108]). The dosage of oral and IV iron in CKD patients are dependent on the presence or absence of inflammatory status of the gut. In Europe and USA, higher doses of IV iron have been used in dialysis patients because of higher inflammation status than in those of Japan. Low doses of IV iron or oral iron have been effective in the Japanese dialysis patients with the same efficacy because inflammation is minimal [109]. Although compared with Western countries, the Japanese guidelines for prescription of IV iron in dialysis patients are more conservative, the outcomes, nevertheless, are as good or better than their American counterparts [110]. Given the potential safety issues with aggressive IV iron treatment, and lack of well-powered studies to examine safety, a more conservative approach to iron therapy should be considered in the US [111].

Intravenous administration is highly efficient at replenishing iron stores, enhancing erythropoiesis and reducing the required ESA dose. This practice is advantageous as high doses of ESA therapy have been associated with negative clinical outcomes [112]. The pitfalls of IV therapy, however, include the invasive method of delivery and increased infection risk [99]. Results from studies of IV iron use and infection have highlighted conflicting results [113,114]. Data from observational, laboratory and animal studies have also indicated that IV iron treatment promotes oxidative stress, atherosclerotic plaque development, infection, hypersensitivity responses and increased cardiovascular mortality [113,115]. Studies involving apolipoprotein E (ApoE) knockout mice have highlighted that elevated iron does not cause atherosclerotic plaque progression, whereas other studies have shown that IV iron sucrose increases superoxide production and monocyte adhesion to the endothelium, instigating atherosclerotic plaque formation [116,117]. IV iron has been found to be effective for functional iron-deficiency anemia in CKD patients with high inflammation but had negative consequences on markers of oxidative stress that could have clinical implications [111]. Moreover, different preparations of IV iron carry different risks. Iron dextran carries a higher risk of adverse reactions, including type 1 hypersensitivity reactions, in comparison to iron sucrose, sodium ferric gluconate and ferric carboxymaltose [118,119]. The recommended adult doses of iron sucrose and sodium ferric gluconate carry lower risks in CKD [120,121]. The Ferumoxytol for Anemia of CKD Trial (FACT), a randomized, phase 4 study [122], reported comparable efficacy and safety of ferumoxytol and iron sucrose in patients with CKD undergoing hemodialysis. However, as clinical trials such as the ferinject assessment in patients with iron-deficiency anemia and non-dialysis-dependent chronic kidney disease (FIND-CKD) and a randomized trial to evaluate intravenous and oral iron in chronic kidney disease (REVOKE) were un-unanimous in their conclusions on IV iron safety, its use remains a subject of continuous debate [112,114]. However, the use of IV iron should be with caution since iron overload has been detected by MRI in hemodialysis patients with relatively low serum ferritin levels [123], suggesting that iron overload can occur in CKD patients receiving standard doses of IV iron. Thus, it was recommended that the dose of IV iron should be reduced to <250 mg/month to avoid iron overload in CKD patients [124]. Recommendations on iron management in CKD patient care are an 'ongoing process' because of limited research evidence.

The outcomes of several randomized controlled trials (RCTs) and observational studies are varied regarding the effectiveness and adverse effects of iron or ESA supplementation. Heterogeneity of confounders have been associated with the study design and can be due to the type, dosage, duration or route of iron administration, population size and the inherent variability within the baseline [125,126] hematological profile of patients.

12. Novel Therapies for the Treatment of Anemia of CKD

Although recent therapies offer benefits to most patients, some patients remain anemic and, therefore, there is a drive to develop novel therapies to address persistent anemic conditions (Table 2).

12.1. Targeting Hepcidin

High levels of hepcidin recorded in CKD patients act to impair absorption and mobilization of iron.

Furthermore, the chronic inflammation which manifests in CKD patients results in the production of pro-inflammatory cytokines including interleukin-6 (IL-6), which has been shown to stimulate the synthesis of hepcidin. Currently, inhibitors of hepcidin production are being investigated. The two main pathways involved in regulating hepcidin expression are the BMP6-HJV-SMAD and the IL-6-STAT3 signalling pathways. Studies have revealed the existence of a cross-talk between the two pathways. In vitro studies have shown that therapies which act to inhibit the BMP pathway by sequestering ligands for the BMP receptor or antagonizing the BMP receptor also inhibit hepcidin expression via the inflammatory IL-6-STAT3 signaling pathway. Inhibitors of this pathway currently being investigated include anti-IL-6 antibodies such as Tocilizumab and IL-6 monoclonal antibodies such as Sultuximab. The safety of using these drugs needs to be verified as sultuximab, despite causing an increase in hemoglobin levels, has been associated with increased infection risk [127]. Dorsomorphin is an inhibitor of the BMP type I serine threonine kinase receptors and targets HJV and IL-6 and thus also dampens down the inflammation-induced expression of hepcidin. However, Dorsomorphin is non-selective and also inhibits the action of AMP kinase. Nonetheless, this highlights the potential therapeutic benefit of developing BMP inhibitors that can have a dual action on both BMP- and IL-6-mediated hepcidin expression [128]. Other potential antagonists or suppressors of hepcidin expression include Atorvastatin, TNFα and TGFγ inhibitors. A 6-month administration of Atorvastatin to CKD patients in a randomized double-blind crossover study revealed a significant decrease in serum hepcidin [129]. This was concomitant with improved haematological parameters. Similarly, Sotatercept and Luspatercept are recombinant soluble activin type-II receptor-IgG-Fc fusion proteins that were reported to increase red blood cell numbers and hemoglobin levels in humans treated for renal anemia [119,130]. An anti-inflammatory Pentoxifylline (PTX)—a phosphodiesterase inhibitor of anti-TNF-alpha activity—has also been proposed as a potential therapy for different disorders, including anemia, and its use in CKD awaits further research [131].

12.2. Hepcidin-Ferroportin Axis

Currently under investigation are newer potential therapies that will target the hepcidin–ferroportin axis in the treatment of anemia in CKD. This axis can be targeted at various points. For example, direct hepcidin antagonists, such as hepcidin antibodies, are currently in clinical trials and are thought to inhibit the action of hepcidin. These antibodies have been shown to bind both human and monkey hepcidin and inhibit its action on ferroportin, and as such, enhance the absorption of dietary iron and promote its mobilization from iron stores for use in erythropoiesis [132]. An additional direct hepcidin antagonist currently under development is hepcidin RNA interference (RNAi), which is predicted to inhibit hepcidin gene expression, to promote FPN function and thereby elevate iron levels [133].

Some therapies are also exploring FPN stabilizers, which make FPN less sensitive to the action of hepcidin, thereby promoting elevated, optimal iron efflux into circulation. These stabilizers tend to reduce hepcidin expression and inhibit its action while preventing FPN degradation, which aid in the treatment of absolute iron deficiency in anemia of CKD. One example of such an FPN stabilizer is the anti-ferroportin monoclonal antibody, which prevents the interaction between hepcidin and FPN [128]. Two other monoclonal antibodies, LY3113593 and LY2928057, targeting BMP6 and ferroportin, respectively, tested in CKD patients resulted in an increase in haemoglobin and reduction in ferritin (compared to the placebo) [134]. Serum iron efflux increased through LY2928057 binding to ferroportin and blocking interactions with hepcidin. In the same vein, LY3113593 blocked BMP6 binding to its receptor to decrease hepcidin expression.

12.3. Targeting Hif1α Inhibitors

The stabilization of HIF via a prolyl hydroxylase inhibitor (HIFα-PHI) system is a novel approach that may also be an effective therapeutic target in the treatment of anemia of CKD as EPO deficiency contributes greatly to this condition. HIF1α regulates renal EPO production and erythropoiesis (described in Section 9). Thus, this approach involves manipulating a physiological regulatory process rather than the conventional EPO administration. Examples of HIF-PHIs that are in clinical trials include Vadustat, Daprodustat and Roxadustat [97,135–138]. Phase II clinical trials of HIF1α stabilizers have concluded the effectiveness and safety for short-term use [128,139]. More recently, a Phase II, randomized, double-blind, placebo-controlled, trial showed a dose-dependent increase in Hb compared to placebo in adult CKD patients with anemia after 6 weeks of Desidustat (ZYAN1) treatment [140]. Desidustat (ZYAN1) is an oral hypoxia-inducible factor prolyl hydroxylase inhibitor (HIF-PHI) that stimulates erythropoiesis. Another novel hypoxia-inducible factor prolyl hydroxylase inhibitor, Molidustat, has the potential to treat anemia of CKD by increasing erythropoietin production and improving iron availability particularly, in non-dialysis patients [141]. However, HIFs have roles in other biological pathways, including in the expression of vascular endothelial growth factor (VEGF), which is associated with retinal disease and cancer [142]. Consequently, the long-term safety of HIF-PHIs, and possibly Hif 2α, needs to be elucidated, in particular, for long-term therapy [143].

12.4. Other Compounds

An additional novel therapeutic strategy in the treatment of anemia in CKD is the development of engineered lipocalins called anticalins, which are able to bind small hydrophobic molecules such as hepcidin and thereby inhibit it from carrying out its function [144]. Anticalin PRS-080#22 has also been shown to sequester hepcidin in a Phase I clinical trial [145]. PRS-080#22 decreased hepcidin and increased serum iron and transferrin saturation in a dose-dependent manner. In mice and in patients with deep vein thrombosis (DVT), administration of the anticoagulant, heparin, caused decreased hepcidin levels and increased mobilization of iron from splenic stores, thereby increasing the circulating iron level [145].

Heparins have been shown to be inhibitors of hepcidin expression in vitro and in vivo [146]. They suppress hepcidin expression via the BMP6/SMAD pathway and are, therefore, promising for the treatment of anemia of CKD that is, in part, exacerbated by high hepcidin levels in the patients [147]. The mechanism by which heparin antagonizes the BMP/SMAD pathways awaits future clarification.

Vitamin D has also been found to reduce hepcidin gene transcription, lower serum levels by 50% in healthy individuals within 24 h, enhance erythropoiesis and reduce inflammation [135,148]. Moreover, in early-stage chronic kidney disease patients, vitamin D3 supplementation decreased hepcidin level after three months of administration [149]. However, the calcitriol form of vitamin D did not reduce serum hepcidin concentrations among individuals with mild to moderate CKD [150]. Similarly, in pregnant women, vitamin D3 supplementation did not influence hepcidin, ferritin, or inflammatory status, indicating no beneficial effect in alleviating iron depletion in the subjects [151]. Further studies are needed to confirm the long-term effect of vitamin D in CKD patients.

Potential New Therapy for Anemia of Chronic Disease in the Future

Recently, the bone-secreted hormone fibroblast growth factor (FGF23) inhibitor has been advocated for the treatment of anemia in CKD patients. FGF23, apart from its canonical functions in bone mineralization for the regulation of phosphate vitamin D homoeostasis exerts a pleiotropic role in iron metabolism in CKD patients [152]. Iron deficiency, inflammation and EPO have been shown to increase FGF23 protein levels and cleavage [153–155], resulting in an increase in the anemic condition in CKD. Conversely, studies have also shown that FGF23 may promote anemia, iron deficiency, and systemic inflammation, particularly in CKD [142,156]. Hence, inhibitors of FGF23 could be employed to stimulate erythropoiesis and treat anemia in CKD patients. Agoro and others [157] reversed anemia and iron deficiency in a mouse model of CKD by inhibiting and blocking the FGF23 signalling pathway with its peptide antagonist. The mice displayed increased erythropoiesis, serum and ferritin levels and reduced erythroid apoptosis and inflammation. Table 2 summarizes the potential novel therapies for anemia in CKD.

Table 2. Summary of potential therapies for anemia of chronic kidney disease (CKD).

Name	Mode of Action	Adverse Effects	References
Hepcidin antagonist, e.g., hepcidin antibodies RNA Interference Atorvastatin, Sotatercept Luspatercept	Inhibit hepcidin action Inhibit hepcidin expression and promote FPN function	Viral delivery system—risk of random genome integration. Unfavorable immunological responses	[121,122,132, 133,144,158]
Hepcidin binding proteins Lipocalin, e.g., Anticalin (PRS-080)	Inhibit hepcidin function	Non-specificity	[159]
Hepcidin production inhibitors BMP inhibitors, e.g., soluble HJV, Dorsomorphin, Anti-BMP6 monoclonal antibody	Inhibit hepcidin expression and the BMP6-HJV-SMAD pathway	Unknown	[134,160]
Anti- IL6 monoclonal antibody, e.g., Siltuximab	Inhibits IL-6 STAT3 signaling cascade	Unknown	[158]
Heparin	Decreases hepcidin levels Increases mobilisation of iron stores	Bleeding Thrombocytopenia Hyperkalaemia Alopecia Osteoporosis	[161]
Vitamin D	Decreases hepcidin gene transcription	In excess causes nausea, vomiting, depression, weakness, and confusion.	[148–150]
FPN stabilizers, e.g., anti-ferroportin monoclonal antibody	Increase ferroportin action	Unknown	[130,134]
HIF-PHDI, e.g., Roxadustat Daprodustat, Vadadustatt, Molidustat,	Increase endogenous EPO expression	Pulmonary hypertension Increase in VEGF Tumour progression	[97,98,134, 136,141]
Anticalin PRS-080#22	Decreases hepcidin levels Increases mobilisation of iron stores	Unknown	[144]
FGF23 inhibitor	Stimulates and promotes erythropoeisis	Unknown	[153,157]

13. Conclusions

Is anemia a symptom, disorder or disease? Iron deficiency occurs insidiously as a symptom or syndrome over a spectrum of severity, with low hemoglobin as a later manifestation of extreme deficiency [11]. Absolute anemia, that manifests after the depletion of iron stores, is a clinical disease condition. However, functional iron-deficiency anemia is a risk factor for several ailments, disorders and diseases. In general, the etiology of anemia is multifactorial and this necessitates diverse therapeutic guidelines in the management of the syndrome. Hence, there are variations in guidelines specifications or consensus statements for the therapy of different stages of iron deficiency and anemia in different disorders. When dietary iron sources are limiting, iron formulations are prescribed as oral supplements. Parenteral or intravenous iron therapy becomes the choice of therapy for iron-deficiency anemia for these patients intolerant or refractory to oral iron administration. However, recommendations to start therapy vary with different conditions. For example, for IBS, CKD or anemia of heart failure, the recommendation to commence therapy is based on a wide range of serum ferritin levels (30–299 ng/mL) and when transferrin saturation is below 20%. A key regulator of iron homeostasis is hepcidin, which contributes to anemia by reducing the absorption of iron from the diet, as well as through diminishing the mobilization of iron from iron stores. One of such anemia is that associated with CKD, which manifests absolute iron deficiency and iron-restricted functional anemia and impaired erythropoiesis. Current therapy is successful in some patients in alleviating the signs and symptoms of anemia such as weakness, headache, vertigo and fatigue; however, despite current intervention, the disorder remains endemic in patients. The current review describes several novel therapies to tackle this devastating condition and correct elevated hepcidin levels in CKD patients not responding to current interventions. However, the efficacy, tolerability and side effect profiles of these novel therapies in CKD patients have not been fully elucidated. It is encouraging that studies are on-going on some of these novel therapeutic approaches that can be translated into clinical applications.

Author Contributions: S.B. and G.O.L.-D. wrote the review." Authorship must be limited to those who have contributed substantially to the work reported.

Funding: This research received no external funding.

Conflicts of Interest: The authors declare no conflict of interest.

Abbreviations

ID	iron deficiency	IDA	Iron-deficiency anaemia
GBD	Global Burden of Disease	CKD	chronic kidney disease
ACD	Anemia of Chronic Disease	IBD	inflammatory bowel disease
IV	intravenous	EPO	erythropoietin
ESA	erythropoietin stimulating agent	rHuEPO	recombinant human erythropoietin
FPN	ferroportin	DMT1	divalent metal transporter
Dcytb	duodenal cytochrome b	MCV	mean corpuscular volume
Hb	haemoglobin	BMP	bone morphogenic protein
HJV	hemojuvelin	SMAD	Mothers Against Decapentaplegic
JAK2	Janus kinase 2	STAT 3	Signal transducer and activator of transcription 3
GDF 15	growth differentiation factor 15	PDGF-BB	platelet-derived growth factor-BB
HIF	hypoxia-inducible factor	VEGF	vascular endothelial growth factor
IL	Interleukin	FCF23	fibroblast growth factor
KDIGO	Kidney Disease: Improving Global Outcomes	CHOIR	Correction of Haemoglobin and Outcomes in Renal Insufficiency
CREATE	Cardiovascular Risk Reduction by Early Anemia Treatment	TREAT	Trial to Reduce Cardiovascular Events with Aranesp
HIF-PHDI	Hypoxia-Inducible factor Prolyl Hydroxylase Inhibitor		

References

1. Kohgo, Y.; Ikuta, K.; Ohtake, T.; Torimoto, Y.; Kato, J. Body iron metabolism and pathophysiology of iron overload. *Int. J. Hematol.* **2008**, *88*, 7–15. [CrossRef] [PubMed]
2. Camaschella, C. New insights into iron deficiency and iron deficiency anemia. *Blood Rev.* **2017**, *31*, 225–233. [CrossRef] [PubMed]
3. GBD 2016. Disease and Injury Incidence and Prevalence Collaborators. Global, regional, and national incidence, prevalence, and years lived with disability for 328 diseases and injuries for 195 countries, 1990–2016: a systematic analysis for the Global Burden of Disease Study 2016. *Lancet* **2017**, *390*, 1211–1259.
4. Kassebaum, N.J.; Jasrasaria, R.; Naghavi, M.; Wulf, S.K.; Johns, N.; Lozano, R.; Regan, M.; Weatherall, D.; Chou, D.P.; Eisele, T.P.; et al. A systematic analysis of global anemia burden from 1990 to 2010. *Blood* **2014**, *123*, 615–624. [CrossRef] [PubMed]
5. Camaschella, C. Iron deficiency. *Blood* **2019**, *133*, 30–39. [CrossRef] [PubMed]
6. Munoz, P.; Humeres, A. Iron deficiency on neuronal function. *Biometals: Int. J. Role Met. Ions Biol. Biochem. Med.* **2012**, *25*, 825–835. [CrossRef]
7. Achebe, M.M.; Gafter-Gvili, A. How I treat anemia in pregnancy: Iron, cobalamin, and folate. *Blood* **2017**, *129*, 940–949. [CrossRef]
8. Koshy, S.M.; Geary, D.F. Anemia in children with chronic kidney disease. *Pediatric Nephrol.* **2008**, *23*, 209–219. [CrossRef]
9. Goodnough, L.T.; Nemeth, E.; Ganz, T. Detection, evaluation, and management of iron-restricted erythropoiesis. *Blood* **2010**, *116*, 4754–4761. [CrossRef]
10. Moreno Chulilla, J.A.; Romero Colas, M.S.; Gutierrez Martin, M. Classification of anemia for gastroenterologists. *World J. Gastroenterol.* **2009**, *15*, 4627–4637. [CrossRef]
11. Camaschella, C. Iron-deficiency anemia. *N. Eng. J. Med.* **2015**, *372*, 1832–1843. [CrossRef] [PubMed]
12. Cappellini, M.D.; Comin-Colet, J.; de Francisco, A.; Dignass, A.; Doehner, W.; Lam, C.S.; Macdougall, I.C.; Rogler, G.; Camaschella, C.; Kadir, R.; et al. Iron deficiency across chronic inflammatory conditions: International expert opinion on definition, diagnosis, and management. *Am. J. Hematol.* **2017**, *92*, 1068–1078. [CrossRef] [PubMed]
13. Latunde-Dada, G.O. Iron metabolism: Microbes, mouse, and man. *BioEssays* **2009**, *31*, 1309–1317. [CrossRef] [PubMed]
14. Huang, H.; Constante, M.; Layoun, A.; Santos, M.M. Contribution of STAT3 and SMAD4 pathways to the regulation of hepcidin by opposing stimuli. *Blood* **2009**, *113*, 3593–3599. [CrossRef] [PubMed]
15. Karafin, M.S.; Koch, K.L.; Rankin, A.B.; Nischik, D.; Rahhal, G.; Simpson, P.; Field, J.J. Erythropoietic drive is the strongest predictor of hepcidin level in adults with sickle cell disease. *Blood Cells Mol. Dis.* **2015**, *55*, 304–307. [CrossRef] [PubMed]
16. Nicolas, G.; Chauvet, C.; Viatte, L.; Danan, J.L.; Bigard, X.; Devaux, I.; Beaumont, C.; Kahn, A.; Vaulont, S. The gene encoding the iron regulatory peptide hepcidin is regulated by anemia, hypoxia, and inflammation. *J. Clin. Investig.* **2002**, *110*, 1037–1044. [CrossRef] [PubMed]
17. Weiss, G.; Ganz, T.; Goodnough, L.T. Anemia of inflammation. *Blood* **2019**, *133*, 40–50. [CrossRef] [PubMed]
18. Aapro, M.; Osterborg, A.; Gascon, P.; Ludwig, H.; Beguin, Y. Prevalence and management of cancer-related anaemia, iron deficiency and the specific role of i.v. iron. *Ann. Oncol.* **2012**, *23*, 1954–1962. [CrossRef] [PubMed]
19. Steegmann, J.L.; Sanchez Torres, J.M.; Colomer, R.; Vaz, A.; Lopez, J.; Jalon, I.; Provencio, M.; Gonzalez-Martin, A.; Perez, M. Prevalence and management of anaemia in patients with non-myeloid cancer undergoing systemic therapy: A Spanish survey. *Clin. Transl. Oncol.* **2013**, *15*, 477–483. [CrossRef]
20. Ludwig, H.; Muldur, E.; Endler, G.; Hubl, W. Prevalence of iron deficiency across different tumors and its association with poor performance status, disease status and anemia. *Ann. Oncol.* **2013**, *24*, 1886–1892. [CrossRef]
21. Ludwig, H.; Aapro, M.; Bokemeyer, C.; Glaspy, J.; Hedenus, M.; Littlewood, T.J.; Osterborg, A.; Rzychon, B.; Mitchell, D.; Beguin, Y. A European patient record study on diagnosis and treatment of chemotherapy-induced anaemia. *Support. Care Cancer* **2014**, *22*, 2197–2206. [CrossRef] [PubMed]

22. Ludwig, H.; Van Belle, S.; Barrett-Lee, P.; Birgegard, G.; Bokemeyer, C.; Gascon, P.; Kosmidis, P.; Krzakowski, M.; Nortier, J.; Olmi, P.; et al. The European Cancer Anaemia Survey (ECAS): A large, multinational, prospective survey defining the prevalence, incidence, and treatment of anaemia in cancer patients. *Eur. J. Cancer* **2004**, *40*, 2293–2306. [CrossRef] [PubMed]
23. Rodgers, G.M.; Gilreath, J.A. The Role of Intravenous Iron in the Treatment of Anemia Associated with Cancer and Chemotherapy. *Acta Haematol.* **2019**, *142*, 13–20. [CrossRef] [PubMed]
24. Felker, G.M.; Adams, K.F., Jr.; Gattis, W.A.; O'Connor, C.M. Anemia as a risk factor and therapeutic target in heart failure. *J. Am. Coll. Cardiol.* **2004**, *44*, 959–966. [CrossRef] [PubMed]
25. Hubert, M.; Gaudriot, B.; Biedermann, S.; Gouezec, H.; Sylvestre, E.; Bouzille, G.; Verhoye, J.P.; Flecher, E.; Ecoffey, C. Impact of Preoperative Iron Deficiency on Blood Transfusion in Elective Cardiac Surgery. *J. Cardiothorac. Vasc. Anesth.* **2019**, *33*, 2141–2150. [CrossRef] [PubMed]
26. Jankowska, E.A.; von Haehling, S.; Anker, S.D.; Macdougall, I.C.; Ponikowski, P. Iron deficiency and heart failure: Diagnostic dilemmas and therapeutic perspectives. *Eur. Heart J.* **2013**, *34*, 816–829. [CrossRef] [PubMed]
27. Yeo, T.J.; Yeo, P.S.; Ching-Chiew Wong, R.; Ong, H.Y.; Leong, K.T.; Jaufeerally, F.; Sim, D.; Santhanakrishnan, R.; Lim, S.L.; Chan, M.M.; et al. Iron deficiency in a multi-ethnic Asian population with and without heart failure: Prevalence, clinical correlates, functional significance and prognosis. *Eur. J. Heart Fail.* **2014**, *16*, 1125–1132. [CrossRef]
28. Tkaczyszyn, M.; Comin-Colet, J.; Voors, A.A.; van Veldhuisen, D.J.; Enjuanes, C.; Moliner-Borja, P.; Rozentryt, P.; Polonski, L.; Banasiak, W.; Ponikowski, P.; et al. Iron deficiency and red cell indices in patients with heart failure. *Eur. J. Heart Fail.* **2018**, *20*, 114–122. [CrossRef]
29. Ponikowski, P.; Voors, A.A.; Anker, S.D.; Bueno, H.; Cleland, J.G.F.; Coats, A.J.S.; Falk, V.; Gonzalez-Juanatey, J.R.; Harjola, V.P.; Jankowska, E.A.; et al. 2016 ESC Guidelines for the diagnosis and treatment of acute and chronic heart failure: The Task Force for the diagnosis and treatment of acute and chronic heart failure of the European Society of Cardiology (ESC) Developed with the special contribution of the Heart Failure Association (HFA) of the ESC. *Eur. Heart J.* **2016**, *37*, 2129–2200. [CrossRef]
30. Van Aelst, L.N.L.; Abraham, M.; Sadoune, M.; Lefebvre, T.; Manivet, P.; Logeart, D.; Launay, J.M.; Karim, Z.; Puy, H.; Cohen-Solal, A. Iron status and inflammatory biomarkers in patients with acutely decompensated heart failure: Early in-hospital phase and 30-day follow-up. *Eur. J. Heart Fail.* **2017**, *19*, 1075–1076. [CrossRef]
31. Eleftheriadis, T.; Pissas, G.; Remoundou, M.; Filippidis, G.; Antoniadi, G.; Oustampasidou, N.; Liakopoulos, V.; Stefanidis, I. Ferroportin in monocytes of hemodialysis patients and its associations with hepcidin, inflammation, markers of iron status and resistance to erythropoietin. *Int. Urol. Nephrol.* **2014**, *46*, 161–167. [CrossRef] [PubMed]
32. Tessitore, N.; Girelli, D.; Campostrini, N.; Bedogna, V.; Pietro Solero, G.; Castagna, A.; Melilli, E.; Mantovani, W.; De Matteis, G.; Olivieri, O.; et al. Hepcidin is not useful as a biomarker for iron needs in haemodialysis patients on maintenance erythropoiesis-stimulating agents. *Nephrol. Dial. Transplant.* **2010**, *25*, 3996–4002. [CrossRef] [PubMed]
33. Musallam, K.M.; Tamim, H.M.; Richards, T.; Spahn, D.R.; Rosendaal, F.R.; Habbal, A.; Khreiss, M.; Dahdaleh, F.S.; Khavandi, K.; Sfeir, P.M.; et al. Preoperative anaemia and postoperative outcomes in non-cardiac surgery: A retrospective cohort study. *Lancet* **2011**, *378*, 1396–1407. [CrossRef]
34. Enko, D.; Wallner, F.; von-Goedecke, A.; Hirschmugl, C.; Auersperg, V.; Halwachs-Baumann, G. The impact of an algorithm-guided management of preoperative anemia in perioperative hemoglobin level and transfusion of major orthopedic surgery patients. *Anemia* **2013**, *2013*, 641876. [CrossRef] [PubMed]
35. Munoz, M.; Acheson, A.G.; Bisbe, E.; Butcher, A.; Gomez-Ramirez, S.; Khalafallah, A.A.; Kehlet, H.; Kietaibl, S.; Liumbruno, G.M.; Meybohm, P.; et al. An international consensus statement on the management of postoperative anaemia after major surgical procedures. *Anaesthesia* **2018**, *73*, 1418–1431. [CrossRef] [PubMed]
36. Butcher, A.; Richards, T. Cornerstones of patient blood management in surgery. *Transfus. Med.* **2018**, *28*, 150–157. [CrossRef]
37. Munoz, M.; Laso-Morales, M.J.; Gomez-Ramirez, S.; Cadellas, M.; Nunez-Matas, M.J.; Garcia-Erce, J.A. Pre-operative haemoglobin levels and iron status in a large multicentre cohort of patients undergoing major elective surgery. *Anaesthesia* **2017**, *72*, 826–834. [CrossRef] [PubMed]

38. Gomez-Ramirez, S.; Bisbe, E.; Shander, A.; Spahn, D.R.; Munoz, M. Management of Perioperative Iron Deficiency Anemia. *Acta Haematol.* **2019**, *142*, 21–29. [CrossRef]
39. Zhou, X.; Xu, Z.; Wang, Y.; Sun, L.; Zhou, W.; Liu, X. Association between storage age of transfused red blood cells and clinical outcomes in critically ill adults: A meta-analysis of randomized controlled trials. *Med. Intensiva* **2018**. [CrossRef]
40. Carson, J.L.; Guyatt, G.; Heddle, N.M.; Grossman, B.J.; Cohn, C.S.; Fung, M.K.; Gernsheimer, T.; Holcomb, J.B.; Kaplan, L.J.; Katz, L.M.; et al. Clinical Practice Guidelines From the AABB: Red Blood Cell Transfusion Thresholds and Storage. *JAMA* **2016**, *316*, 2025–2035. [CrossRef]
41. Lasocki, S.; Krauspe, R.; von Heymann, C.; Mezzacasa, A.; Chainey, S.; Spahn, D.R. PREPARE: The prevalence of perioperative anaemia and need for patient blood management in elective orthopaedic surgery: A multicentre, observational study. *Eur. J. Anaesthesiol.* **2015**, *32*, 160–167. [CrossRef] [PubMed]
42. Nielsen, O.H.; Soendergaard, C.; Vikner, M.E.; Weiss, G. Rational Management of Iron-Deficiency Anaemia in Inflammatory Bowel Disease. *Nutrients* **2018**, *10*. [CrossRef] [PubMed]
43. Goldberg, N.D. Iron deficiency anemia in patients with inflammatory bowel disease. *Clin. Exp. Gastroenterol.* **2013**, *6*, 61–70. [CrossRef] [PubMed]
44. Eriksson, C.; Henriksson, I.; Brus, O.; Zhulina, Y.; Nyhlin, N.; Tysk, C.; Montgomery, S.; Halfvarson, J. Incidence, prevalence and clinical outcome of anaemia in inflammatory bowel disease: A population-based cohort study. *Aliment. Pharmacol. Ther.* **2018**, *48*, 638–645. [CrossRef] [PubMed]
45. Portela, F.; Lago, P.; Cotter, J.; Goncalves, R.; Vasconcelos, H.; Ministro, P.; Lopes, S.; Eusebio, M.; Morna, H.; Cravo, M.; et al. Anaemia in Patients with Inflammatory Bowel Disease—A Nationwide Cross-Sectional Study. *Digestion* **2016**, *93*, 214–220. [CrossRef]
46. Mitchell, A.; Guyatt, G.; Singer, J.; Irvine, E.J.; Goodacre, R.; Tompkins, C.; Williams, N.; Wagner, F. Quality of life in patients with inflammatory bowel disease. *J. Clin. Gastroenterol.* **1988**, *10*, 306–310. [CrossRef] [PubMed]
47. World Health Organization, Centers for Disease Control and Prevention. *Assessing the Iron Status of Populations*, 2nd ed.; WHO: Geneva, Switzerland, 2007.
48. Beutler, E.; Waalen, J. The definition of anemia: What is the lower limit of normal of the blood hemoglobin concentration? *Blood* **2006**, *107*, 1747–1750. [CrossRef]
49. Nielsen, O.H.; Ainsworth, M.; Coskun, M.; Weiss, G. Management of Iron-Deficiency Anemia in Inflammatory Bowel Disease: A Systematic Review. *Medicine* **2015**, *94*, e963. [CrossRef]
50. Dignass, A.U.; Gasche, C.; Bettenworth, D.; Birgegard, G.; Danese, S.; Gisbert, J.P.; Gomollon, F.; Iqbal, T.; Katsanos, K.; Koutroubakis, I.; et al. European consensus on the diagnosis and management of iron deficiency and anaemia in inflammatory bowel diseases. *J. Crohn's Colitis* **2015**, *9*, 211–222. [CrossRef]
51. Basak, T.B.; Talukder, S.I. Anemia of chronic disease in rheumatoid arthritis and its relationship with disease activities. *Dinajpur. Med. Col.* **2013**, *6*, 113–122.
52. Demirag, M.D.; Haznedaroglu, S.; Sancak, B.; Konca, C.; Gulbahar, O.; Ozturk, M.A.; Goker, B. Circulating hepcidin in the crossroads of anemia and inflammation associated with rheumatoid arthritis. *Intern. Med.* **2009**, *48*, 421–426. [CrossRef] [PubMed]
53. Ostgard, R.D.; Glerup, H.; Jurik, A.G.; Kragstrup, T.W.; Stengaard-Pedersen, K.; Hetland, M.L.; Horslev-Petersen, K.; Junker, P.; Deleuran, B.W. Hepcidin plasma levels are not associated with changes in haemoglobin in early rheumatoid arthritis patients. *Scand. J. Rheumatol.* **2017**, *46*, 441–445. [CrossRef] [PubMed]
54. Sahebari, M.; Rezaieyazdi, Z.; Hashemy, S.I.; Khorasani, S.; Shahgordi, S.; Alizadeh, M.K.; Ghaeni, A.; Khodashahi, M. Serum hepcidin level and rheumatoid arthritis disease activity. *Eur. J. Rheumatol.* **2018**, *6*, 76–80. [CrossRef] [PubMed]
55. Sabău, A.; Crăciun, A.M.; Gabriela, C.; Bolosiu, H.D.; Rednic, S.; Damian, L.; Siao-pin, S.; Florin, A.A.; Sabau, E. Association between acute phase reactant levels, and disease activity score (DAS28), in patients with rheumatoid arthritis and anemia. Revista Română de Rheumatologie. *Rom. J. Rheumatol.* **2011**, *20*, 225–229.
56. Khalaf, W.; Al-Rubaie, H.A.; Shihab, S. Studying anemia of chronic disease and iron deficiency in patients with rheumatoid arthritis by iron status and circulating hepcidin. *Hematol. Rep.* **2019**, *11*, 7708. [CrossRef] [PubMed]

57. Cojocaru, M.; Cojocaru, I.M.; Silosi, I.; Vrabie, C.D.; Tanasescu, R. Extra-articular Manifestations in Rheumatoid Arthritis. *Maedica* **2010**, *5*, 286–291. [PubMed]
58. Wilson, A.; Yu, H.T.; Goodnough, L.T.; Nissenson, A.R. Prevalence and outcomes of anemia in rheumatoid arthritis: A systematic review of the literature. *Am. J. Med.* **2004**, *116* (Suppl. 7A), 50s–57s. [CrossRef]
59. Marti-Carvajal, A.J.; Agreda-Perez, L.H.; Sola, I.; Simancas-Racines, D. Erythropoiesis-stimulating agents for anemia in rheumatoid arthritis. *Cochrane Database Syst. Rev.* **2013**. [CrossRef] [PubMed]
60. Paul, S.K.; Montvida, O.; Best, J.H.; Gale, S.; Pethoe-Schramm, A.; Sarsour, K. Effectiveness of biologic and non-biologic antirheumatic drugs on anaemia markers in 153,788 patients with rheumatoid arthritis: New evidence from real-world data. *Semin. Arthritis Rheum.* **2018**, *47*, 478–484. [CrossRef] [PubMed]
61. Babitt, J.L.; Lin, H.Y. Mechanisms of anemia in CKD. *J. Am. Soc. Nephrol.* **2012**, *23*, 1631–1634. [CrossRef]
62. Estrella, M.M.; Astor, B.C.; Kottgen, A.; Selvin, E.; Coresh, J.; Parekh, R.S. Prevalence of kidney disease in anaemia differs by GFR-estimating method: The Third National Health and Nutrition Examination Survey (1988-94). *Nephrol. Dial. Transplant.* **2010**, *25*, 2542–2548. [CrossRef] [PubMed]
63. Macdougall, I.C. Anemia of chronic kidney disease. *Medicine* **2007**, *35*, 457–460. [CrossRef]
64. Vera-Aviles, M.; Vantana, E.; Kardinasari, E.; Koh, N.L.; Latunde-Dada, G.O. Protective Role of Histidine Supplementation Against Oxidative Stress Damage in the Management of Anemia of Chronic Kidney Disease. *Pharmaceutical* **2018**, *11*. [CrossRef] [PubMed]
65. Jelkmann, W. Regulation of erythropoietin production. *J. Physiol.* **2011**, *589*, 1251–1258. [CrossRef] [PubMed]
66. Atkinson, M.A.; Warady, B.A. Anemia in chronic kidney disease. *Pediatric Nephrol.* **2018**, *33*, 227–238. [CrossRef] [PubMed]
67. Maxwell, P.H.; Osmond, M.K.; Pugh, C.W.; Heryet, A.; Nicholls, L.G.; Tan, C.C.; Doe, B.G.; Ferguson, D.J.; Johnson, M.H.; Ratcliffe, P.J. Identification of the renal erythropoietin-producing cells using transgenic mice. *Kidney Int.* **1993**, *44*, 1149–1162. [CrossRef] [PubMed]
68. Paliege, A.; Rosenberger, C.; Bondke, A.; Sciesielski, L.; Shina, A.; Heyman, S.N.; Flippin, L.A.; Arend, M.; Klaus, S.J.; Bachmann, S. Hypoxia-inducible factor-2alpha-expressing interstitial fibroblasts are the only renal cells that express erythropoietin under hypoxia-inducible factor stabilization. *Kidney Int.* **2010**, *77*, 312–318. [CrossRef] [PubMed]
69. Rankin, E.B.; Biju, M.P.; Liu, Q.; Unger, T.L.; Rha, J.; Johnson, R.S.; Simon, M.C.; Keith, B.; Haase, V.H. Hypoxia-inducible factor-2 (HIF-2) regulates hepatic erythropoietin in vivo. *J. Clin. Investig.* **2007**, *117*, 1068–1077. [CrossRef] [PubMed]
70. Rosenberger, C.; Mandriota, S.; Jurgensen, J.S.; Wiesener, M.S.; Horstrup, J.H.; Frei, U.; Ratcliffe, P.J.; Maxwell, P.H.; Bachmann, S.; Eckardt, K.U. Expression of hypoxia-inducible factor-1alpha and -2alpha in hypoxic and ischemic rat kidneys. *J. Am. Soc. Nephrol.* **2002**, *13*, 1721–1732. [CrossRef]
71. Gruber, M.; Hu, C.J.; Johnson, R.S.; Brown, E.J.; Keith, B.; Simon, M.C. Acute postnatal ablation of Hif-2alpha results in anemia. *Proc. Natl. Acad. Sci. USA* **2007**, *104*, 2301–2306. [CrossRef]
72. Haase, V.H. Regulation of erythropoiesis by hypoxia-inducible factors. *Blood Rev.* **2013**, *27*, 41–53. [CrossRef] [PubMed]
73. Ghosh, M.C.; Zhang, D.L.; Jeong, S.Y.; Kovtunovych, G.; Ollivierre-Wilson, H.; Noguchi, A.; Tu, T.; Senecal, T.; Robinson, G.; Crooks, D.R.; et al. Deletion of iron regulatory protein 1 causes polycythemia and pulmonary hypertension in mice through translational derepression of HIF2alpha. *Cell Metab.* **2013**, *17*, 271–281. [CrossRef] [PubMed]
74. Anderson, S.A.; Nizzi, C.P.; Chang, Y.I.; Deck, K.M.; Schmidt, P.J.; Galy, B.; Damnernsawad, A.; Broman, A.T.; Kendziorski, C.; Hentze, M.W.; et al. The IRP1-HIF-2alpha axis coordinates iron and oxygen sensing with erythropoiesis and iron absorption. *Cell Metab.* **2013**, *17*, 282–290. [CrossRef] [PubMed]
75. Zimmer, M.; Ebert, B.L.; Neil, C.; Brenner, K.; Papaioannou, I.; Melas, A.; Tolliday, N.; Lamb, J.; Pantopoulos, K.; Golub, T.; et al. Small-molecule inhibitors of HIF-2a translation link its 5′UTR iron-responsive element to oxygen sensing. *Mol. Cell* **2008**, *32*, 838–848. [CrossRef] [PubMed]
76. Suzuki, T.; Abe, T. Crossroads of metabolism and CKD. *Kidney Int.* **2018**, *94*, 242–243. [CrossRef] [PubMed]
77. Eleftheriadis, T.; Pissas, G.; Antoniadi, G.; Liakopoulos, V.; Stefanidis, I. Kynurenine, by activating aryl hydrocarbon receptor, decreases erythropoietin and increases hepcidin production in HepG2 cells: A new mechanism for anemia of inflammation. *Exp. Hematol.* **2016**, *44*, 60–67. [CrossRef] [PubMed]

78. Hamano, H.; Ikeda, Y.; Watanabe, H.; Horinouchi, Y.; Izawa-Ishizawa, Y.; Imanishi, M.; Zamami, Y.; Takechi, K.; Miyamoto, L.; Ishizawa, K.; et al. The uremic toxin indoxyl sulfate interferes with iron metabolism by regulating hepcidin in chronic kidney disease. *Nephrol. Dial. Transplant.* **2018**, *33*, 586–597. [CrossRef]
79. Asai, H.; Hirata, J.; Watanabe-Akanuma, M. Indoxyl glucuronide, a protein-bound uremic toxin, inhibits hypoxia-inducible factordependent erythropoietin expression through activation of aryl hydrocarbon receptor. *Biochem. Biophys. Res. Commun.* **2018**, *504*, 538–544. [CrossRef]
80. Besarab, A.; Ayyoub, F. Anemia in renal disease. In *Diseases of the Kidney and Urinary Tract*; Schrier, R.W., Ed.; Lippincott Williams and Wilkins: Philadelphia, PA, USA, 2007.
81. Wish, J.B.; Aronoff, G.R.; Bacon, B.R.; Brugnara, C.; Eckardt, K.U.; Ganz, T.; Macdougall, I.C.; Nunez, J.; Perahia, A.J.; Wood, J.C. Positive Iron Balance in Chronic Kidney Disease: How Much is Too Much and How to Tell? *Am. J. Nephrol.* **2018**, *47*, 72–83. [CrossRef]
82. Korolnek, T.; Hamza, I. Macrophages and iron trafficking at the birth and death of red cells. *Blood* **2015**, *125*, 2893–2897. [CrossRef]
83. Koury, M.J.; Haase, V.H. Anaemia in kidney disease: Harnessing hypoxia responses for therapy. *Nat. Rev. Nephrol.* **2015**, *11*, 394–410. [CrossRef] [PubMed]
84. Srai, S.K.; Chung, B.; Marks, J.; Pourvali, K.; Solanky, N.; Rapisarda, C.; Chaston, T.B.; Hanif, R.; Unwin, R.J.; Debnam, E.S.; et al. Erythropoietin regulates intestinal iron absorption in a rat model of chronic renal failure. *Kidney Int.* **2010**, *78*, 660–667. [CrossRef] [PubMed]
85. Babitt, J.L.; Lin, H.Y. Molecular mechanisms of hepcidin regulation: Implications for the anemia of CKD. *Am. J. Kidney Dis.* **2010**, *55*, 726–741. [CrossRef] [PubMed]
86. Del Vecchio, L.; Longhi, S.; Locatelli, F. Safety concerns about intravenous iron therapy in patients with chronic kidney disease. *Clin. Kidney J.* **2016**, *9*, 260–267. [CrossRef] [PubMed]
87. Nemeth, E.; Tuttle, M.S.; Powelson, J.; Vaughn, M.B.; Donovan, A.; Ward, D.M.; Ganz, T.; Kaplan, J. Hepcidin regulates cellular iron efflux by binding to ferroportin and inducing its internalization. *Science* **2004**, *306*, 2090–2093. [CrossRef] [PubMed]
88. Wang, H.E.; Gamboa, C.; Warnock, D.G.; Muntner, P. Chronic kidney disease and risk of death from infection. *Am. J. Nephrol.* **2011**, *34*, 330–336. [CrossRef] [PubMed]
89. Nicolas, G.; Bennoun, M.; Devaux, I.; Beaumont, C.; Grandchamp, B.; Kahn, A.; Vaulont, S. Lack of hepcidin gene expression and severe tissue iron overload in upstream stimulatory factor 2 (USF2) knockout mice. *Proc. Natl. Acad. Sci. USA* **2001**, *98*, 8780–8785. [CrossRef] [PubMed]
90. Nemeth, E.; Valore, E.V.; Territo, M.; Schiller, G.; Lichtenstein, A.; Ganz, T. Hepcidin, a putative mediator of anemia of inflammation, is a type II acute-phase protein. *Blood* **2003**, *101*, 2461–2463. [CrossRef] [PubMed]
91. Zumbrennen-Bullough, K.; Babitt, J.L. The iron cycle in chronic kidney disease (CKD): From genetics and experimental models to CKD patients. *Nephrol. Dial. Transplant.* **2014**, *29*, 263–273. [CrossRef]
92. Pinto, J.P.; Ribeiro, S.; Pontes, H.; Thowfeequ, S.; Tosh, D.; Carvalho, F.; Porto, G. Erythropoietin mediates hepcidin expression in hepatocytes through EPOR signaling and regulation of C/EBPalpha. *Blood* **2008**, *111*, 5727–5733. [CrossRef]
93. Kautz, L.; Jung, G.; Valore, E.V.; Rivella, S.; Nemeth, E.; Ganz, T. Identification of erythroferrone as an erythroid regulator of iron metabolism. *Nat. Genet.* **2014**, *46*, 678–684. [CrossRef] [PubMed]
94. Pigeon, C.; Ilyin, G.; Courselaud, B.; Leroyer, P.; Turlin, B.; Brissot, P.; Loreal, O. A new mouse liver-specific gene, encoding a protein homologous to human antimicrobial peptide hepcidin, is overexpressed during iron overload. *J. Biol. Chem.* **2001**, *276*, 7811–7819. [CrossRef] [PubMed]
95. Besarab, A.; Coyne, D.W. Iron supplementation to treat anemia in patients with chronic kidney disease. *Nat. Rev. Nephrol.* **2010**, *6*, 699–710. [CrossRef] [PubMed]
96. National Institute for Health and Care Excellence. *Chronic Kidney Disease: Managing Anaemia*; NICE guideline: London, UK, 2015.
97. Gupta, N.; Wish, J.B. Hypoxia-Inducible Factor Prolyl Hydroxylase Inhibitors: A Potential New Treatment for Anemia in Patients With CKD. *Am. J. Kidney Dis.* **2017**, *69*, 815–826. [CrossRef] [PubMed]
98. Hayat, A.; Haria, D.; Salifu, M.O. Erythropoietin stimulating agents in the management of anemia of chronic kidney disease. *Patient Prefer. Adherence* **2008**, *2*, 195–200. [PubMed]
99. KDIGO. Use of ESAs and other agents to treat anemia in CKD. *Kidney Int. Sup.* **2012**, *2*, 299–310. [CrossRef] [PubMed]

100. Nikhoul, G.; Simon, F. Anemia of chronic kidney disease: Treat it, but not to aggressively. *Clevel. Clin. J. Med.* **2016**, *83*, 613–624. [CrossRef] [PubMed]
101. de Francisco, A.L.; Stenvinkel, P.; Vaulont, S. Inflammation and its impact on anaemia in chronic kidney disease: From haemoglobin variability to hyporesponsiveness. *Ndt Plus* **2009**, *2*, i18–i26. [CrossRef] [PubMed]
102. Silverstein, D.M. Inflammation in chronic kidney disease: Role in the progression of renal and cardiovascular disease. *Pediatric Nephrol.* **2009**, *24*, 1445–1452. [CrossRef] [PubMed]
103. Atkinson, M.A.; White, C.T. Hepcidin in anemia of chronic kidney disease: Review for the pediatric nephrologist. *Pediatric Nephrol.* **2012**, *27*, 33–40. [CrossRef] [PubMed]
104. Jelkmann, W. Proinflammatory cytokines lowering erythropoietin production. *J. Interferon Cytokine Res.* **1998**, *18*, 555–559. [CrossRef] [PubMed]
105. Wagner, M.; Alam, A.; Zimmermann, J.; Rauh, K.; Koljaja-Batzner, A.; Raff, U.; Wanner, C.; Schramm, L. Endogenous erythropoietin and the association with inflammation and mortality in diabetic chronic kidney disease. *Clin. J. Am. Soc. Nephrol.* **2011**, *6*, 1573–1579. [CrossRef] [PubMed]
106. Horl, W.H. Clinical aspects of iron use in the anemia of kidney disease. *J. Am. Soc. Nephrol.* **2007**, *18*, 382–393. [CrossRef] [PubMed]
107. Pisani, A.; Riccio, E.; Sabbatini, M.; Andreucci, M.; Del Rio, A.; Visciano, B. Effect of oral liposomal iron versus intravenous iron for treatment of iron deficiency anaemia in CKD patients: A randomized trial. *Nephrol. Dial. Transplant.* **2015**, *30*, 645–652. [CrossRef] [PubMed]
108. Latunde-Dada, G.O.; Pereira, D.I.; Tempest, B.; Ilyas, H.; Flynn, A.C.; Aslam, M.F.; Simpson, R.J.; Powell, J.J. A nanoparticulate ferritin-core mimetic is well taken up by HuTu 80 duodenal cells and its absorption in mice is regulated by body iron. *J. Nutr.* **2014**, *144*, 1896–1902. [CrossRef] [PubMed]
109. Ueda, N.; Takasawa, K. Impact of Inflammation on Ferritin, Hepcidin and the Management of Iron Deficiency Anemia in Chronic Kidney Disease. *Nutrients* **2018**, *10*. [CrossRef] [PubMed]
110. Vaziri, N.D. Understanding iron: Promoting its safe use in patients with chronic kidney failure treated by hemodialysis. *Am. J. Kidney Dis.* **2013**, *61*, 992–1000. [CrossRef]
111. Susantitaphong, P.; Alqahtani, F.; Jaber, B.L. Efficacy and safety of intravenous iron therapy for functional iron deficiency anemia in hemodialysis patients: A meta-analysis. *Am. J. Nephrol.* **2014**, *39*, 130–141. [CrossRef]
112. Macdougall, I.C. Special issue: iron therapy in patients with chronic kidney disease. *Clincal Kidney J.* **2017**, *10*, 1–12. [CrossRef]
113. Litton, E.; Xiao, J.; Ho, K.M. Safety and efficacy of intravenous iron therapy in reducing requirement for allogeneic blood transfusion: Systematic review and meta-analysis of randomised clinical trials. *BMJ* **2013**, *347*, f4822. [CrossRef]
114. Agarwal, R.; Kusek, J.W.; Pappas, M.K. A randomized trial of intravenous and oral iron in chronic kidney disease. *Kidney Int.* **2015**, *88*, 905–914. [CrossRef] [PubMed]
115. Leaf, D.E.; Swinkels, D.W. Catalytic iron and acute kidney injury. *Am. J. Physiol.* **2016**, *311*, F871–F876. [CrossRef] [PubMed]
116. Kautz, L.; Gabayan, V.; Wang, X.; Wu, J.; Onwuzurike, J.; Jung, G.; Qiao, B.; Lusis, A.J.; Ganz, T.; Nemeth, E. Testing the iron hypothesis in a mouse model of atherosclerosis. *Cell Rep.* **2013**, *5*, 1436–1442. [CrossRef] [PubMed]
117. Kuo, K.L.; Hung, S.C.; Lee, T.S.; Tarng, D.C. Iron sucrose accelerates early atherogenesis by increasing superoxide production and upregulating adhesion molecules in CKD. *J. Am. Soc. Nephrol.* **2014**, *25*, 2596–2606. [CrossRef] [PubMed]
118. Bailie, G.R.; Clark, J.A.; Lane, C.E.; Lane, P.L. Hypersensitivity reactions and deaths associated with intravenous iron preparations. *Nephrol. Dial. Transplant.* **2005**, *20*, 1443–1449. [CrossRef] [PubMed]
119. Macdougall, I.C.; Bock, A.H.; Carrera, F.; Eckardt, K.U.; Gaillard, C.; Van Wyck, D.; Roubert, B.; Nolen, J.G.; Roger, S.D. FIND-CKD: A randomized trial of intravenous ferric carboxymaltose versus oral iron in patients with chronic kidney disease and iron deficiency anaemia. *Nephrol. Dial. Transplant.* **2014**, *29*, 2075–2084. [CrossRef] [PubMed]
120. Aronoff, G.R.; Bennett, W.M.; Blumenthal, S.; Charytan, C.; Pennell, J.P.; Reed, J.; Rothstein, M.; Strom, J.; Wolfe, A.; Van Wyck, D.; et al. Iron sucrose in hemodialysis patients: Safety of replacement and maintenance regimens. *Kidney Int.* **2004**, *66*, 1193–1198. [CrossRef] [PubMed]

121. Michael, B.; Coyne, D.W.; Folkert, V.W.; Dahl, N.V.; Warnock, D.G. Sodium ferric gluconate complex in haemodialysis patients: a prospective evaluation of long-term safety. *Nephrol. Dial. Transplant.* **2004**, *19*, 1576–1580. [CrossRef] [PubMed]
122. Macdougall, I.C.; Strauss, W.E.; Dahl, N.V.; Bernard, K.; Li, Z. Ferumoxytol for iron deficiency anemia in patients undergoing hemodialysis. The FACT randomized controlled trial. *Clin. Nephrol.* **2019**, *91*, 237–245. [CrossRef] [PubMed]
123. Rostoker, G.; Griuncelli, M.; Loridon, C.; Magna, T.; Machado, G.; Drahi, G.; Dahan, H.; Janklewicz, P.; Cohen, Y. Reassessment of Iron Biomarkers for Prediction of Dialysis Iron Overload: An MRI Study. *PLoS ONE* **2015**, *10*, e0132006. [CrossRef]
124. Rostoker, G.; Griuncelli, M.; Loridon, C.; Magna, T.; Janklewicz, P.; Drahi, G.; Dahan, H.; Cohen, Y. Maximal standard dose of parenteral iron for hemodialysis patients: An MRI-based decision tree learning analysis. *PLoS ONE* **2014**, *9*, e115096. [CrossRef] [PubMed]
125. Macdougall, I.C. Intravenous iron therapy in patients with chronic kidney disease: Recent evidence and future directions. *Clin. Kidney J.* **2017**, *10*, i16–i24. [CrossRef] [PubMed]
126. Macdougall, I.C.; Bircher, A.J.; Eckardt, K.U.; Obrador, G.T.; Pollock, C.A.; Stenvinkel, P.; Swinkels, D.W.; Wanner, C.; Weiss, G.; Chertow, G.M. Iron management in chronic kidney disease: Conclusions from a "Kidney Disease: Improving Global Outcomes" (KDIGO) Controversies Conference. *Kidney Int.* **2016**, *89*, 28–39. [CrossRef] [PubMed]
127. Lang, V.R.; Englbrecht, M.; Rech, J.; Nusslein, H.; Manger, K.; Schuch, F.; Tony, H.P.; Fleck, M.; Manger, B.; Schett, G.; et al. Risk of infections in rheumatoid arthritis patients treated with tocilizumab. *Rheumatology* **2012**, *51*, 852–857. [CrossRef] [PubMed]
128. Fung, E.; Sugianto, P.; Hsu, J.; Damoiseaux, R.; Ganz, T.; Nemeth, E. High-throughput screening of small molecules identifies hepcidin antagonists. *Mol. Pharmacol.* **2013**, *83*, 681–690. [CrossRef] [PubMed]
129. Masajtis-Zagajewska, A.; Nowicki, M. Effect of atorvastatin on iron metabolism regulation in patients with chronic kidney disease—A randomized double blind crossover study. *Ren. Fail.* **2018**, *40*, 700–709. [CrossRef]
130. Jelkmann, W. Activin receptor ligand traps in chronic kidney disease. *Curr. Opin. Nephrol. Hypertens.* **2018**, *27*, 351–357. [CrossRef] [PubMed]
131. Sasu, B.J.; Cooke, K.S.; Arvedson, T.L.; Plewa, C.; Ellison, A.R.; Sheng, J.; Winters, A.; Juan, T.; Li, H.; Begley, C.G.; et al. Antihepcidin antibody treatment modulates iron metabolism and is effective in a mouse model of inflammation-induced anemia. *Blood* **2010**, *115*, 3616–3624. [CrossRef] [PubMed]
132. Bolignano, D.; D'Arrigo, G.; Pisano, A.; Coppolino, G. Pentoxifylline for Anemia in Chronic Kidney Disease: A Systematic Review and Meta-Analysis. *PLoS ONE* **2015**, *10*, e0134104. [CrossRef]
133. Wang, J.; Lu, Z.; Wientjes, M.G.; Au, J.L. Delivery of siRNA therapeutics: Barriers and carriers. *Aaps J.* **2010**, *12*, 492–503. [CrossRef]
134. Sheetz, M.; Barrington, P.; Callies, S.; Berg, P.H.; McColm, J.; Marbury, T.; Decker, B.; Dyas, G.L.; Truhlar, S.M.E.; Benschop, R.; et al. Targeting the hepcidin-ferroportin pathway in anaemia of chronic kidney disease. *Br. J. Clin. Pharmacol.* **2019**, *85*, 935–948. [CrossRef] [PubMed]
135. Besarab, A.; Provenzano, R.; Hertel, J.; Zabaneh, R.; Klaus, S.J.; Lee, T.; Leong, R.; Hemmerich, S.; Yu, K.H.; Neff, T.B. Randomized placebo-controlled dose-ranging and pharmacodynamics study of roxadustat (FG-4592) to treat anemia in nondialysis-dependent chronic kidney disease (NDD-CKD) patients. *Nephrol. Dial. Transplant.* **2015**, *30*, 1665–1673. [CrossRef] [PubMed]
136. Provenzano, R.; Besarab, A.; Wright, S.; Dua, S.; Zeig, S.; Nguyen, P.; Poole, L.; Saikali, K.G.; Saha, G.; Hemmerich, S.; et al. Roxadustat (FG-4592) Versus Epoetin Alfa for Anemia in Patients Receiving Maintenance Hemodialysis: A Phase 2, Randomized, 6- to 19-Week, Open-Label, Active-Comparator, Dose-Ranging, Safety and Exploratory Efficacy Study. *Am. J. Kidney Dis.* **2016**, *67*, 912–924. [CrossRef] [PubMed]
137. Chen, N.; Qian, J.; Chen, J.; Yu, X.; Mei, C.; Hao, C.; Jiang, G.; Lin, H.; Zhang, X.; Zuo, L.; et al. Phase 2 studies of oral hypoxia-inducible factor prolyl hydroxylase inhibitor FG-4592 for treatment of anemia in China. *Nephrol. Dial. Transplant.* **2017**, *32*, 1373–1386. [CrossRef] [PubMed]
138. Akizawa, T.; Tsubakihara, Y.; Nangaku, M.; Endo, Y.; Nakajima, H.; Kohno, T.; Imai, Y.; Kawase, N.; Hara, K.; Lepore, J.; et al. Effects of Daprodustat, a Novel Hypoxia-Inducible Factor Prolyl Hydroxylase Inhibitor on Anemia Management in Japanese Hemodialysis Subjects. *Am. J. Nephrol.* **2017**, *45*, 127–135. [CrossRef] [PubMed]

139. Brigandi, R.A.; Johnson, B.; Oei, C.; Westerman, M.; Olbina, G.; de Zoysa, J.; Roger, S.D.; Sahay, M.; Cross, N.; McMahon, L.; et al. A Novel Hypoxia-Inducible Factor-Prolyl Hydroxylase Inhibitor (GSK1278863) for Anemia in CKD: A 28-Day, Phase 2A Randomized Trial. *Am. J. Kidney Dis.* **2016**, *67*, 861–871. [CrossRef]
140. Parmar, D.V.; Kansagra, K.A.; Patel, J.C.; Joshi, S.N.; Sharma, N.S.; Shelat, A.D.; Patel, N.B.; Nakrani, V.B.; Shaikh, F.A.; Patel, H.V. Outcomes of Desidustat Treatment in People with Anemia and Chronic Kidney Disease: A Phase 2 Study. *Am. J. Nephrol.* **2019**, *49*, 470–478. [CrossRef]
141. Akizawa, T.; Macdougall, I.C.; Berns, J.S.; Yamamoto, H.; Taguchi, M.; Iekushi, K.; Bernhardt, T. Iron Regulation by Molidustat, a Daily Oral Hypoxia-Inducible Factor Prolyl Hydroxylase Inhibitor, in Patients with Chronic Kidney Disease. *Nephron* **2019**, 1–12. [CrossRef]
142. Kurihara, T.; Westenskow, P.D.; Friedlander, M. Hypoxia-inducible factor (HIF)/vascular endothelial growth factor (VEGF) signaling in the retina. *Adv. Exp. Med. Biol.* **2014**, *801*, 275–281. [CrossRef]
143. Kular, D.; Macdougall, I.C. HIF stabilizers in the management of renal anemia: From bench to bedside to pediatrics. *Pediatric Nephrol.* **2019**, *34*, 365–378. [CrossRef]
144. Rothe, C.; Skerra, A. Anticalin((R)) Proteins as Therapeutic Agents in Human Diseases. *Biodrugs* **2018**, *32*, 233–243. [CrossRef] [PubMed]
145. Renders, L.; Budde, K.; Rosenberger, C.; van Swelm, R.; Swinkels, D.; Dellanna, F.; Feuerer, W.; Wen, M.; Erley, C.; Bader, B.; et al. First-in-human Phase I studies of PRS-080#22, a hepcidin antagonist, in healthy volunteers and patients with chronic kidney disease undergoing hemodialysis. *PLoS ONE* **2019**, *14*, e0212023. [CrossRef]
146. Poli, M.; Asperti, M.; Ruzzenenti, P.; Mandelli, L.; Campostrini, N.; Martini, G.; Di Somma, M.; Maccarinelli, F.; Girelli, D.; Naggi, A.; et al. Oversulfated heparins with low anticoagulant activity are strong and fast inhibitors of hepcidin expression in vitro and in vivo. *Biochem. Pharmacol.* **2014**, *92*, 467–475. [CrossRef] [PubMed]
147. Asperti, M.; Naggi, A.; Esposito, E.; Ruzzenenti, P.; Di Somma, M.; Gryzik, M.; Arosio, P.; Poli, M. High Sulfation and a High Molecular Weight Are Important for Anti-hepcidin Activity of Heparin. *Front. Pharmacol.* **2015**, *6*, 316. [CrossRef] [PubMed]
148. Bacchetta, J.; Zaritsky, J.; Lisse, T.; Sea, J.; Chun, R.; Nemeth, E.; Ganz, T.; Westerman, M.; Hewison, M. Vitamin D as a New Regulator of Iron Metabolism: Vitamin D Suppresses Hepcidin in Vitro and In Vivo. *J. Am. Soc. Nephrol.* **2011**, *22*, 564–572.
149. Zughaier, S.M.; Alvarez, J.A.; Sloan, J.H.; Konrad, R.J.; Tangpricha, V. The role of vitamin D in regulating the iron-hepcidin-ferroportin axis in monocytes. *J. Clin. Transl. Endocrinol.* **2014**, *1*, 19–25. [CrossRef]
150. Panwar, B.; McCann, D.; Olbina, G.; Westerman, M.; Gutierrez, O.M. Effect of calcitriol on serum hepcidin in individuals with chronic kidney disease: A randomized controlled trial. *BMC Nephrol.* **2018**, *19*, 35. [CrossRef]
151. Braithwaite, V.S.; Crozier, S.R.; D'Angelo, S.; Prentice, A.; Cooper, C.; Harvey, N.C.; Jones, K.S. The Effect of Vitamin D Supplementation on Hepcidin, Iron Status, and Inflammation in Pregnant Women in the United Kingdom. *Nutrients* **2019**, *11*. [CrossRef]
152. Edmonston, D.; Wolf, M. FGF23 at the crossroads of phosphate, iron economy and erythropoiesis. *Nat. Rev. Nephrol.* **2019**. [CrossRef]
153. Hanudel, M.R.; Eisenga, M.F.; Rappaport, M.; Chua, K.; Qiao, B.; Jung, G.; Gabayan, V.; Gales, B.; Ramos, G.; de Jong, M.A.; et al. Effects of erythropoietin on fibroblast growth factor 23 in mice and humans. *Nephrol. Dial. Transplant.* **2018**. [CrossRef]
154. Hanudel, M.R.; Laster, M.; Salusky, I.B. Non-renal-Related Mechanisms of FGF23 Pathophysiology. *Curr. Osteoporos. Rep.* **2018**, *16*, 724–729. [CrossRef] [PubMed]
155. David, V.; Martin, A.; Isakova, T.; Spaulding, C.; Qi, L.; Ramirez, V.; Zumbrennen-Bullough, K.B.; Sun, C.C.; Lin, H.Y.; Babitt, J.L.; et al. Inflammation and functional iron deficiency regulate fibroblast growth factor 23 production. *Kidney Int.* **2016**, *89*, 135–146. [CrossRef] [PubMed]
156. Singh, S.; Grabner, A.; Yanucil, C.; Schramm, K.; Czaya, B.; Krick, S.; Czaja, M.J.; Bartz, R.; Abraham, R.; Di Marco, G.S.; et al. Fibroblast growth factor 23 directly targets hepatocytes to promote inflammation in chronic kidney disease. *Kidney Int.* **2016**, *90*, 985–996. [CrossRef] [PubMed]
157. Agoro, R.; Montagna, A.; Goetz, R.; Aligbe, O.; Singh, G.; Coe, L.M.; Mohammadi, M.; Rivella, S.; Sitara, D. Inhibition of fibroblast growth factor 23 (FGF23) signaling rescues renal anemia. *Faseb J.* **2018**, *32*, 3752–3764. [CrossRef] [PubMed]

158. Song, S.N.; Tomosugi, N.; Kawabata, H.; Ishikawa, T.; Nishikawa, T.; Yoshizaki, K. Down-regulation of hepcidin resulting from long-term treatment with an anti-IL-6 receptor antibody (tocilizumab) improves anemia of inflammation in multicentric Castleman disease. *Blood* **2010**, *116*, 3627–3634. [CrossRef] [PubMed]
159. Hohlbaum, A.M.; Gille, H.; Trentmann, S.; Kolodziejczyk, M.; Rattenstetter, B.; Laarakkers, C.M.; Katzmann, G.; Christian, H.J.; Andersen, N.; Allersdorfer, A.; et al. Sustained plasma hepcidin suppression and iron elevation by Anticalin-derived hepcidin antagonist in cynomolgus monkey. *Br. J. Pharmacol.* **2018**, *175*, 1054–1065. [CrossRef] [PubMed]
160. Andriopoulos, B., Jr.; Corradini, E.; Xia, Y.; Faasse, S.A.; Chen, S.; Grgurevic, L.; Knutson, M.D.; Pietrangelo, A.; Vukicevic, S.; Lin, H.Y.; et al. BMP6 is a key endogenous regulator of hepcidin expression and iron metabolism. *Nat. Genet.* **2009**, *41*, 482–487. [CrossRef]
161. Poli, M.; Girelli, D.; Campostrini, N.; Maccarinelli, F.; Finazzi, D.; Luscieti, S.; Nai, A.; Arosio, P. Heparin: A potent inhibitor of hepcidin expression in vitro and in vivo. *Blood* **2011**, *117*, 997–1004. [CrossRef] [PubMed]

© 2019 by the authors. Licensee MDPI, Basel, Switzerland. This article is an open access article distributed under the terms and conditions of the Creative Commons Attribution (CC BY) license (http://creativecommons.org/licenses/by/4.0/).

MDPI
St. Alban-Anlage 66
4052 Basel
Switzerland
Tel. +41 61 683 77 34
Fax +41 61 302 89 18
www.mdpi.com

Nutrients Editorial Office
E-mail: nutrients@mdpi.com
www.mdpi.com/journal/nutrients

www.ingramcontent.com/pod-product-compliance
Lightning Source LLC
LaVergne TN
LVHW070656100526
838202LV00013B/973